The heART

ATLAS OF CARDIOLOGY

JUAN CARLOS JIMÉNEZ DE LA PUERTA

Warning:
Veterinary science is constantly evolving, as are pharmacology and the other sciences. Inevitably, it is therefore the responsibility of the veterinary clinician to determine and verify the dosage, the method of administration, the duration of treatment and any possible contraindications to the treatments given to each individual patient, based on his or her professional experience. Neither the publisher nor the author can be held liable for any damage or harm caused to people, animals or properties resulting from the correct or incorrect application of the information contained in this book.

This book has been published originally in Spanish under the title:
The heART. Atlas de cardiología

ISBN Spanish edition: 978-84-941389-8-0

For this English edition:

Plaza Antonio Beltrán Martínez nº 1, planta 8 - letra I
(Centro empresarial El Trovador)
50002 Zaragoza - Spain

Translation:
Grupo Asís Biomedia, S.L.

Design and layout:
Servet editorial - Grupo Asís Biomedia, S.L.
www.grupoasis.com
info@grupoasis.com

ISBN: 978-84-941389-7-3
D.L.: Z 1638-2013

Printed in Spain

This book is dedicated to all the people who love me and who have supported me with great patience and, why not say it, who have put up with me before and during the preparation of this book. You know perfectly who you are and how much I love you.

ACKNOWLEDGEMENTS

I must thank many professionals for contributing with their knowledge and help to the creation of this book. Some of them, unfortunately, are not here anymore, such as Professor Julio Escalona Zapata, whom I met when he was the Head of the Pathological Anatomy Service of the Gregorio Marañón Hospital while I was writing my doctoral thesis; he was able to transmit part of his know-how and enthusiasm for research to me.

I would like to thank my former colleagues at CEVETSA (Manuel Villagrasa, José Capacés, José Figueroa, José Miguel Sánchez and Fernando Aguado), who encouraged me when I started in the field of cardiology.

I would also like to thank some of the people who have worked by my side every day, such as Carmen Marín Carreño, Ramón López Quiroga and Esther Rey Valls.

I would like to express my gratitude to Dr. Alberto Montoya for his support and enthusiasm for this project, and for helping me to organise my first exhibition of photographs of the heart (Valves), which eventually gave rise to the idea of creating this book.

I wish to thank Dr. Larry P. Tilley, whom I met at this first photographic exhibition; his appreciation of the work I presented greatly encouraged me.

Finally, I thank all the colleagues who have referred cardiology patients to me, as this has allowed me to keep records of more cases.

AUTHOR

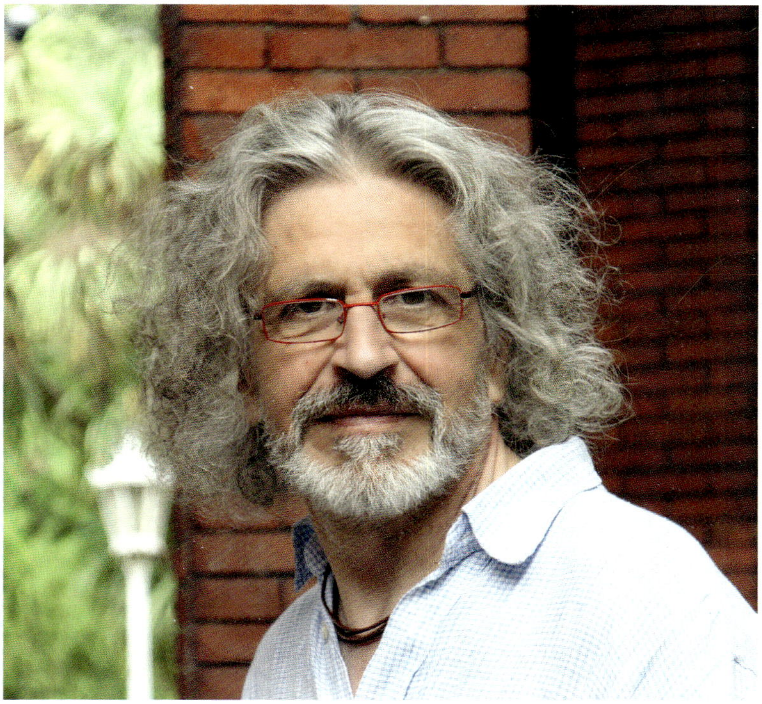

[JUAN CARLOS JIMÉNEZ DE LA PUERTA]

He graduated in Veterinary Medicine from the Complutense University of Madrid in 1978. He obtained his PhD in Veterinary Medicine in 1993. He obtained a diploma in Vascular and Nerve Microsurgery from the University of Extremadura in 1987, as well as a diploma in Microsurgery from the Gregorio Marañón Hospital in 1988. He received a scholarship from the Madrid College of Veterinary Surgeons to complete an internship at the Department of Medicine and Experimental Surgery of the Gregorio Marañón Hospital in 1988, and another from the Centre for Industrial Technological Development to work at the Department of Cardiovascular Pharmacology of ALTER Laboratories (1989-1992). He obtained a diploma in Echocardiography from the University of Murcia in 1996. In 1998 he won the AVEPA prize for scientific photography and was awarded the Miguel Luera prize in 2000. He is the author of several publications and papers in national and international journals and congresses.

He has been working as a clinical veterinary surgeon since 1981 and has specialised in cardiology since 1988.

He has organised several scientific and artistic photography exhibitions.

PROLOGUE

The heART by Juan Carlos Jiménez is a photographic atlas of normal and clinical cardiac anatomy that every veterinarian and veterinary technician should have. As an author and educator, I can say that the close-up photographic images are of the highest quality for continuing education. Dr. Jiménez has undertaken the challenge of bringing together his expertise in photography and pathological knowledge for a wonderful view of cardiac anatomy. The book provides a quick illustrative guide for the common cardiac disorders and normal cardiac anatomy that will facilitate client communication, with a very easy-to-use format. For all these reasons, Juan Carlos Jiménez's book is worth the highest merit since the reader will easily understand in a more accurate manner normal and abnormal cardiac anatomy and apply it on a clinical basis. Every veterinary student, resident, technician, and veterinarian should have this cardiology photographic atlas and it undoubtedly deserves to be in every personal library.

Larry P. Tilley, DVM
Diplomate, ACVIM (Internal Medicine)
VetMed Consultants, Inc.
Comparative Cardiology Division
Santa Fe, New Mexico, USA

PREFACE

Transmitting your knowledge, which you have usually acquired over long periods of time, is not an easy task; this is why I have always admired those good teachers who, in an apparently simple manner, managed to attract their students' attention and make them leave the classroom with clear ideas and enthusiasm and desire to know more.

Part of the success in this transmission, in addition to eloquence or, when required, good writing skills, lies in visual transmission. Charts, diagrams and images, which are important to complement the information given, are usually used for this purpose. The saying "A picture is worth a thousand words" is often perfectly true. Rather sooner than later, my passion for cardiology met my interest in photography, where light and shadows, volumes and colours become a valuable source of expression.

A photographic archive of anatomical structures and cardiac lesions progressively grew. What started as a simple database from which I occasionally obtained a picture for a conference or publication soon became a source of fun. With the lighting and somewhat unconventional perspectives, I tried to make the pictures speak by themselves and not only show structures or lesions, but beauty too.

A first photographic exhibition –Valves– arose from these pictures, which aimed at showing an attractive and different visual aspect of an organ with a complex morphology and functioning, rather than a didactic view of it.

This new photographic atlas is the result of more than 25 years of dedication to this specialty; this time I have tried to mix the scientific and didactic part with a presentation that is aesthetically pleasing to the eyes.

I am aware that among the pictures included in this book, some show more a play of light and volumes than a clear view of a specific structure, while, on the other hand, the view of this structure is predominant in other pictures that may thus not be as visually strong; however, I hope that the final objective of giving a clear idea of the anatomy of the heart and of its most common diseases has been achieved.

We cannot forget that science, learning and art are three concepts that are sometimes difficult to combine.

Juan Carlos Jiménez

INDEX OF CONTENTS

The heART

ATLAS OF CARDIOLOGY

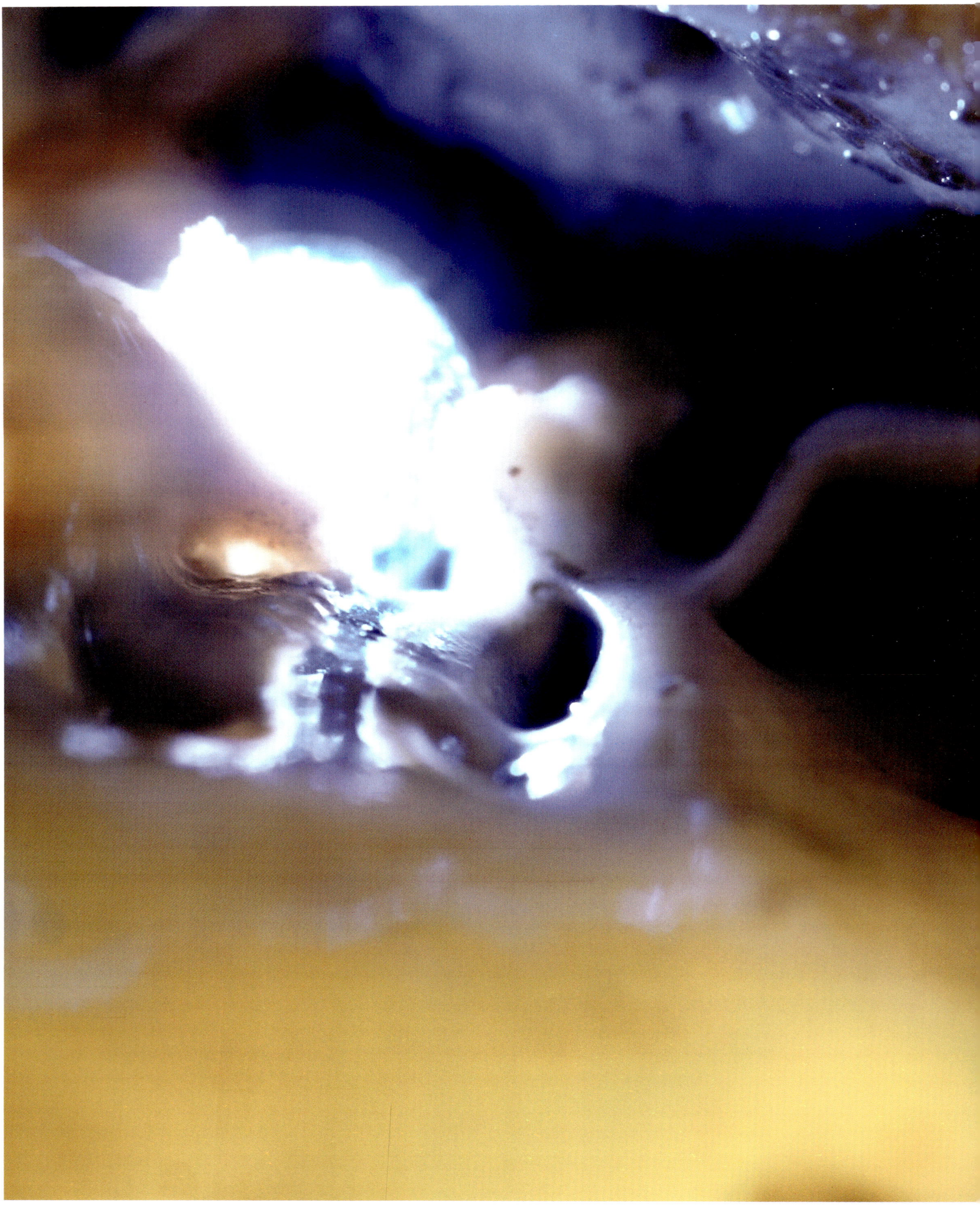

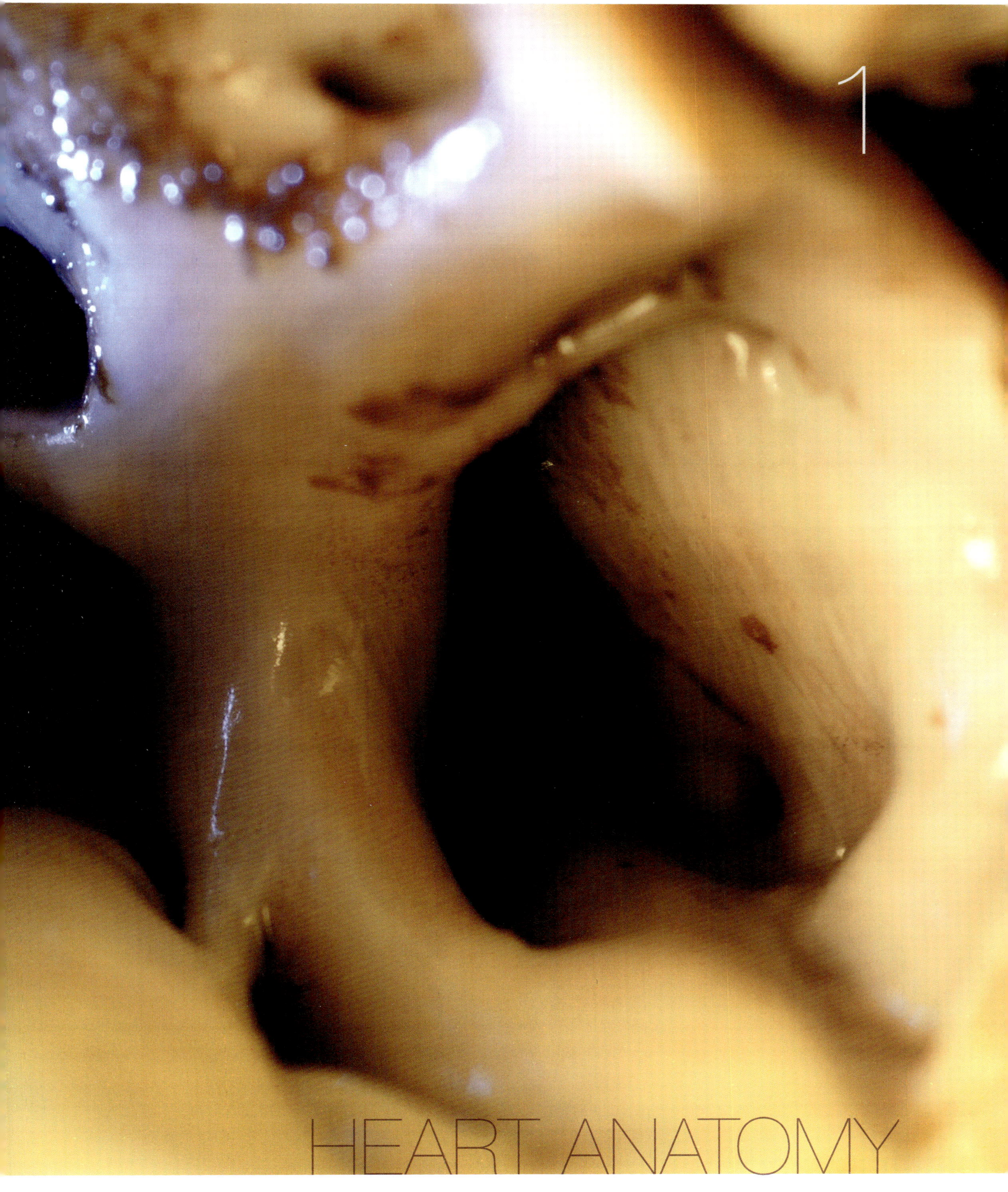

1

HEART ANATOMY

ORIENTATION AND LOCATION IN THE THORACIC CAVITY

The heart is the aspirating and impelling muscular pump of the cardiovascular system. It is cone-shaped and its base lies in dorsocranial position, while its apex is located in ventrocaudal position. Its axis forms an oblique line; only in dogs with a deep thorax such as Greyhounds is the apex almost ventral to the base.

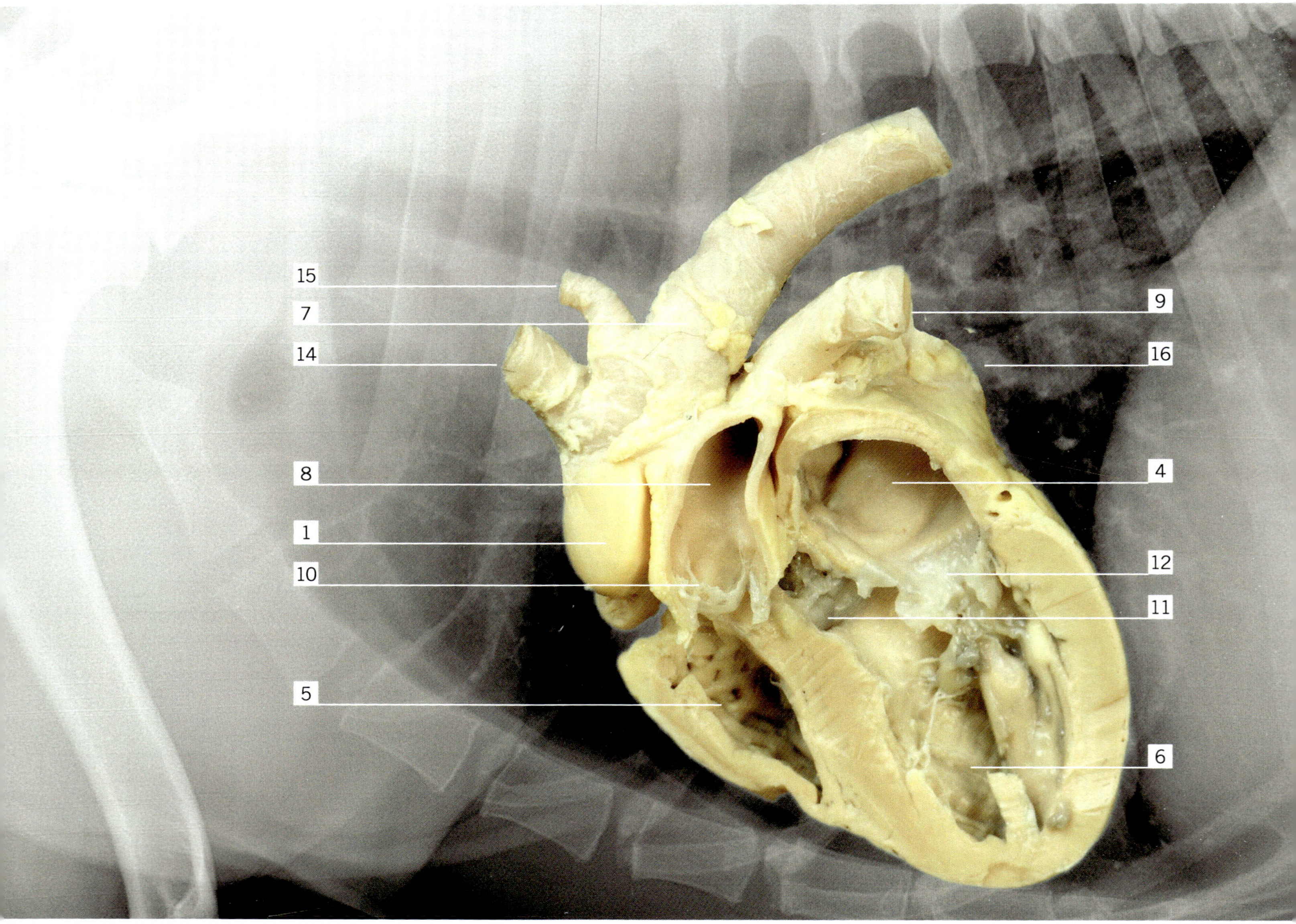

Figure 1. Location in the thoracic cavity.

This organ is located in the mediastinum and most of its surface is surrounded by the lungs. Its ventral region partially lies on the sternum and its cranial region just above the base is related to the trachea, main bronchi, lymph nodes and oesophagus. Part of its caudal area is in contact with the diaphragm.

[1 Right atrial appendage]
[2 Left atrial appendage]
[3 Right atrium]
[4 Left atrium]
[5 Right ventricle]
[6 Left ventricle]
[7 Aorta]
[8 Pulmonary trunk]
[9 Left pulmonary artery]
[10 Pulmonary valve]
[11 Aortic valve]
[12 Mitral valve]
[13 Tricuspid valve]
[14 Brachiocephalic trunk]
[15 Left subclavian artery]
[16 Caudal vena cava]

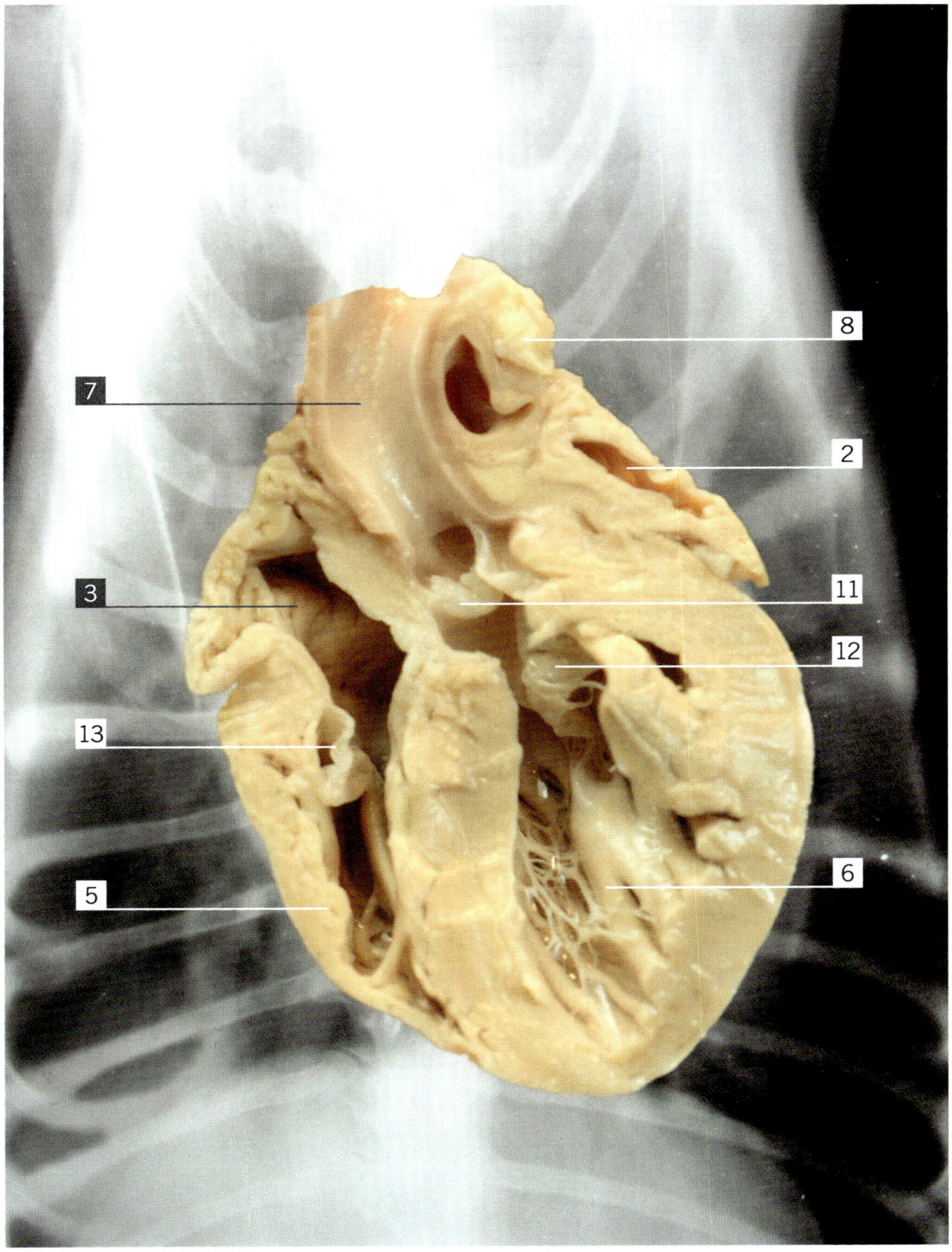

Figure 2. Location in the thoracic cavity.

SIZE OF THE HEART

The heart of an adult dog weighs on average 8.10 g/kg in males and 7.92 g/kg in females. Cats have a considerably smaller heart, with an average weight of 3.3 g/kg.

The left ventricle weighs, in dogs, about 3 times more than the right ventricle (considering the septum as part of the left ventricle); while in cats it weighs about 3.5 times more.

PERICARDIUM

The pericardium is a serofibrous sac that surrounds the heart. It is divided into two parts, the fibrous pericardium and the serous pericardium:

- The **fibrous pericardium** is the outer layer that inserts into the adventitia of the great vessels at the base of the heart and into the diaphragm in the area of its apex, thus forming the phrenicopericardial ligament.
- The **serous pericardium** has two layers: one related to the inner side of the fibrous pericardium, the parietal pericardium, and another in direct contact with the heart, the epicardium or visceral pericardium. The pericardial cavity is formed between these two layers of serous pericardium and is hydrated and lubricated by a small amount of fluid secreted by the cells of the serous pericardium. Both layers join at the base of the heart and form an undulated line known as the pericardial reflection.

A part of the pericardium, the transverse sinus of the pericardium, goes through the base of the heart caudally to the origin of the aorta and pulmonary trunk.

The left and right phrenic nerves run in craniocaudal direction along the left and right surface of the pericardium; the ventral vagal trunk runs along the left surface, closer to the aorta.

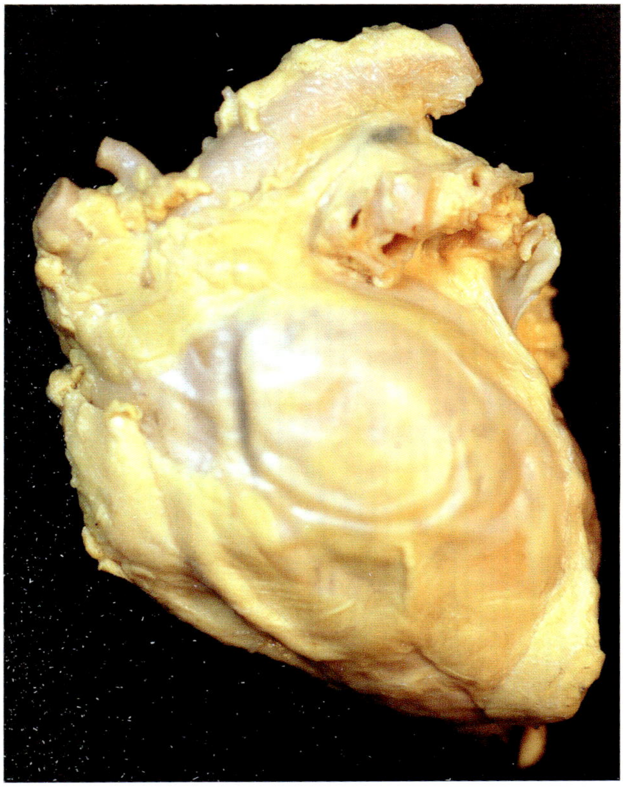

Figure 3. Pericardial sac surrounding the heart, the origin of the phrenicopericardial ligament can be observed in the area of the apex.

[1 Fibrous pericardium]

[2 Parietal layer of the serous pericardium]

[3 Visceral layer of the serous pericardium]

[4 Pericardial cavity]

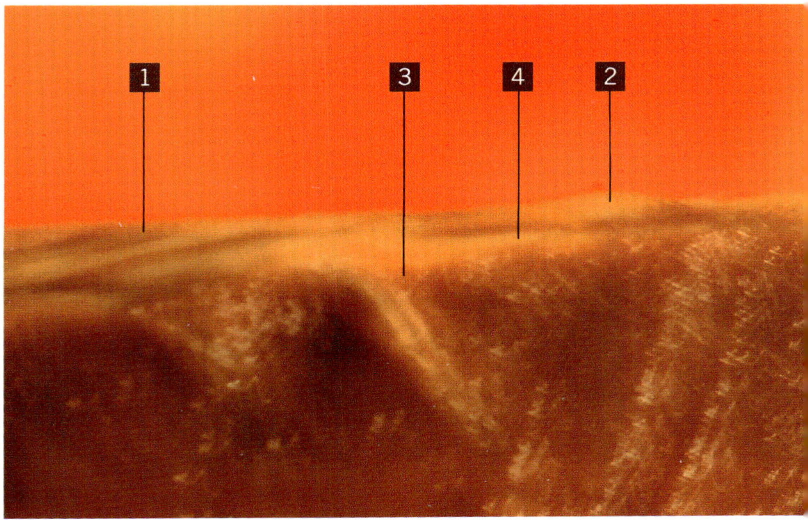

Figure 4. Layers of the pericardium. The outermost layer is the fibrous pericardium. The parietal layer of the serous pericardium is intimately attached to the internal surface of the fibrous pericardium, while the visceral layer of the serous pericardium is in direct contact with the heart. The pericardial cavity can be seen between the two layers of the serous pericardium.

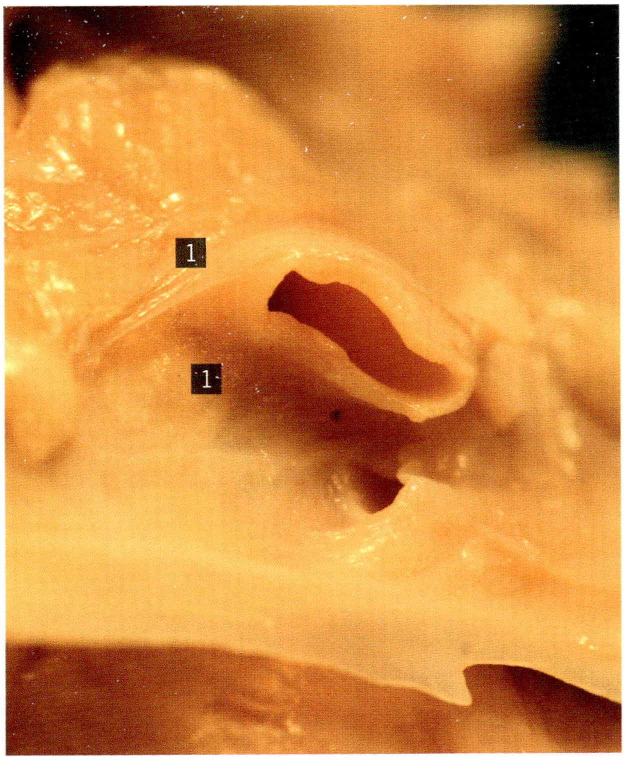

Figure 5. Attachment of the fibrous pericardium to the adventitia of the left pulmonary artery (1).

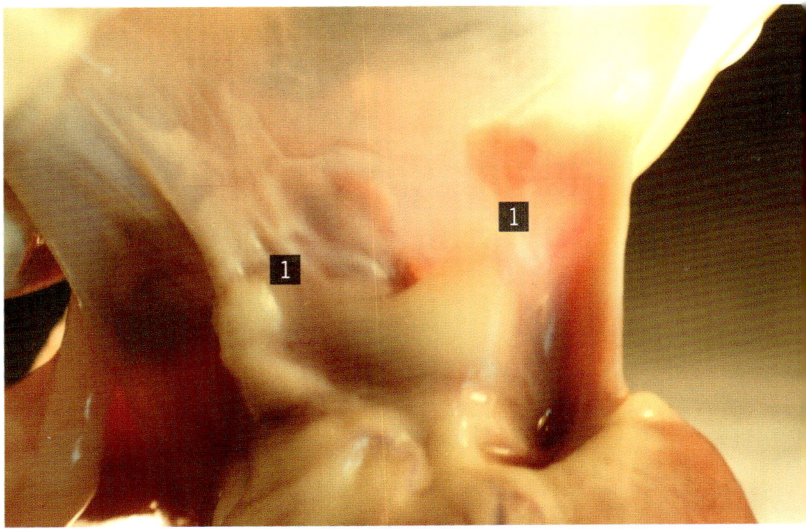

Figure 6. Attachment of the pericardium to the base of the heart (1). The pericardium has been sectioned and reflected dorsally so the attachment could be observed.

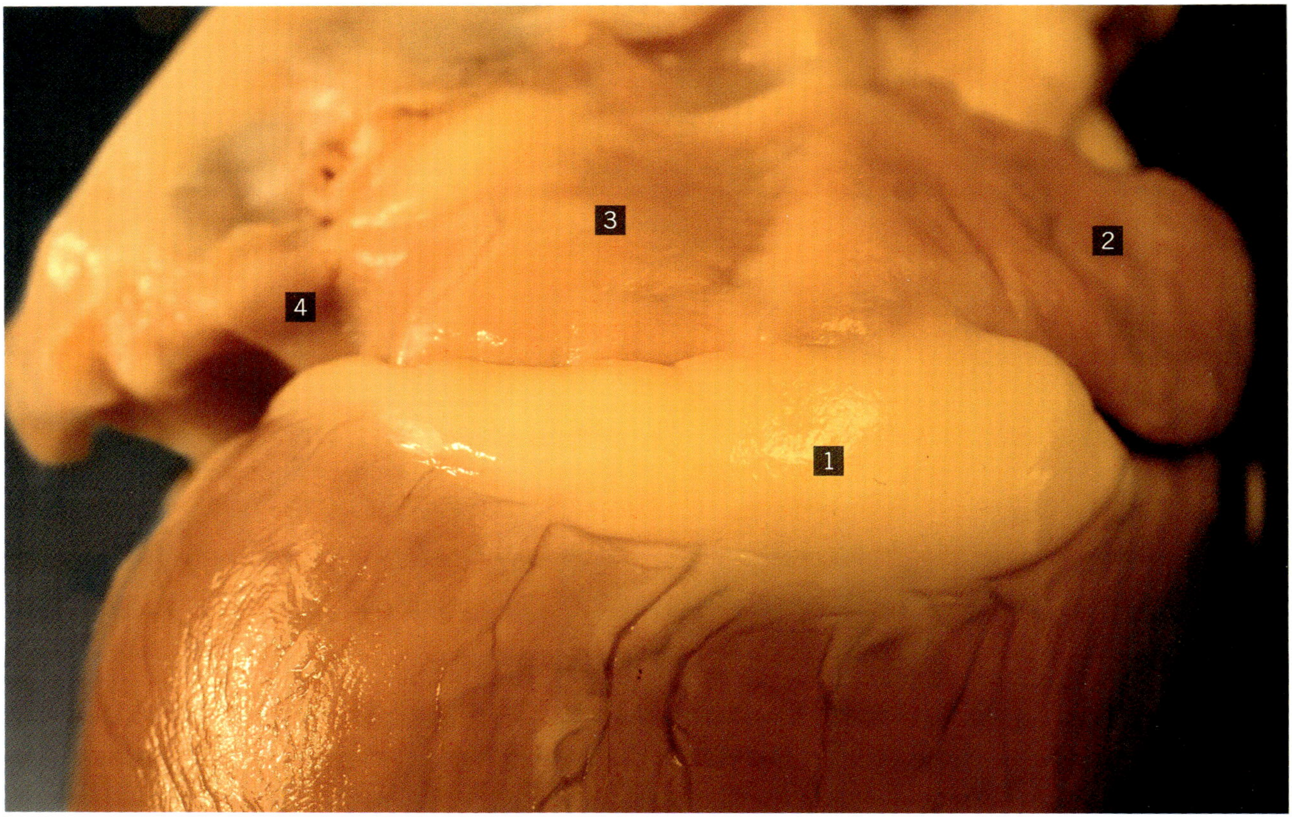

Figure 7. Right coronary sulcus, which marks the boundary between the atrium and ventricle. As can be observed, it is usually rich in fatty tissue. In this case, the right coronary artery and small cardiac vein run along it.

[1 Coronary sulcus] [2 Right atrial appendage] [3 Right atrium] [4 Caudal vena cava]

CARDIAC SURFACE AND MAIN BLOOD VESSELS

The coronary sulcus (sulcus coronarius) marks, on the cardiac surface, the boundary between the atria and the ventricles. This sulcus, which completely encircles the heart, except in the area that corresponds to the outflow tract of the right ventricle, is rich in fatty tissue and contains the right and left circumflex coronary arteries and cardiac veins.

The interventricular grooves originate from the coronary sulcus and run along the interventricular septum, making the division between the left and right ventricles.

Figure 8. The coronary sulcus is absent in the area corresponding to the outflow tract of the right ventricle.

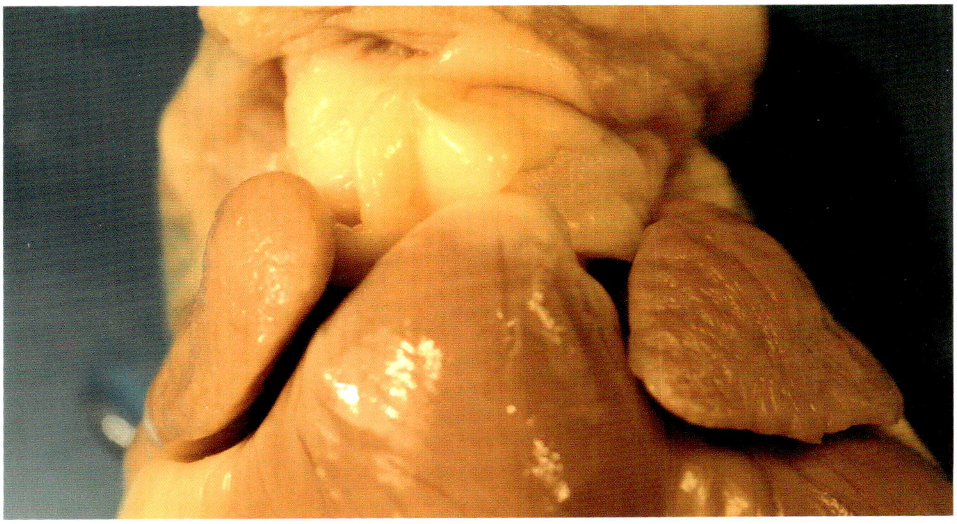

Figure 9. If the right atrial appendage is displaced dorsally, it is possible to see the origin of the right coronary sulcus, which corresponds to the exit of the right coronary artery from the aorta.

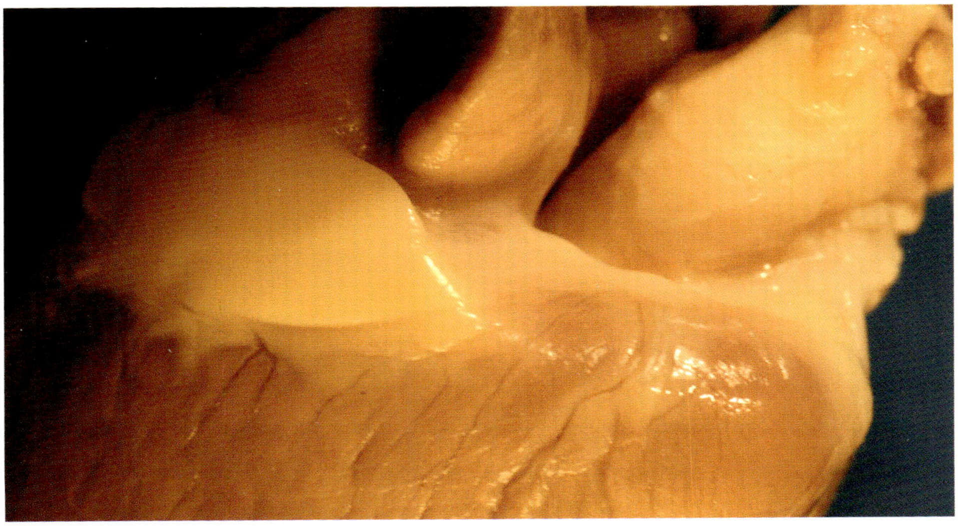

Figure 10. Origin of the left coronary artery from the aorta and division into the paraconal branch and circumflex branch.

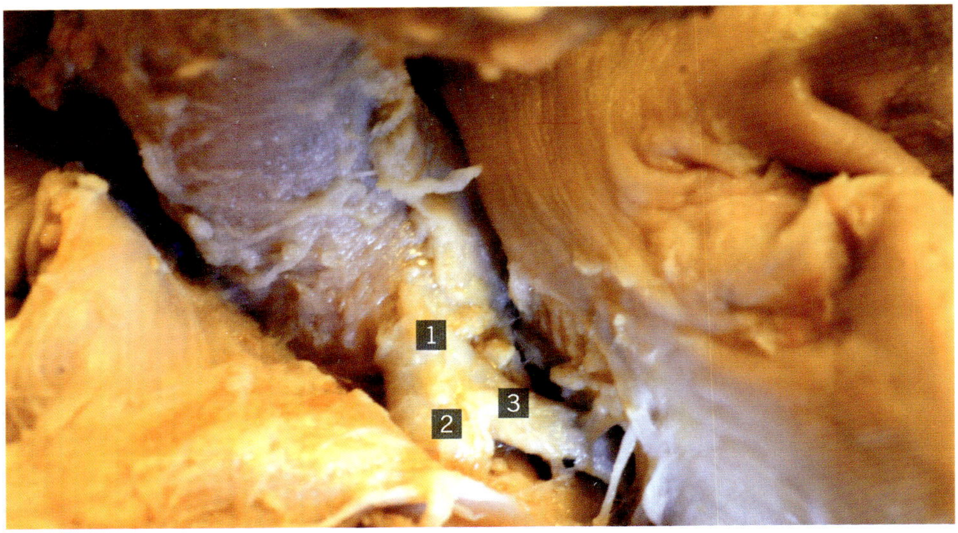

[1 Left coronary artery]

[2 Left paraconal artery]

[3 Left circumflex artery]

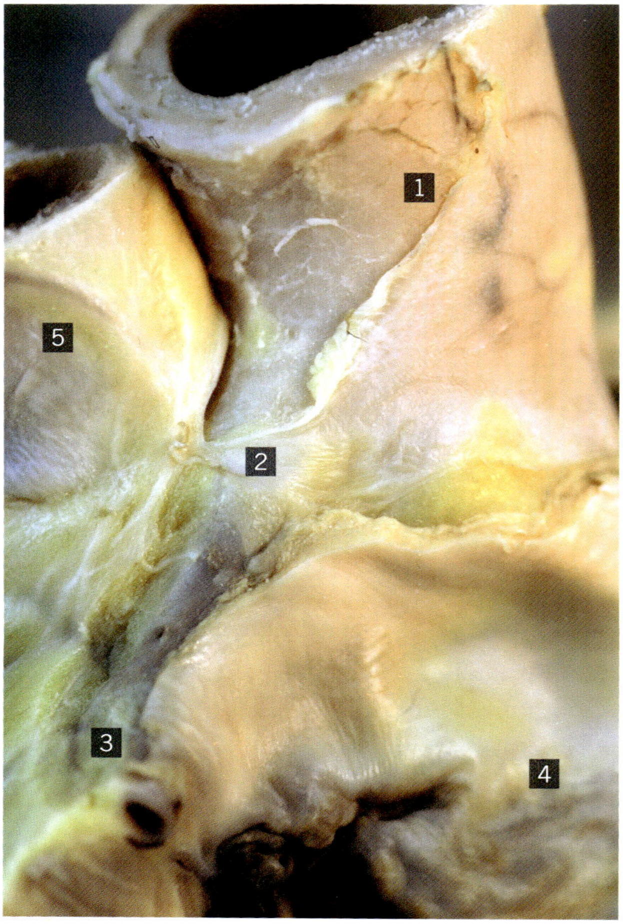

Figure 11. Origin of the left coronary artery from the aorta and left circumflex artery in the left coronary sulcus. The left atrium has been removed and the pulmonary trunk has been displaced cranially for a better view.

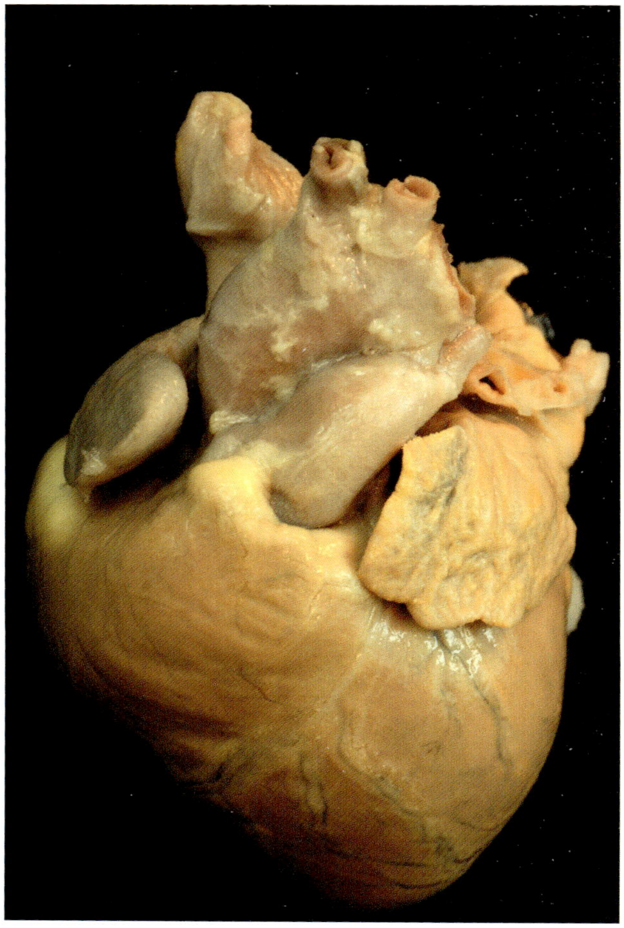

Figure 12. Paraconal interventricular groove; it marks the separation between the right and left ventricles. The paraconal coronary artery descends along this groove while the great cardiac vein ascends along it before encircling the heart in the coronary sulcus. It then empties into the coronary sinus.

[1 Aorta] [2 Left coronary artery] [3 Left circumflex coronary artery] [4 Mitral valve] [5 Pulmonary trunk]

The paraconal interventricular groove goes across the cranioventral surface obliquely. The paraconal branch of the left coronary artery descends along this groove while the great cardiac vein ascends along it before encircling the heart in the coronary sulcus.

The subsinuosal interventricular groove is much less marked than the previous one. The caudal interventricular branch of the left circumflex artery descends along this groove, while the middle cardiac vein ascends along it.

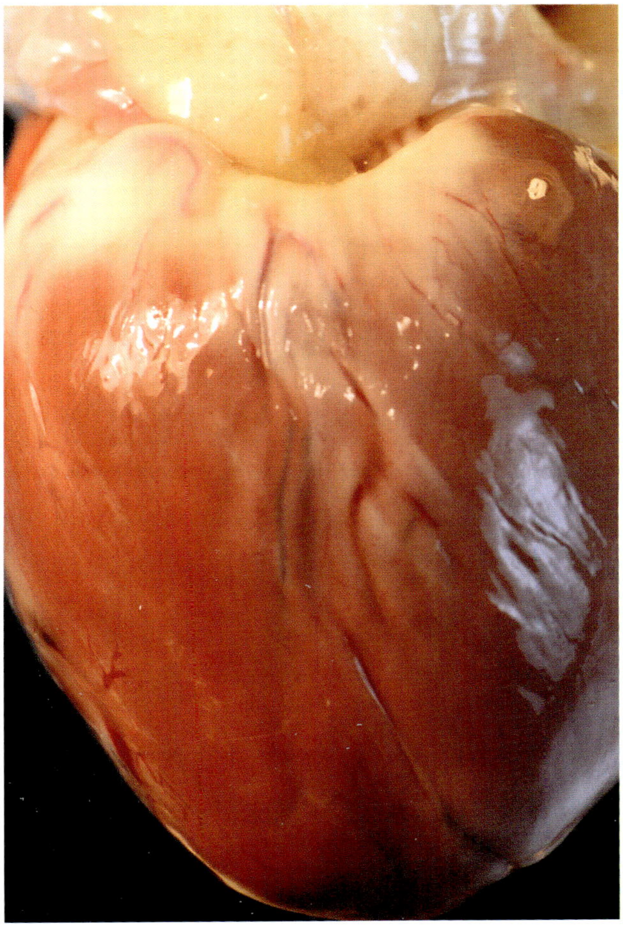

Figure 13. Subsinuosal interventricular groove. The caudal interventricular branch of the left circumflex artery descends along this groove, while the middle cardiac vein ascends along it.

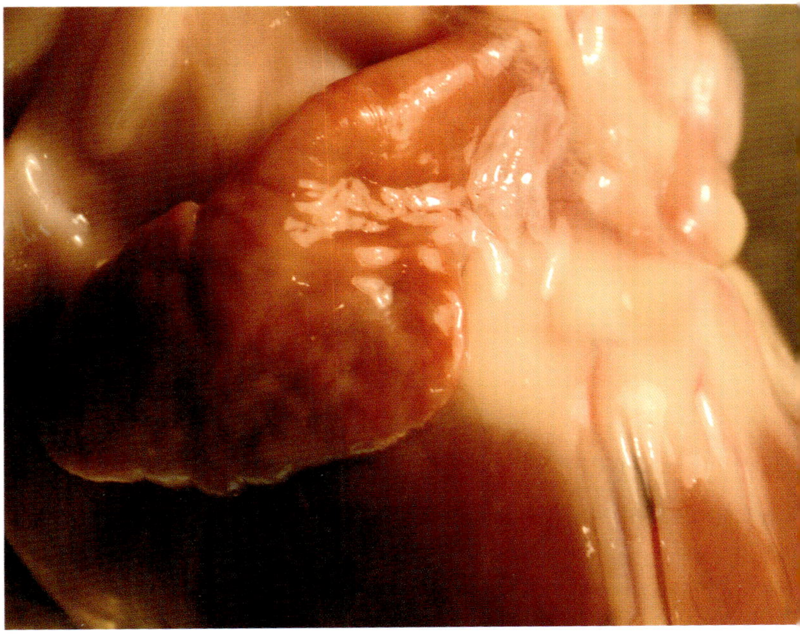

Figure 14. Left ventricular artery.

For the orientation of the different structures on the cardiac surface, we will bear in mind the fact that the outflow tract of the right ventricle is delimited by the two atrial appendages and that it is cranial and runs, in an ascending manner, from right to left to the origin of the pulmonary trunk. The atria are located caudal to the atrial appendages. The ventricles are located ventral to the corresponding atrium; the right ventricle mostly occupies the right surface of the heart, but it ascends cranially and towards the left surface where it joins the pulmonary trunk; the surface of the left ventricle occupies part of the left and caudal surface of the heart, although its apex also occupies the most ventral area of the right surface of the heart.

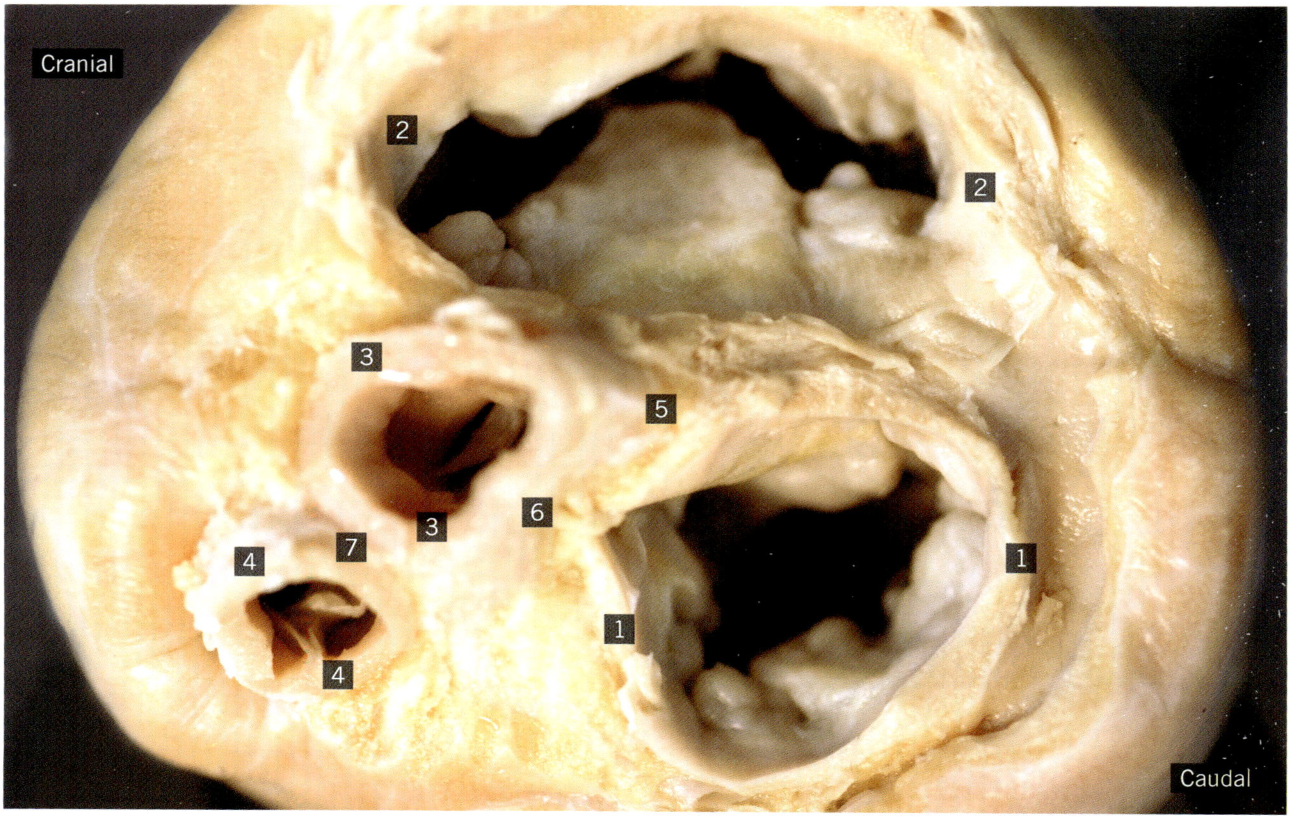

Figure 15. Fibrous skeleton of the heart.

FIBROUS SKELETON

The fibrous skeleton is the fibrocartilaginous base that supports the four heart valves and separates the thin atrial muscle from the much thicker ventricular muscle. This isolates them electrically, so that only an area of special neuromuscular tissue, the atrioventricular node, which lies in the interior of this fibrous base, and the bundle of His, which goes through it, maintain a "continuity" between the atria and ventricles.

It is formed by two thin fibrous rings that both surround an atrioventricular orifice and two arterial annuli:

- The **aortic valve annulus** is the most developed ring and forms the central base of the structure. It is formed by a triangular area located between the non-coronary cusp of the aortic valve, the septal leaflet of the tricuspid valve and the cranial or aortic leaflet of the mitral valve, named the right fibrous trigone, which is pierced by the bundle of His, and a smaller area, formed by the caudal wall of the aorta and the left atrioventricular ring, named left fibrous trigone.
- The **pulmonary valve annulus**, which is much less developed, is connected with the aortic valve annulus through a band of collagen fibres, the conus ligament.

[1 Mitral atrioventricular annulus]

[2 Tricuspid atrioventricular annulus]

[3 Aortic valve annulus]

[4 Pulmonary valve annulus]

[5 Right fibrous trigone]

[6 Left fibrous trigone]

[7 Conus ligament]

[1 Right atrial appendage]

[2 Left atrial appendage]

[3 Cranially displaced aorta and pulmonary trunk]

[4 Cranial vena cava]

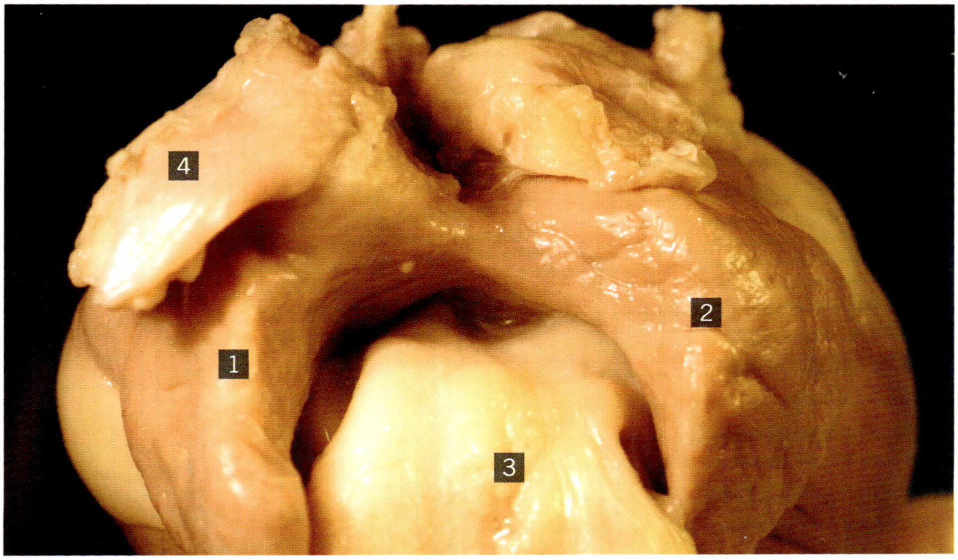

Figure 16. Craniodorsal view of the atrial appendages. The aorta and pulmonary trunk have been displaced cranially so the outer continuity of the atrial appendages can be observed.

[1 Terminal crest (site of origin of the atrial appendage)]

[2 Mouth of the cranial vena cava]

[3 Right atrial appendage (pectinate muscles)]

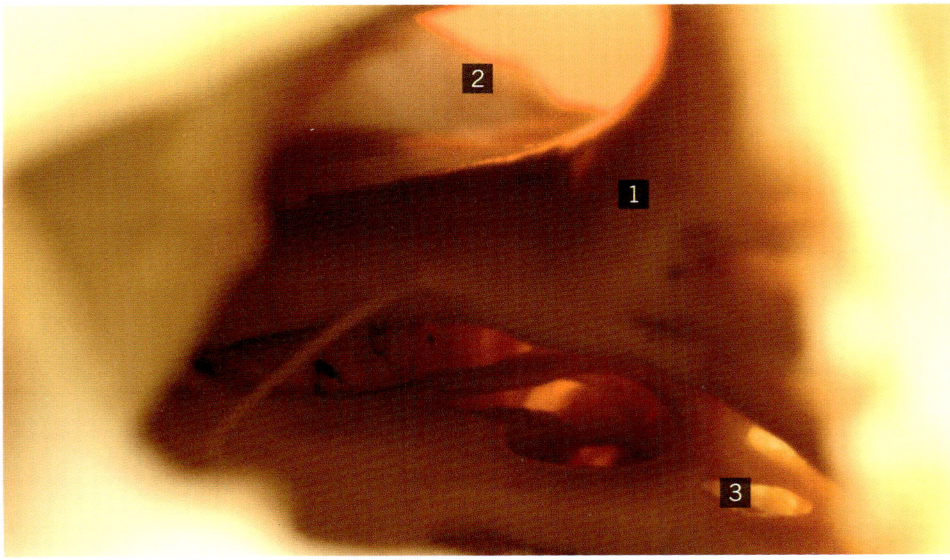

Figure 17. View of the right atrial appendage from the body of the atrium.

RIGHT ATRIUM

It is the chamber that receives the systemic venous blood. It is divided into two parts, a main part, the sinus venarum cavarum (sinus of the vena cava) or body of the atrium and a blind pouch that projects cranially, the right atrial appendage. While the internal part of the body of the atrium is smooth, the atrial appendage has a dense network of muscular bands, the pectinate muscles, which radiate from the terminal crest. This crest is a thick band of tissue located between the entrance of the cranial vena cava and the atrioventricular orifice.

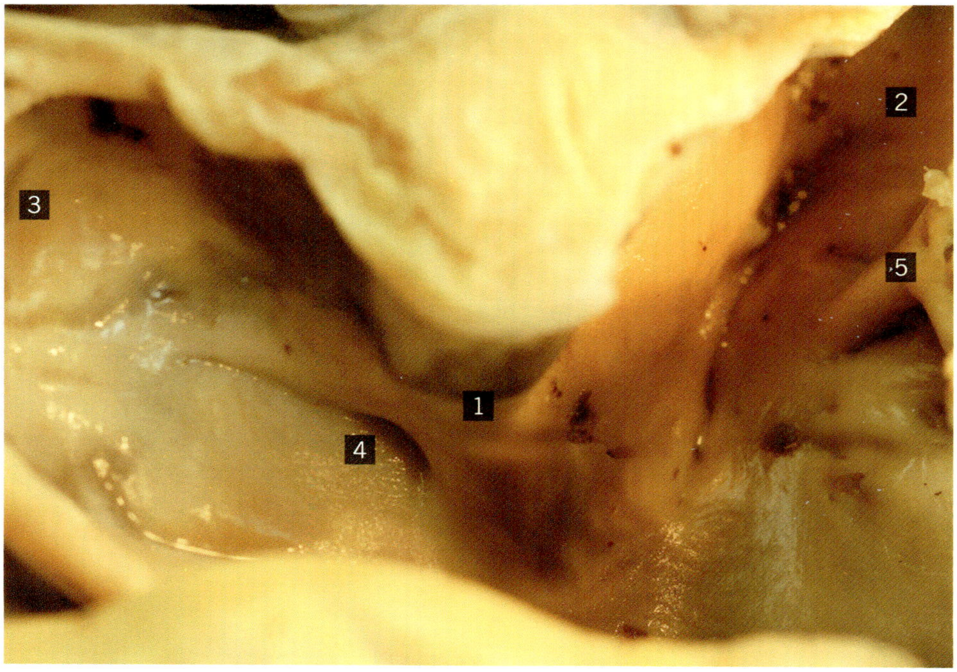

[1 Intervenous tubercle]

[2 Opening of the cranial vena cava]

[3 Opening of the caudal vena cava]

[4 Fossa ovalis]

[5 Terminal crest]

Figure 18. Right atrium.

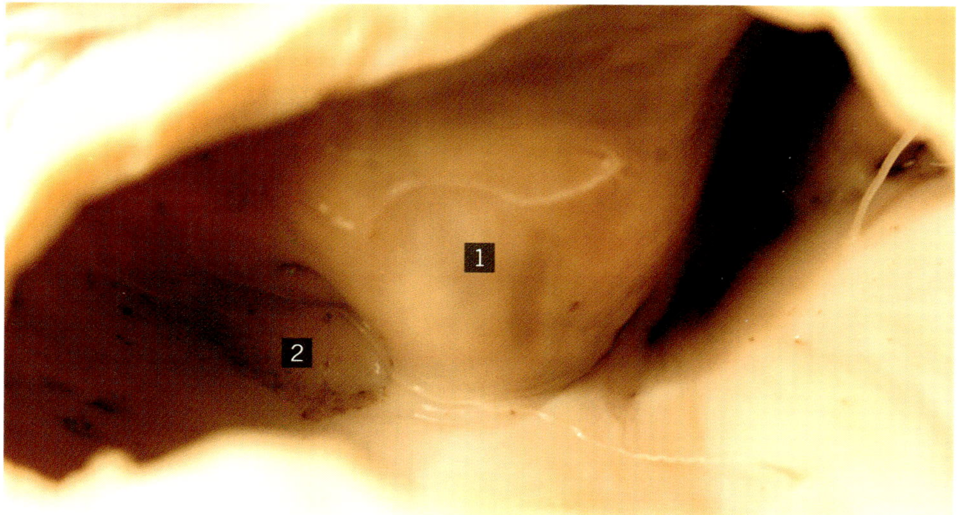

[1 Intervenous tubercle]

[2 Fossa ovalis]

Figure 19. Right atrium. The size of the intervenous tubercle may considerably vary from one animal to another.

There is another thick band of tissue, the intervenous tubercle, in the central area of the interatrial septum, between the entrance of the cranial vena cava and the entrance of the caudal vena cava. The fossa ovalis is located caudal to the intervenous tubercle.

In addition to the entrances of the cranial and caudal venae cavae, there is another orifice of entrance into the right atrium, the coronary sinus, located ventral to the caudal vena cava and dorsocaudal and to the left of the septal leaflet of the tricuspid valve.

The azygos vein empties into the cranial vena cava, close to the site of entry of this latter into the right atrium.

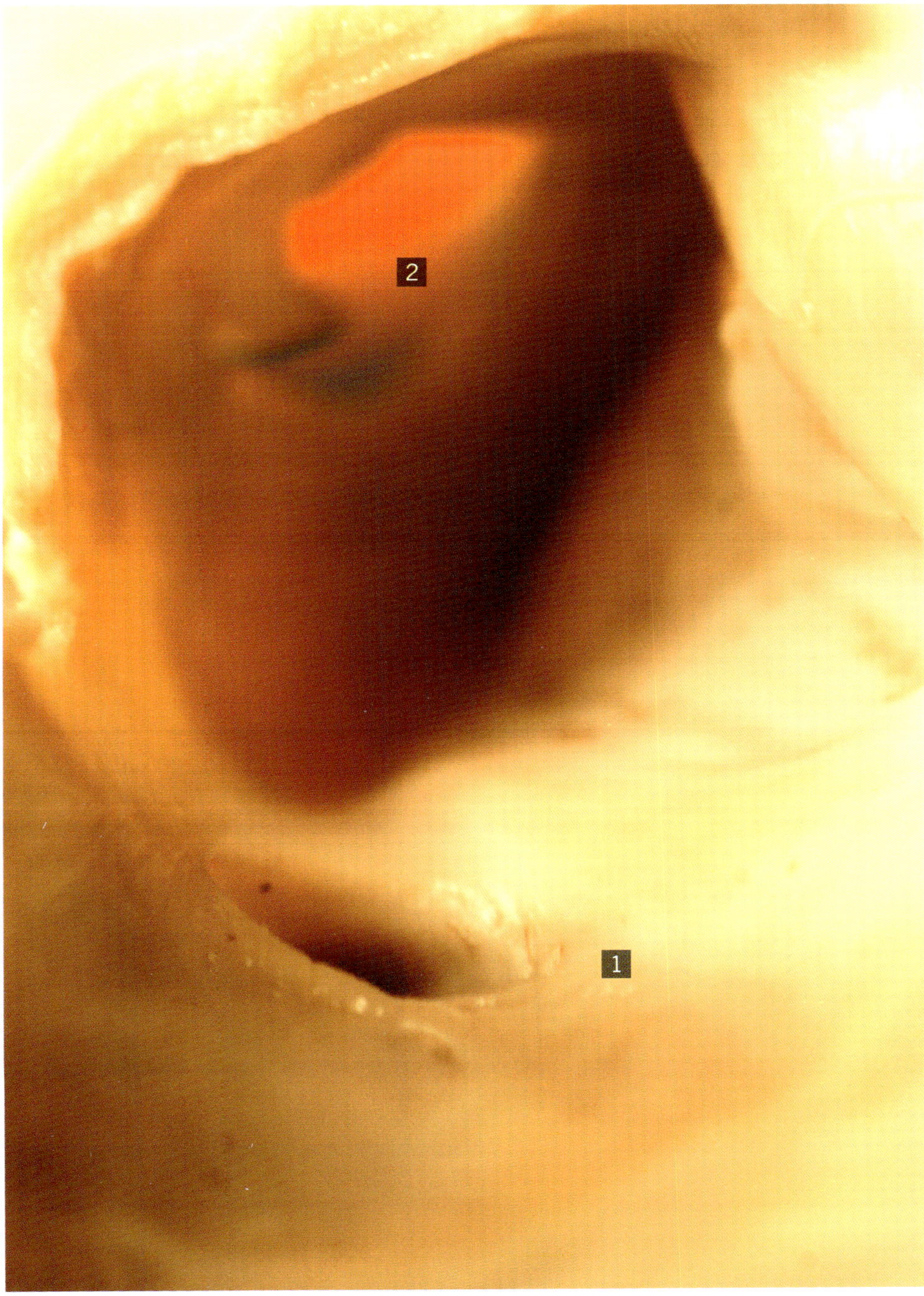

Figure 20. Coronary sinus; opening of the cardiac veins into the right atrium.

[1 Coronary sinus] [2 Opening of the caudal vena cava]

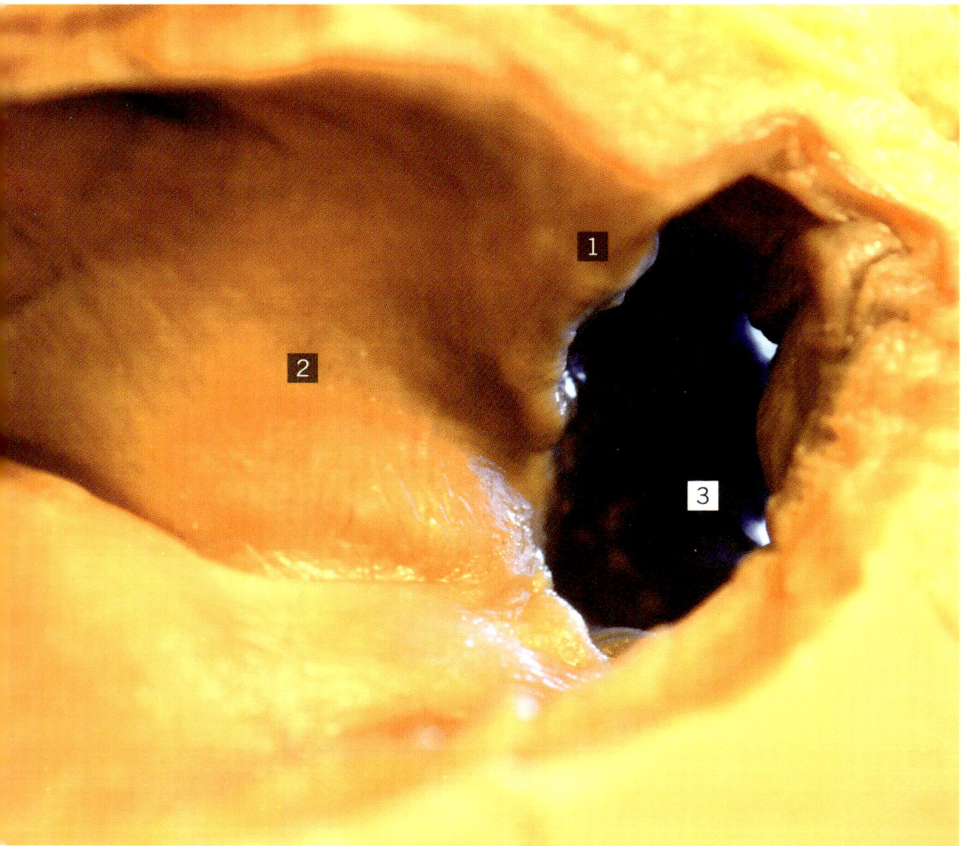

Figure 21. Supraventricular crest; it separates the outflow tract or infundibulum from the ventricle.

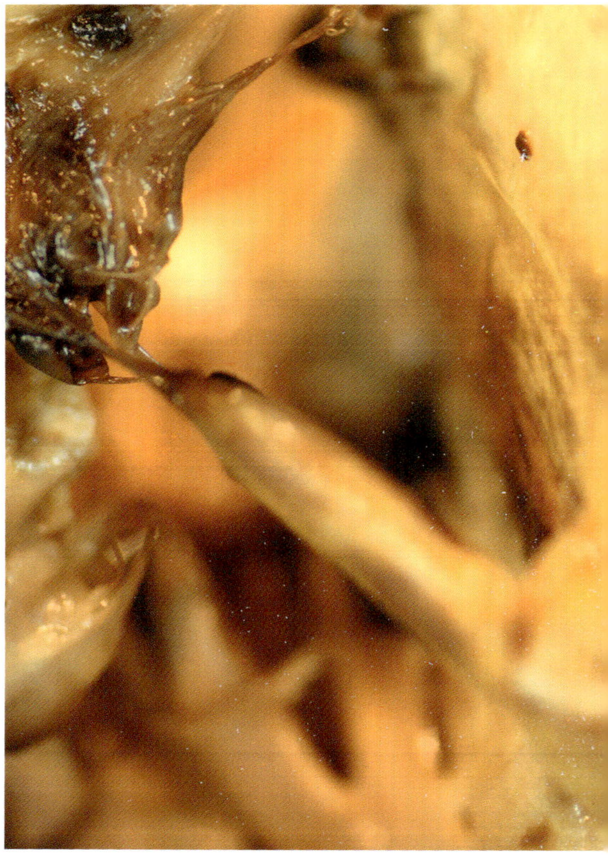

Figure 22. Papillary muscles.

[1 Interventricular crest] [2 Body of the ventricle] [3 Infundibulum]

RIGHT VENTRICLE

The right ventricle receives the systemic blood from the right atrium and pumps it to the lungs through the pulmonary trunk. Its walls are thinner and have less muscle mass than those of the left ventricle, which it partially surrounds in cranioventral direction.

It can be divided into two parts: the body of the ventricle, located immediately below the tricuspid valve, and the outflow tract or infundibulum, which runs cranially to the left. The ventricle and infundibulum are separated by a band of tissue, the supraventricular crest.

The papillary muscles are located in the body of the ventricle and usually originate from the apical third of the interventricular septum. Three main papillary muscles can normally be found, although there can be many variations. The papillary muscle closest to the outflow tract is generally the largest one. A small papillary muscle, the papillary muscle of the conus, can be observed immediately ventral to the terminal crest.

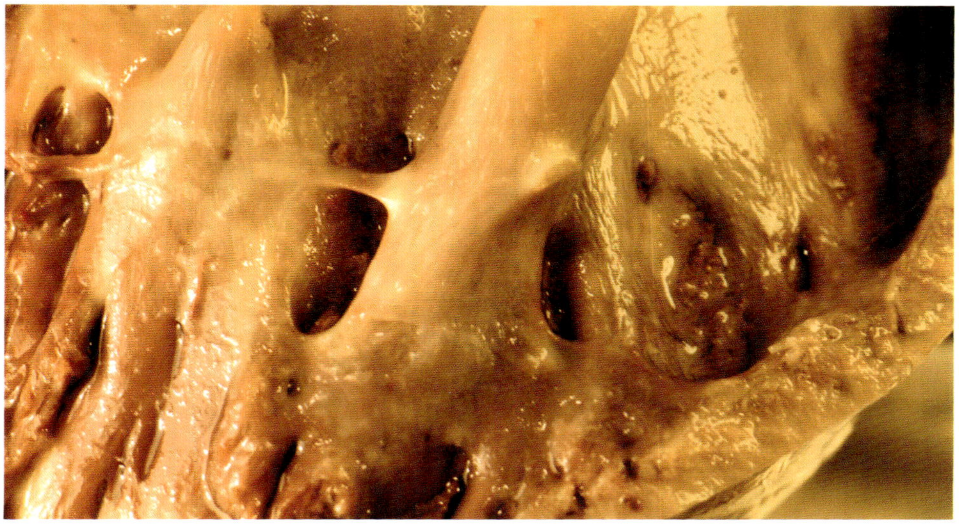

Figure 23. Papillary muscles. Note how the wall of the septum has many trabeculae below its insertion, as opposed to its upper part and towards the infundibulum.

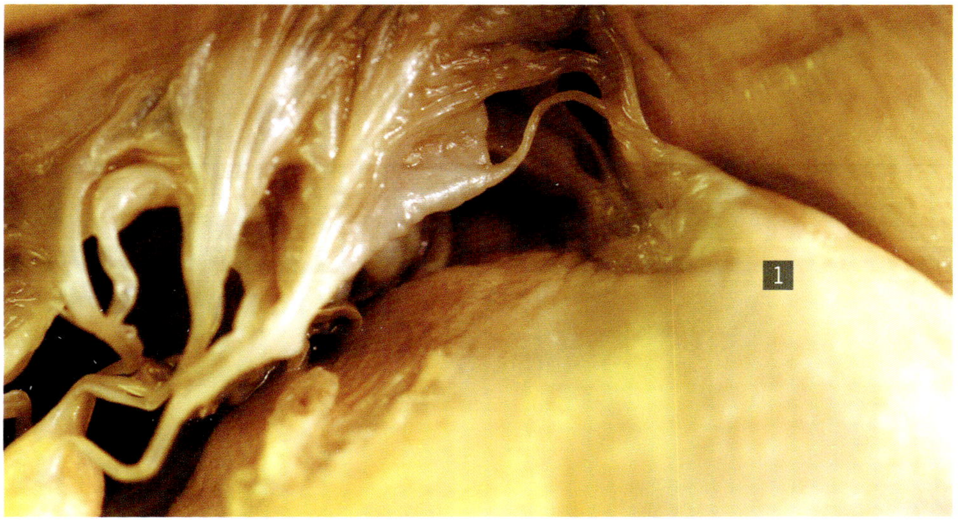

Figure 24. Papillary muscle of the conus (1).

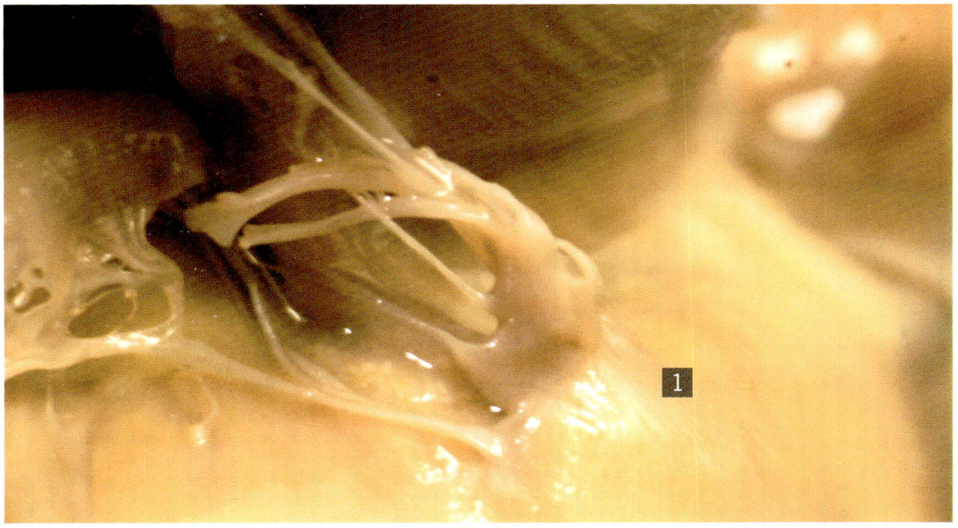

Figure 25. Papillary muscle of the conus (1). As can be observed, the morphology of the papillary muscles, including that of the papillary muscle of the conus, is very varied.

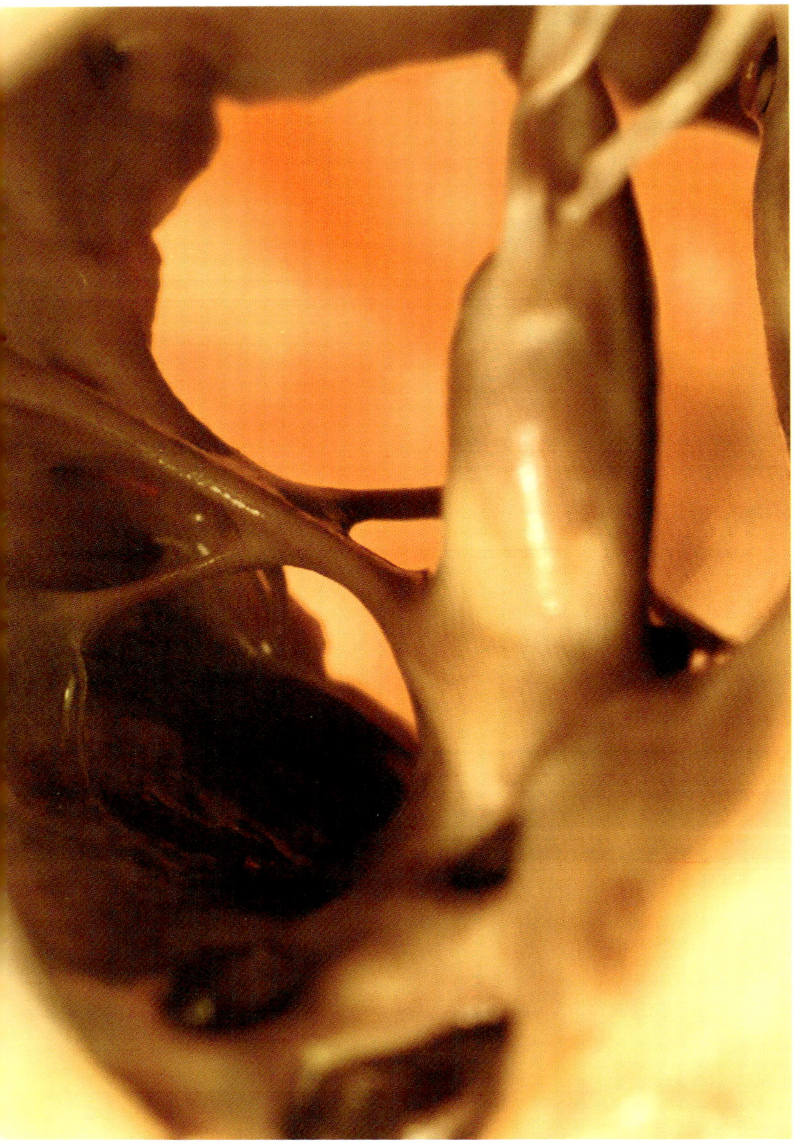

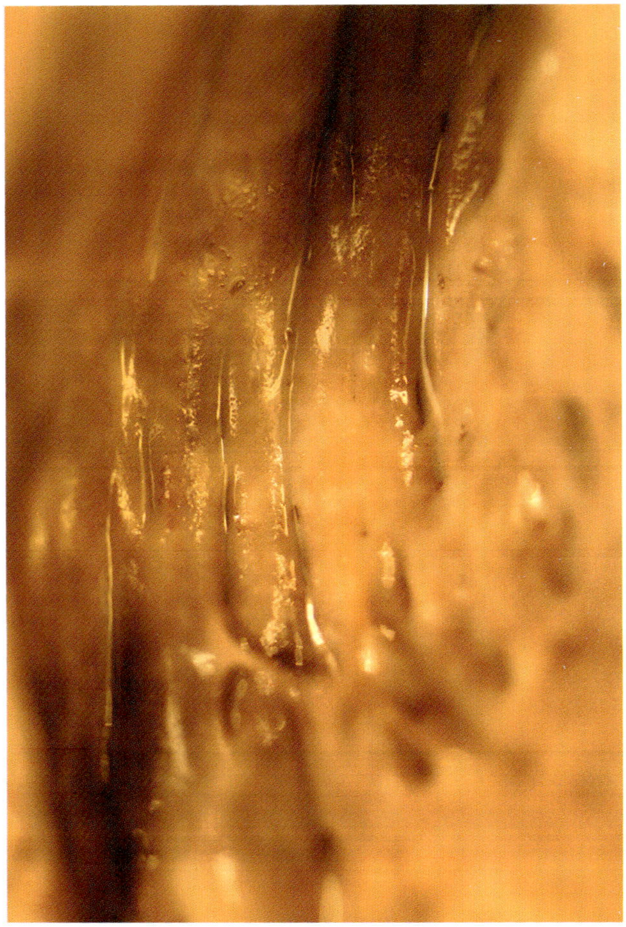

Figure 27. Trabeculae carnae in the free wall of the right ventricle.

Figure 26. Septomarginal trabecula and moderator bands.

The interventricular septum is smooth in the area dorsal to the papillary muscles, and only has small muscular "papillae", which are the origin of the chordae tendineae of the septal leaflet of the tricuspid valve. The area of the septum that is ventral to the papillary muscles has many trabeculae (trabeculae carneae), just like the free wall that surrounds the whole ventricle. The function of these trabeculae seems to be that of contributing to a more efficient ventricular pumping.

A thin muscle band, the septomarginal trabecula, originates in the interventricular septum, close to the main base of the main papillary muscle, and runs to the free wall of the ventricle. This septomarginal trabecula carries the right bundle branch from the bundle of His to the fibres of Purkinje of the free wall of the ventricle. The trabecula usually divides and gives moderator bands of anastomosis.

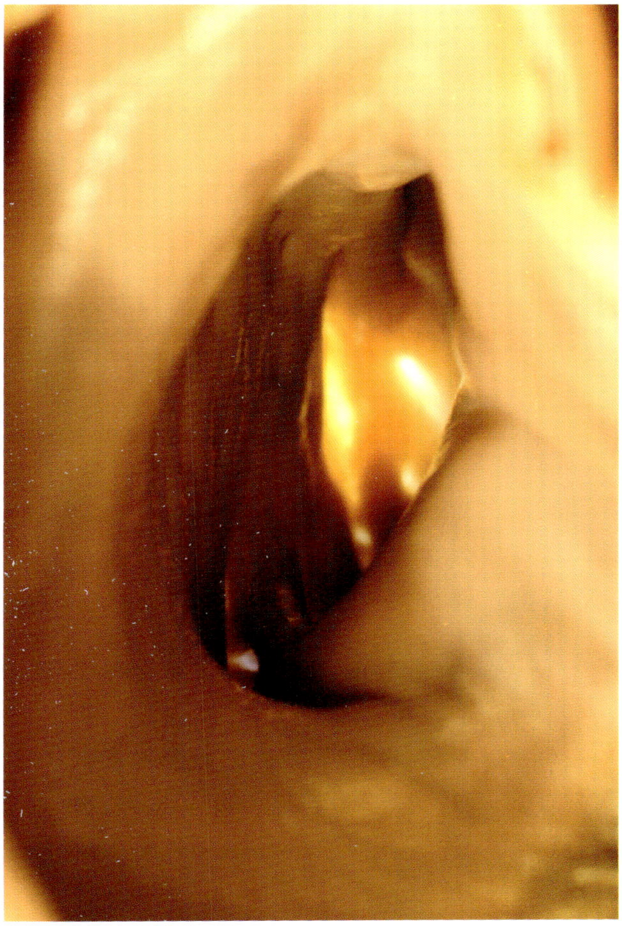

Figure 28. View of the left atrial appendage from the atrium where pectinate muscles may be observed, as in the right atrial appendage. These are absent in the body of the atrium.

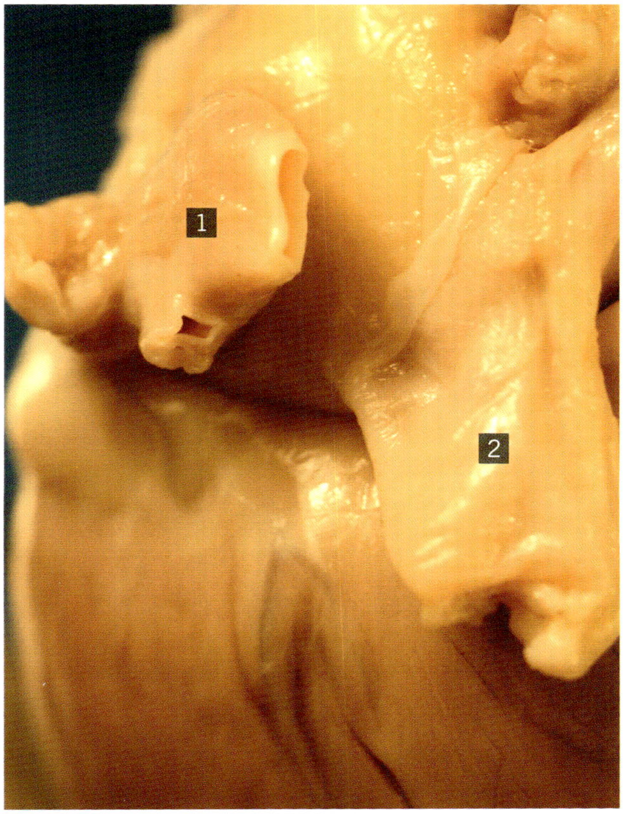

Figure 29. Entrance of the left pulmonary veins into the caudodorsal area of the atrium.

[1 The three veins come from the left lung]

[2 Caudal vena cava]

LEFT ATRIUM

It is the chamber that receives the blood from the pulmonary veins. It occupies the left dorsocaudal area of tne base of the heart. It is divided into the body of the atrium and the left atrial appendage. The left atrium is located immediately below the carina of the trachea. The atrial appendage projects cranially and is located ventral to the pulmonary trunk. Numerous trabeculae (pectinate muscles) can be found in it, as in the right atrial appendage. The body of the left atrium is completely smooth. Its five or six openings are the openings of the pulmonary veins into the atrium: the two or three veins from the right lung empty into the craniodorsal part of the chamber and the three veins from the left lung do so in the caudodorsal part. We can sometimes find a small flap of tissue on the cranial part of the septal wall, which corresponds to the remnants of the valve of the foramen ovale.

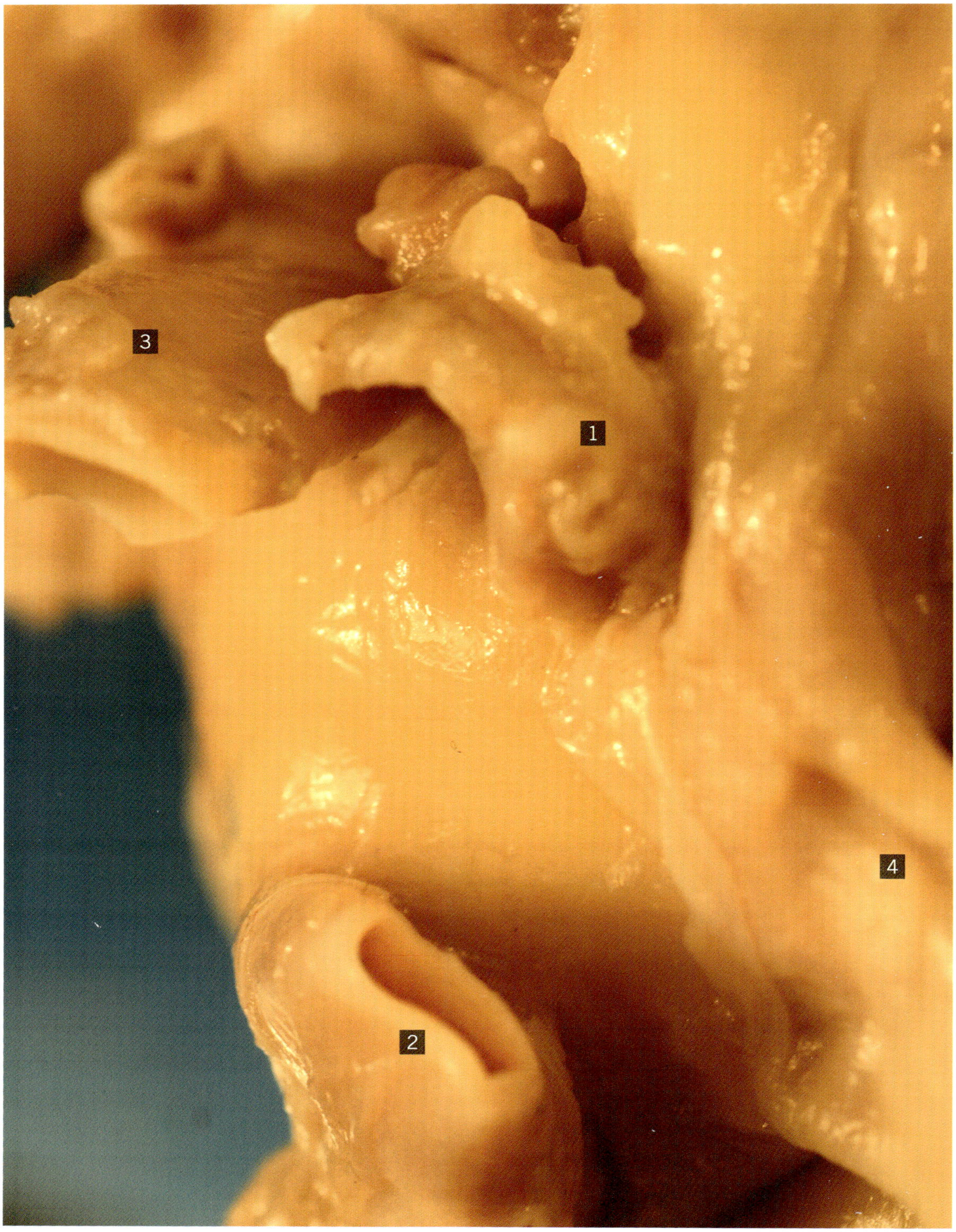

Figure 30. Entrance of the right pulmonary veins into the craniodorsal part of the body of the atrium.

[1 Right pulmonary veins] [3 Left pulmonary artery]

[2 Left pulmonary veins] [4 Caudal vena cava]

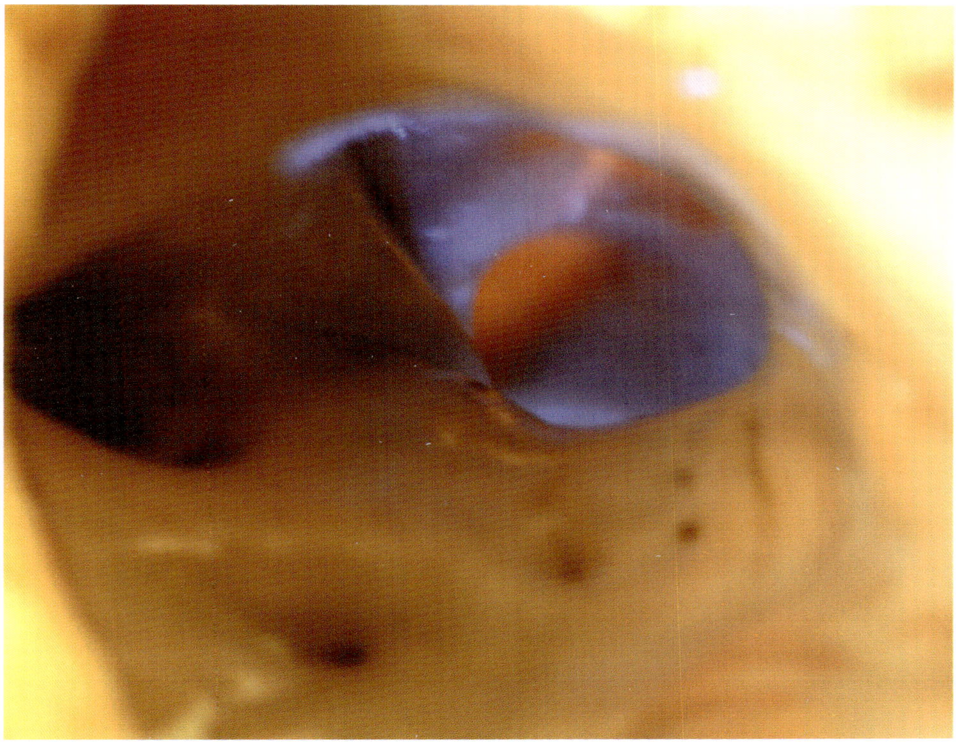

Figure 31. Entrance of the left pulmonary veins; view from the floor of the left atrium.

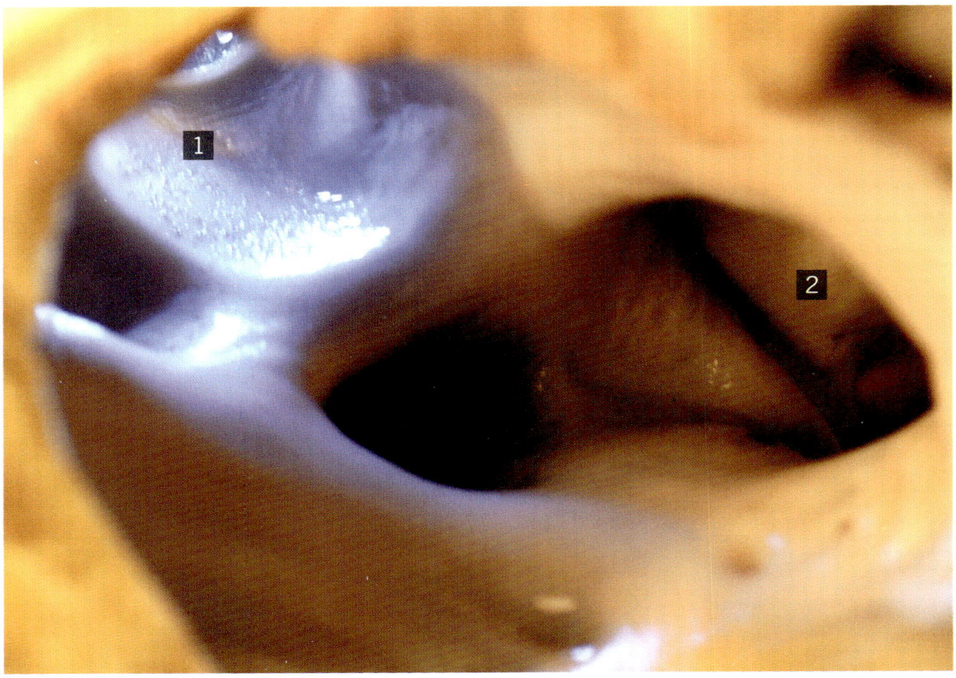

Figure 32. Entrance of the pulmonary veins seen from the floor of the left atrium.

[1 Right pulmonary veins] [2 Left pulmonary veins]

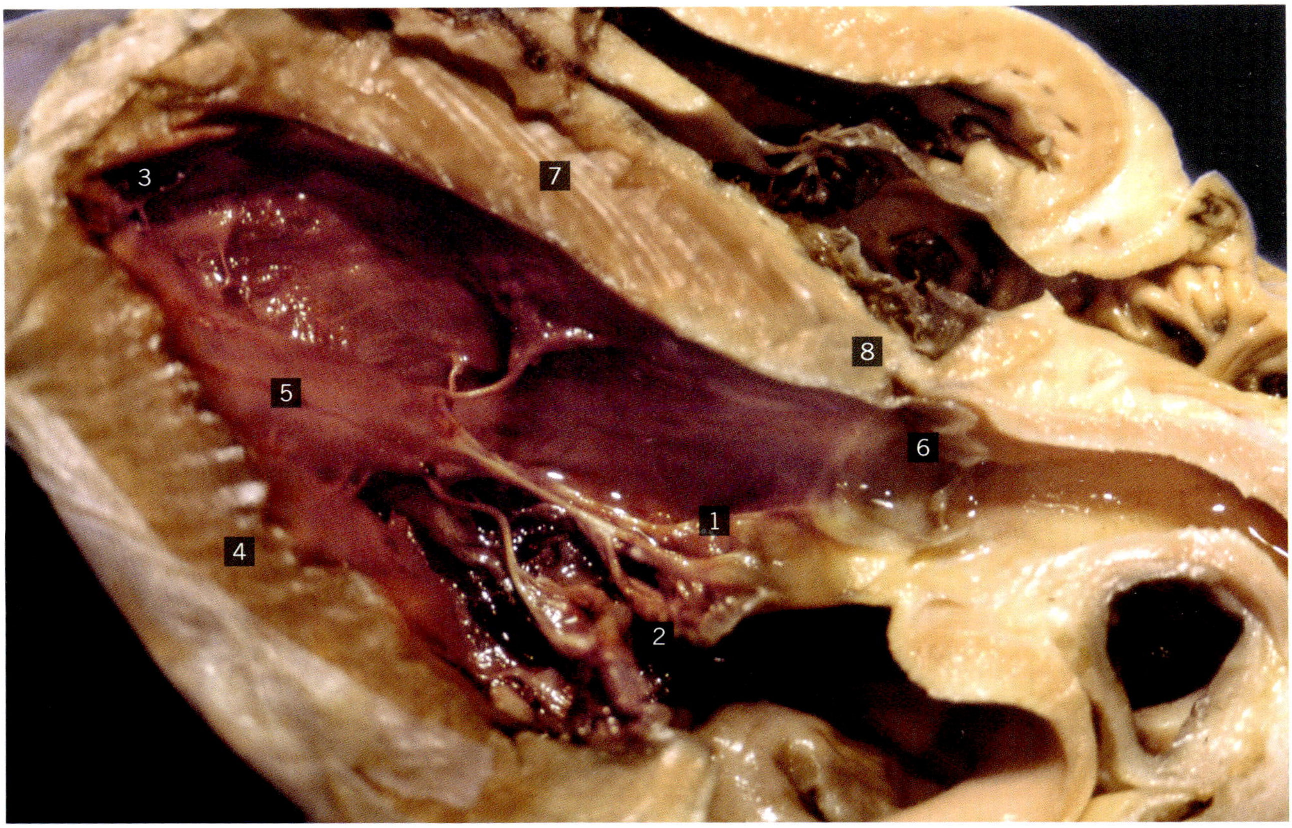

Figure 33. Longitudinal section of the left ventricle. The aortic leaflet of the mitral valve (1) divides the ventricle into two areas, the area of entrance, which goes from the mitral valve (2) to the apex (3) and is delimited by the free wall of the ventricle (4) and the papillary muscles (5), and the exit area, which goes from the apex (3) to the aortic ostium (6) and is essentially delimited by the interventricular septum (7). Membranous part of the interventricular septum (8).

LEFT VENTRICLE

It is the greater structure of the heart. It is located ventral to the left atrium, is cone-shaped and its tip forms the apex of the heart. It receives oxygenated blood from the lungs and pumps it into the systemic circulation through the aorta. Its main characteristic is its thick wall, which is 3 or 4 times thicker than that of the right ventricle. The cranial or aortic leaflet of the open mitral valve divides the left ventricle in two areas: the area of entrance, which goes from the mitral valve orifice to the apex and is formed by the free wall of the ventricle and the papillary muscles, and the exit area, which goes from the apex to the aortic ostium and is essentially delimited by the interventricular septum.

The two papillary muscles of the left ventricle originate from its free wall. The muscle that originates closest to the subsinuosal interventricular groove is termed "dorsal" and the one closest to the paraconal interventricular groove is termed "ventral".

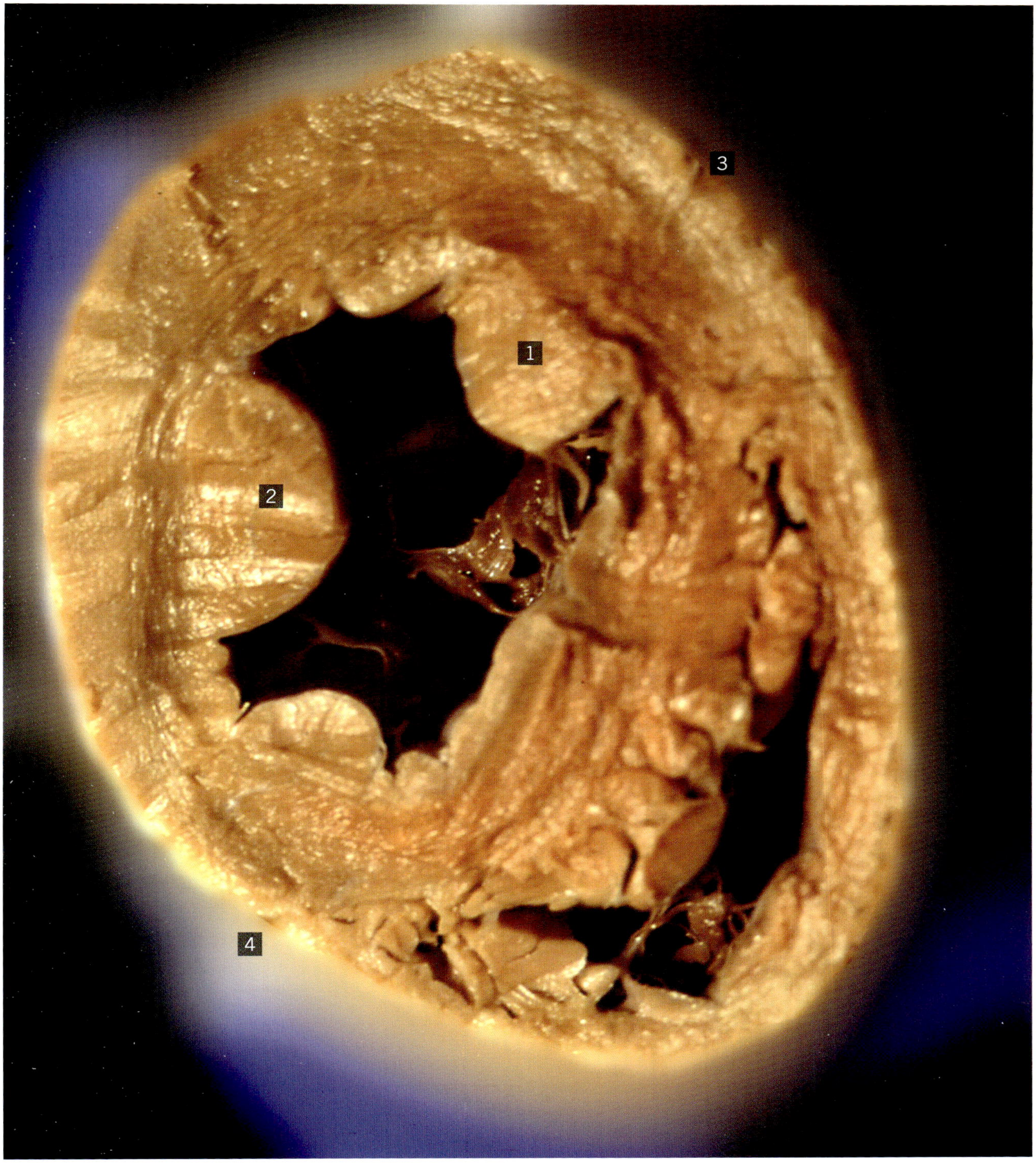

Figure 34. Cross-section of both ventricles.

[1 Dorsal papillary muscle] [3 Subsinuosal interventricular groove]

[2 Ventral papillary muscle] [4 Paraconal interventricular groove]

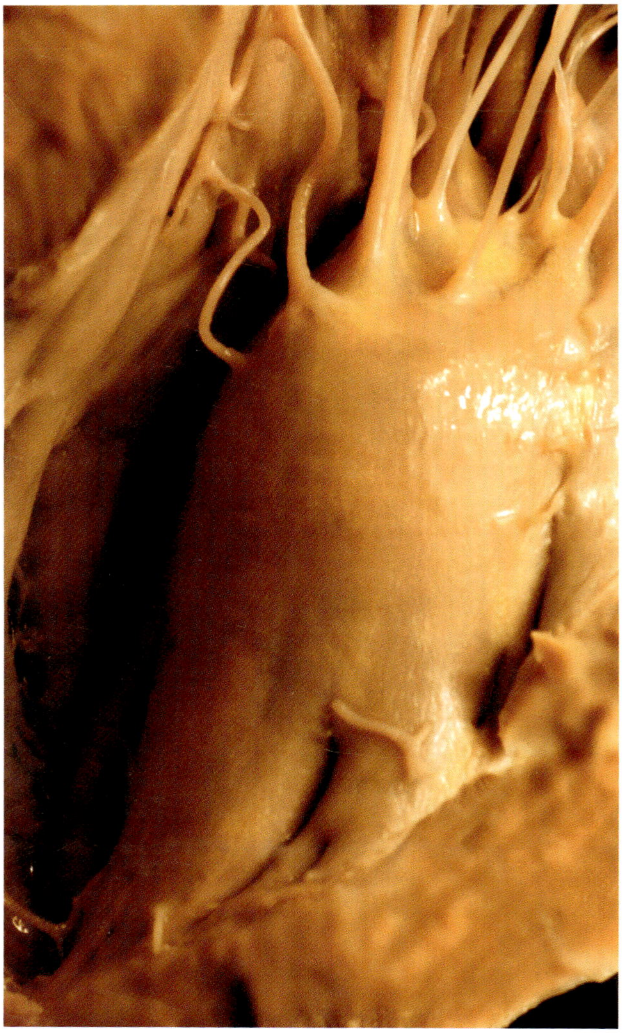

Figure 35. Dorsal papillary muscle.

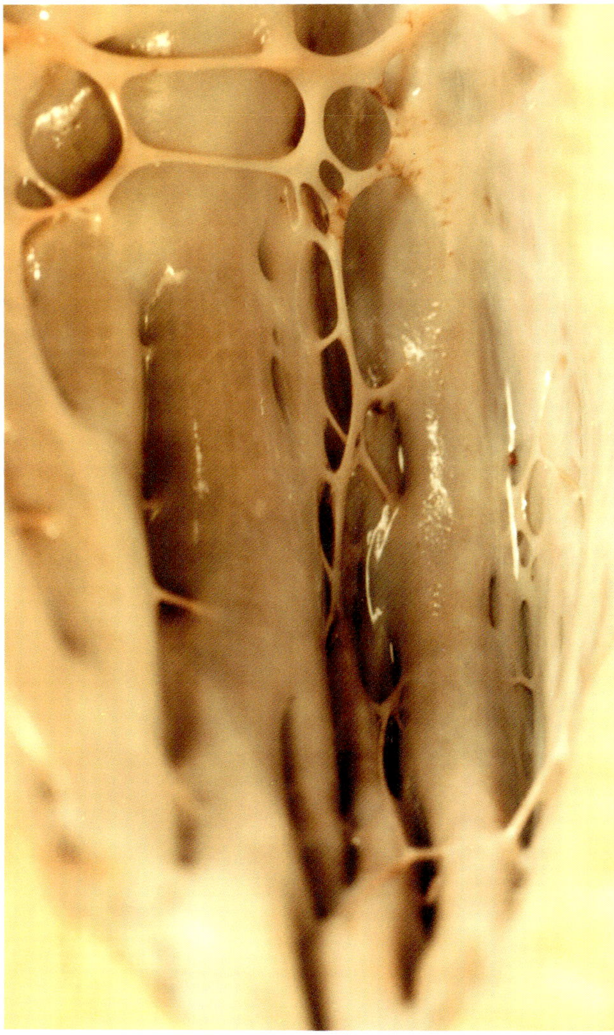

Figure 36. It is sometimes possible to observe trabeculae carnae in the left ventricle.

The interventricular septum is formed by two parts: a small portion, located just below the attachment of the non-coronary cusp, which is the membranous part of the septum and joins the other part, the muscular part of the septum, formed by the union of the myocardium of the septa of both ventricles.

The left ventricle also has trabeculae (trabeculae carneae), although their amount is smaller and they are much less marked than in the right ventricle.

The presence of a moderator band that crosses the ventricular cavity may sometimes be observed.

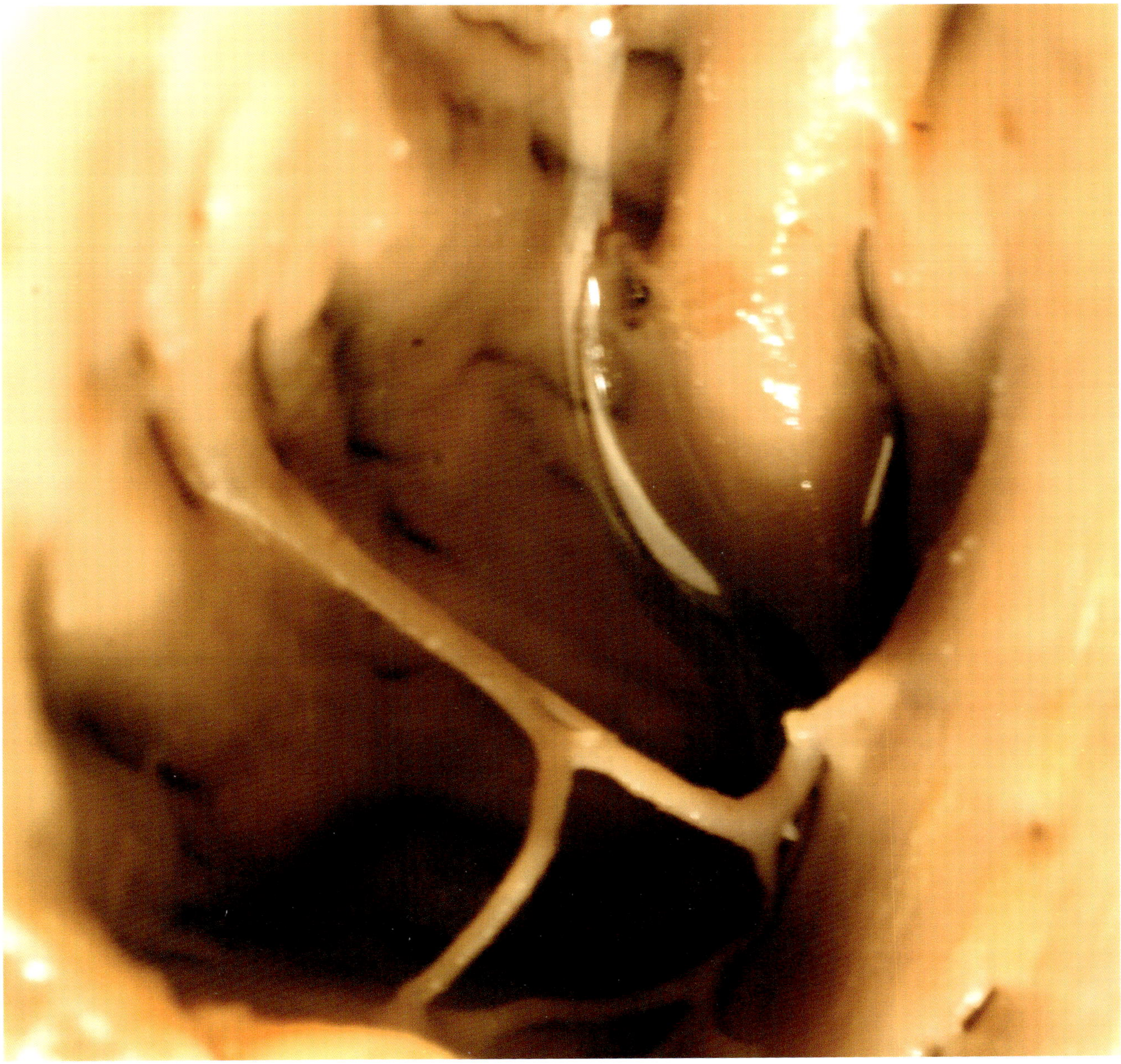

Figure 37. It is also sometimes possible to observe moderator bands that pass across the ventricular cavity in the left ventricle.

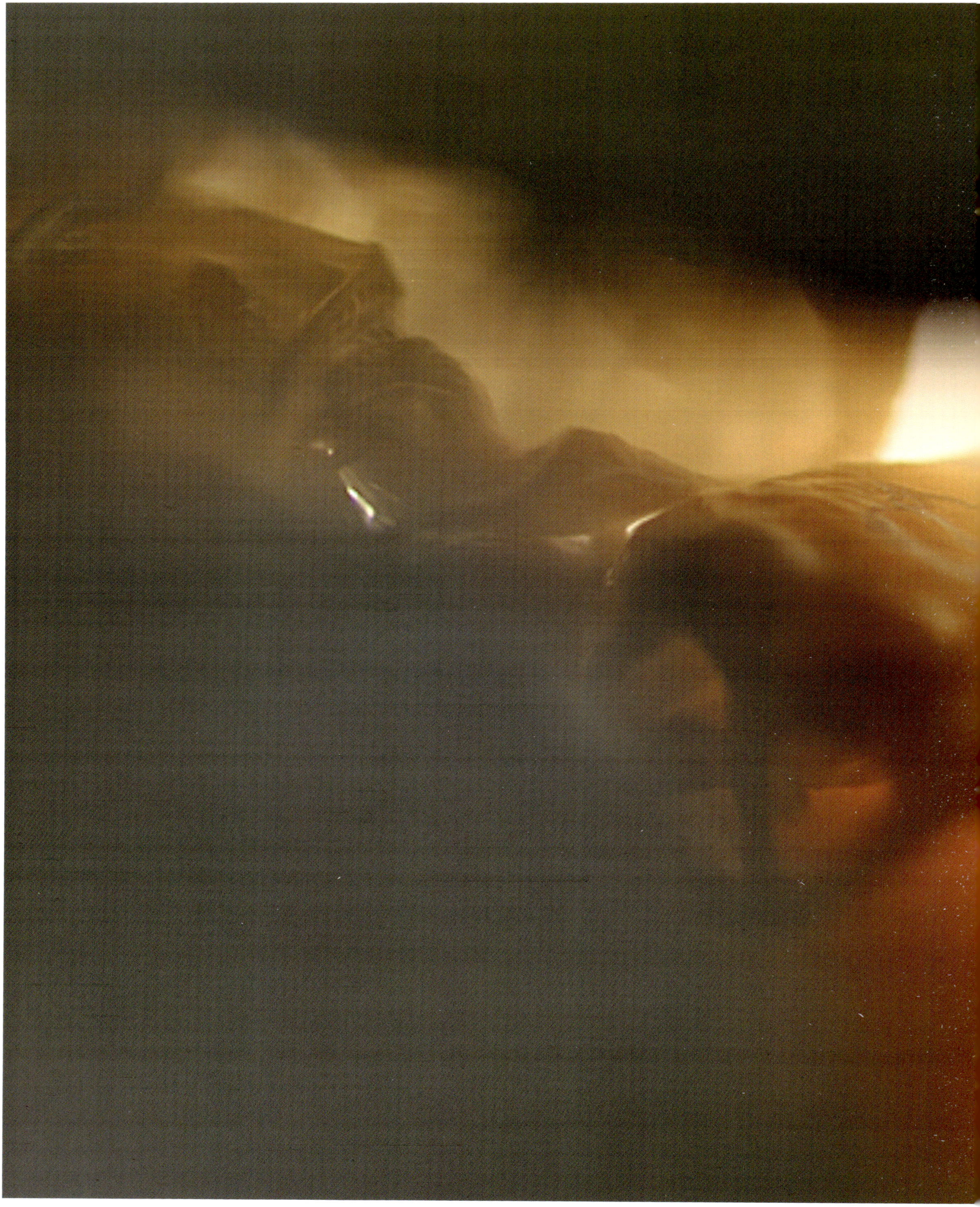

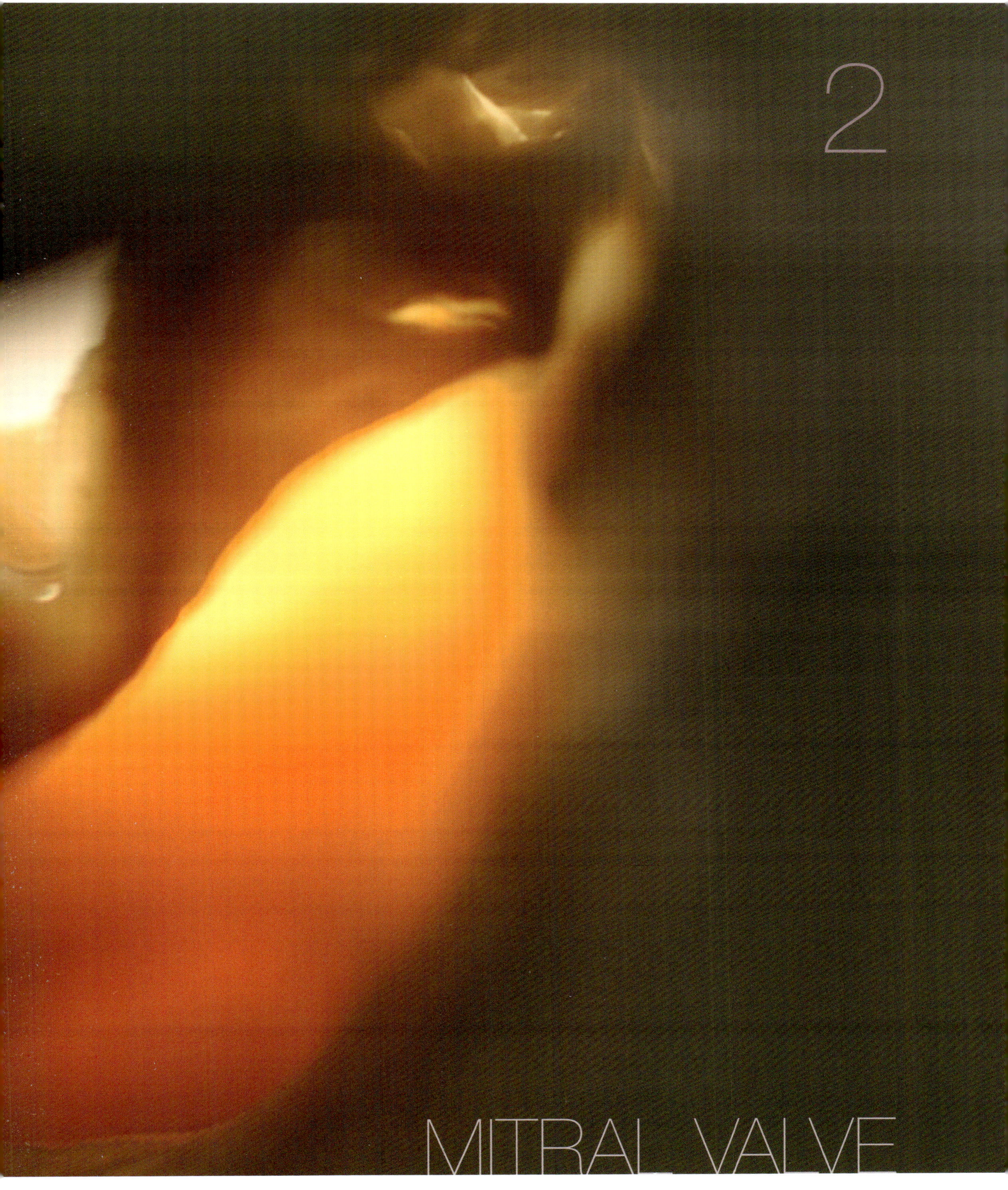

2

MITRAL VALVE

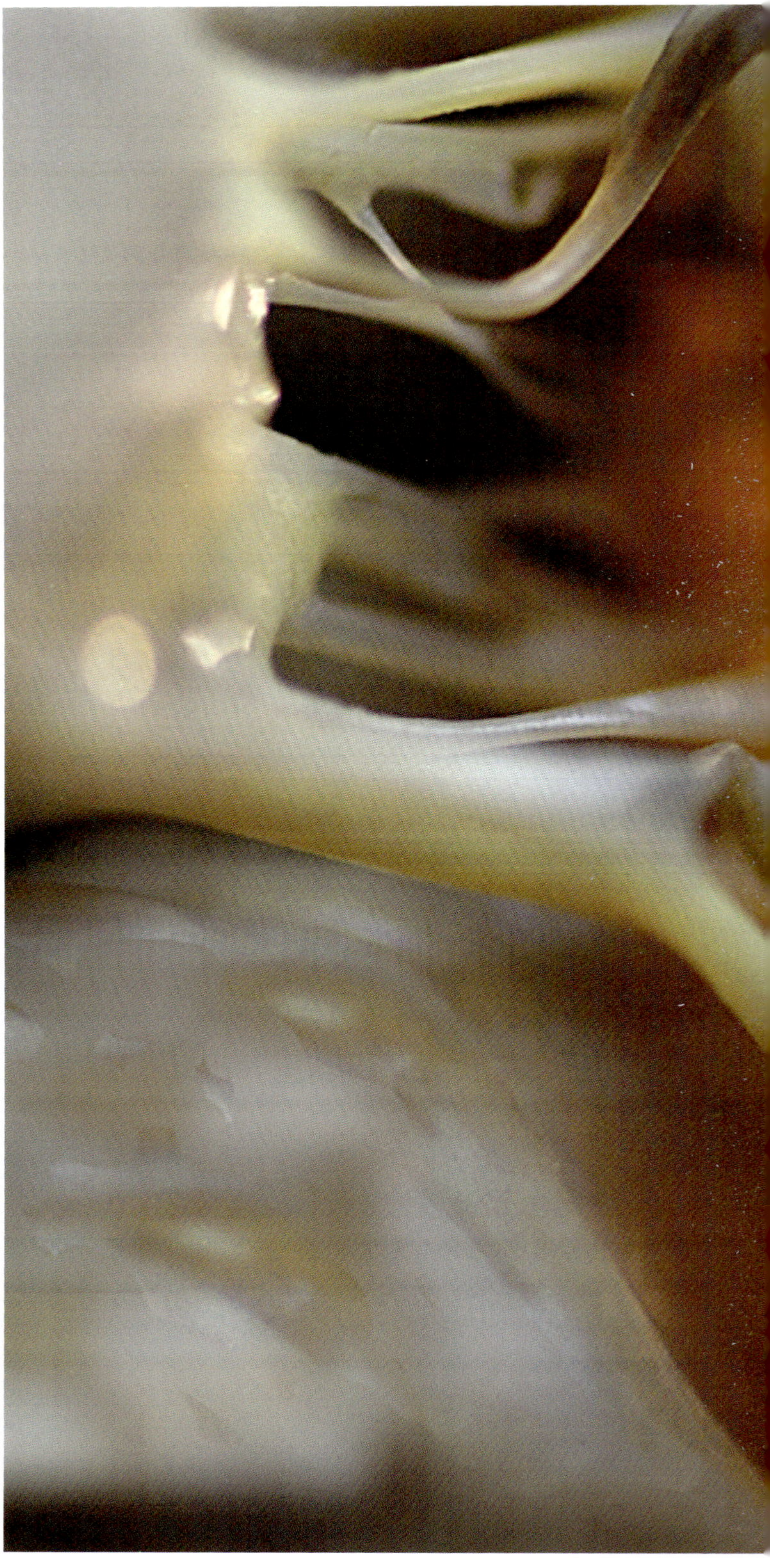

It seems that it was Andreas Vesalius who first used the name "mitral valve" to refer to the valve that lies between the left atrium and ventricle, due to its resemblance to a bishop's mitre.

The main function of this valve is to prevent backflow into the left atrium during ventricular systole.

The mitral valve apparatus is formed by:

- The mitral valve annulus.
- Leaflets, or cusps.
- Chordae tendinae.
- Papillary muscles.

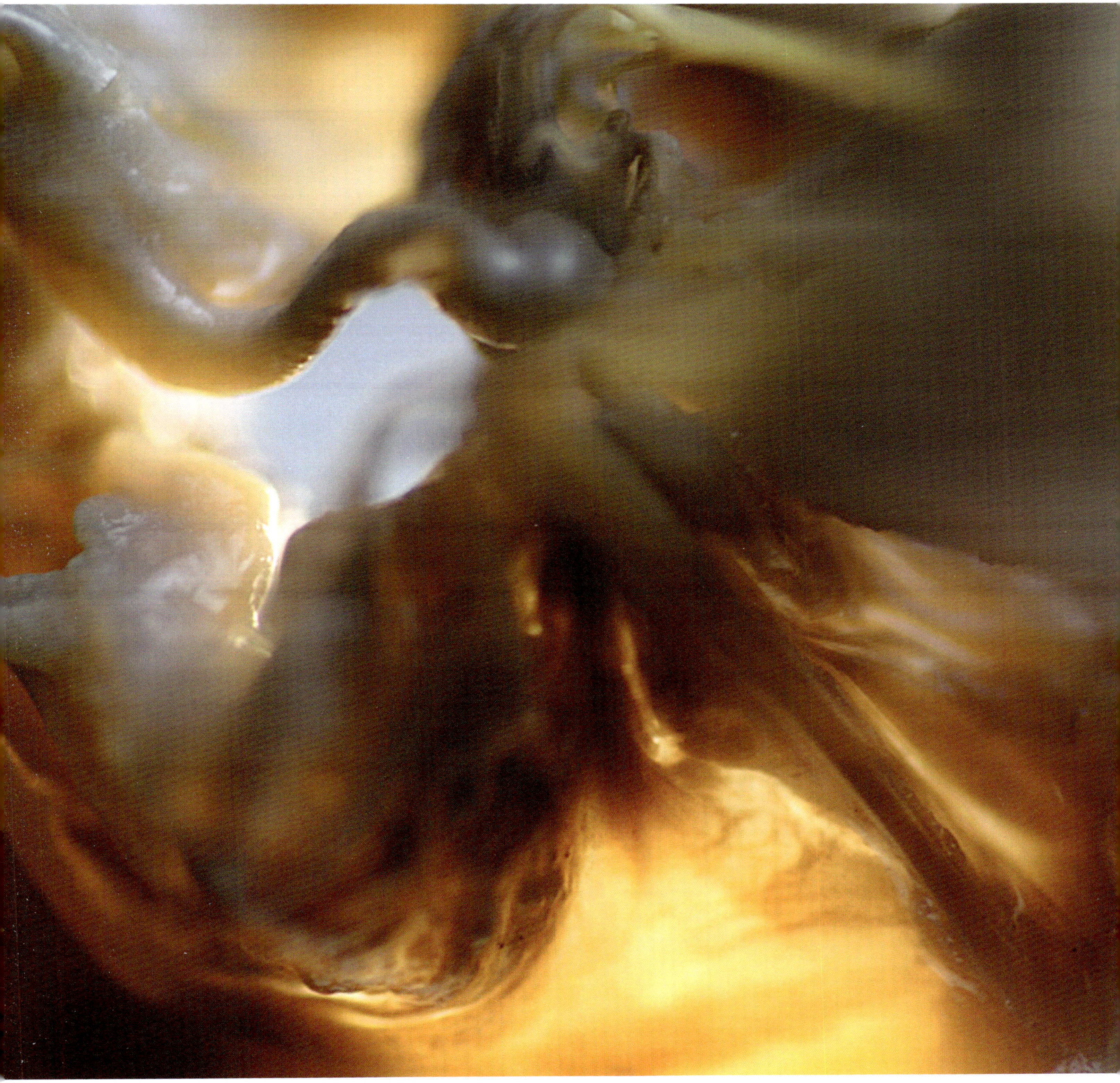

Figure 1. Mitral valve apparatus.

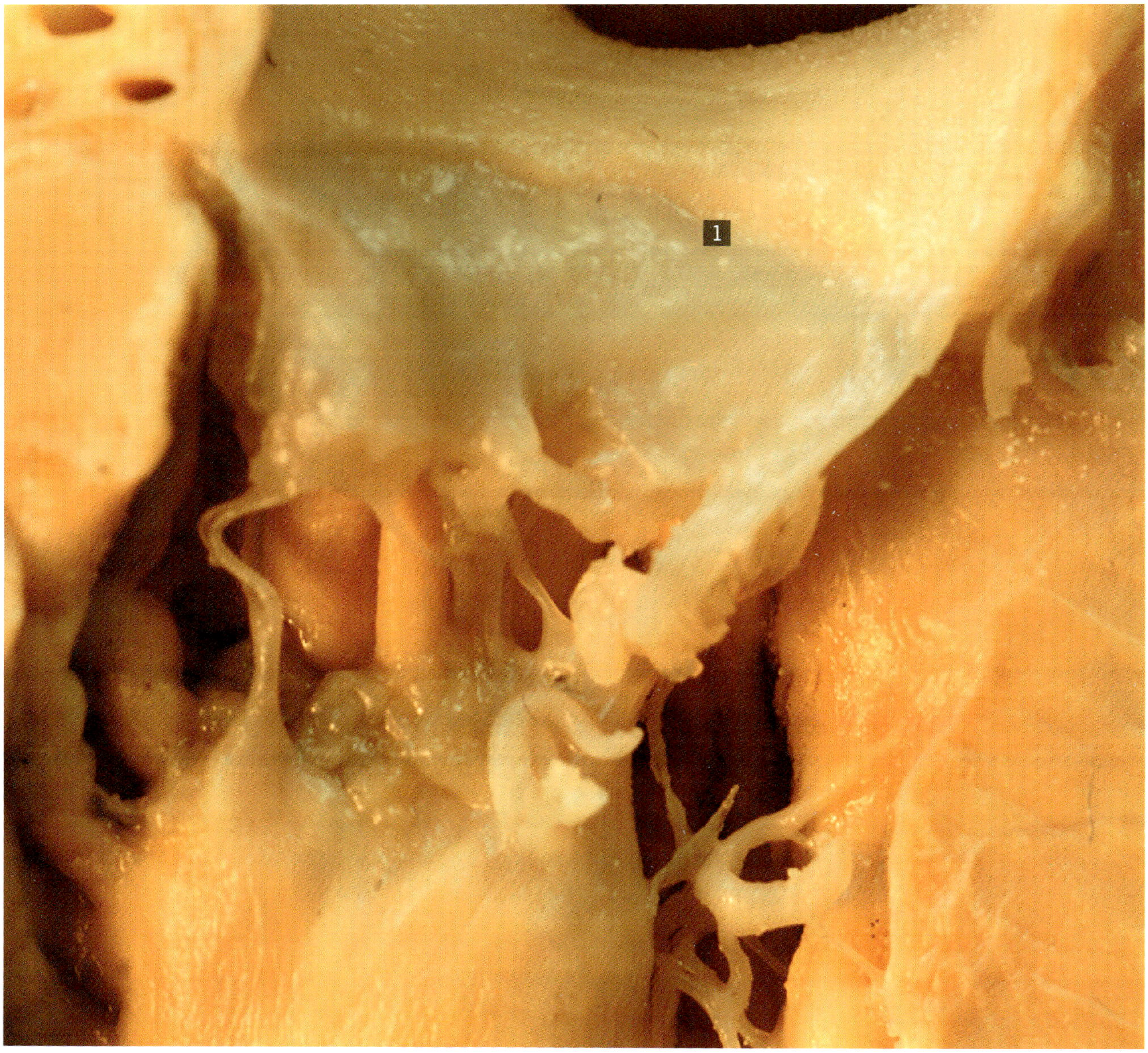

Figure 2. Caudal leaflet.

MITRAL VALVE ANNULUS

[1 Annulus]

The annulus marks the hinge line of the leaflets. In this region, the aortic valve lies adjacent to the cranial leaflet, an area where the left and right fibrous trigones expand, thus contributing to a great extent to the formation of the annulus. The atrial myocardium lies above it.

The circumflex coronary artery courses along its lateral and caudal part and the interatrial septum can be found medial to it.

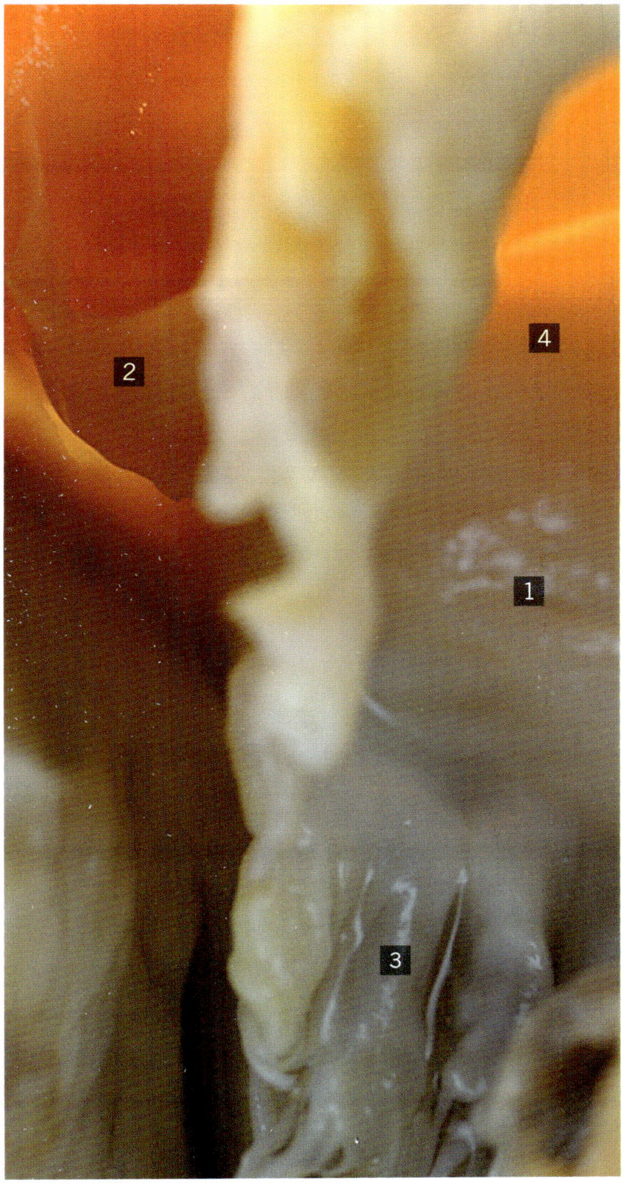

Figure 3. Cranial leaflet.

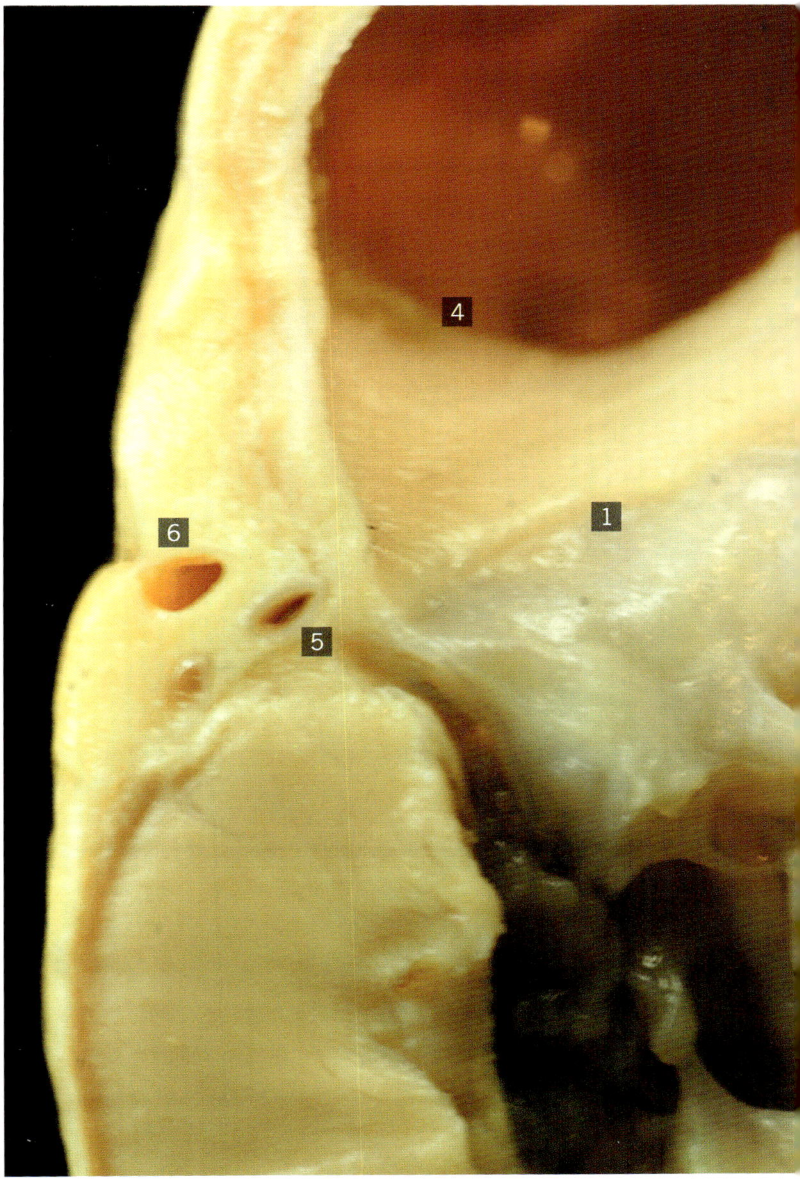

Figure 4. Annulus, caudal leaflet.

[1 Annulus]

[2 Aortic cusp]

[3 Cranial leaflet]

[4 Left atrium]

[5 Left circumflex artery]

[6 Main coronary vein]

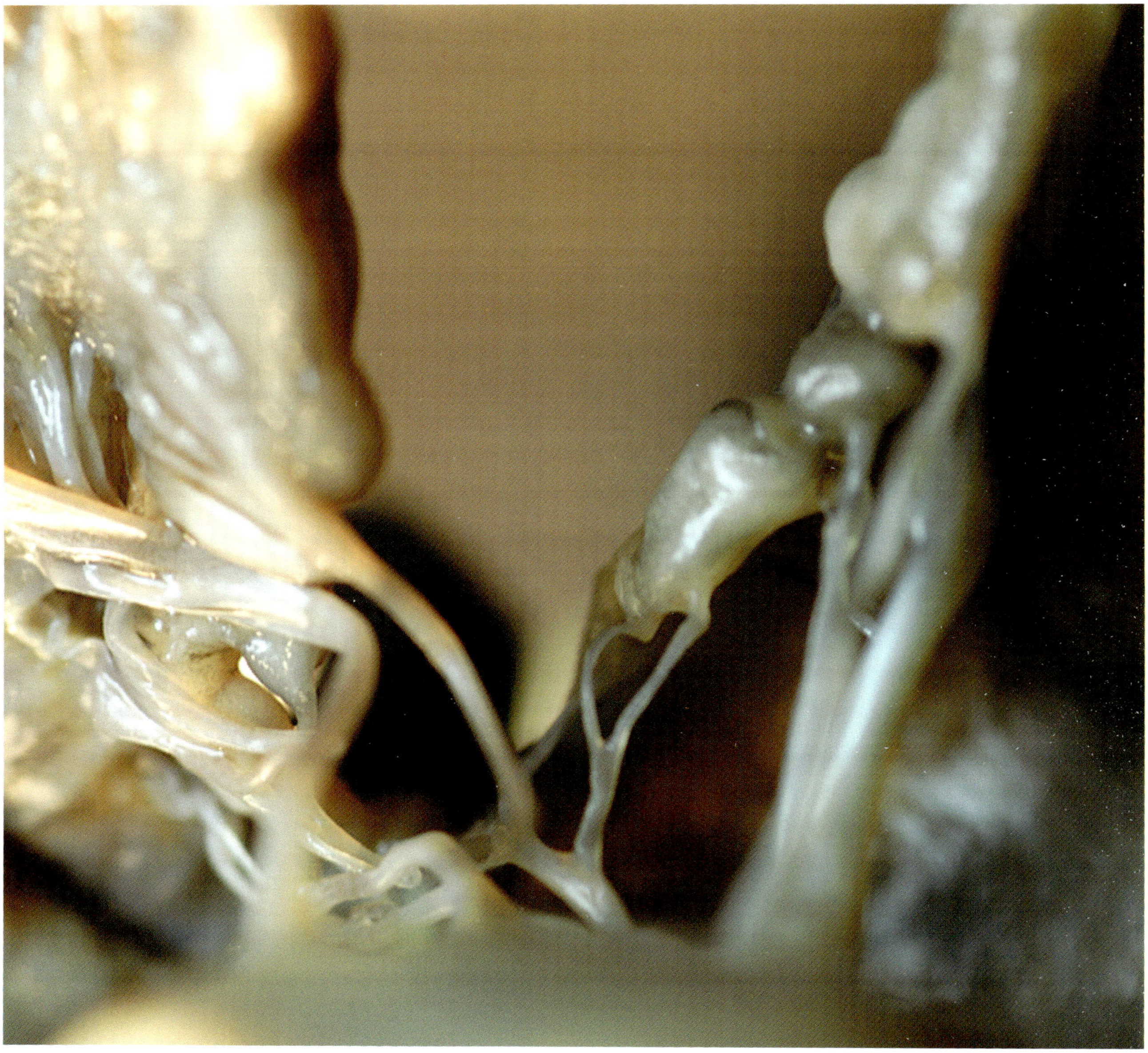

Figure 5. Cranial and caudal leaflets seen from the ventricular cavity.

LEAFLETS

Two leaflets form the mitral valve. The cranial (aortic) leaflet, which is closely related to the aorta, marks the aortic outflow tract together with the interventricular septum; the caudal or mural leaflet is related to the free wall of the ventricle and is more sensitive to morphological changes than the left atrium. They could be defined as thin and flexible. They are smooth and soft on their atrial surface and the chordae tendineae insert into their ventricular surface, giving rise to morphological changes. Close to their free edges they are more irregular and have small, normal nodular thickenings.

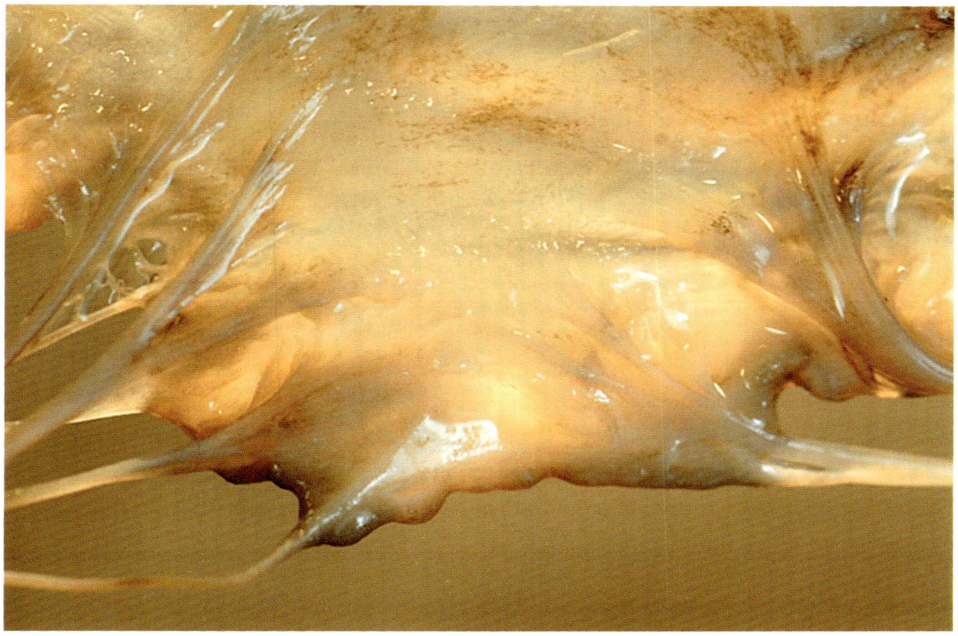

Figure 6. Cranial leaflet, view of the ventricular surface.

[1 Caudal leaflet]

[2 Cranial leaflet]

[3 Aortic outflow tract]

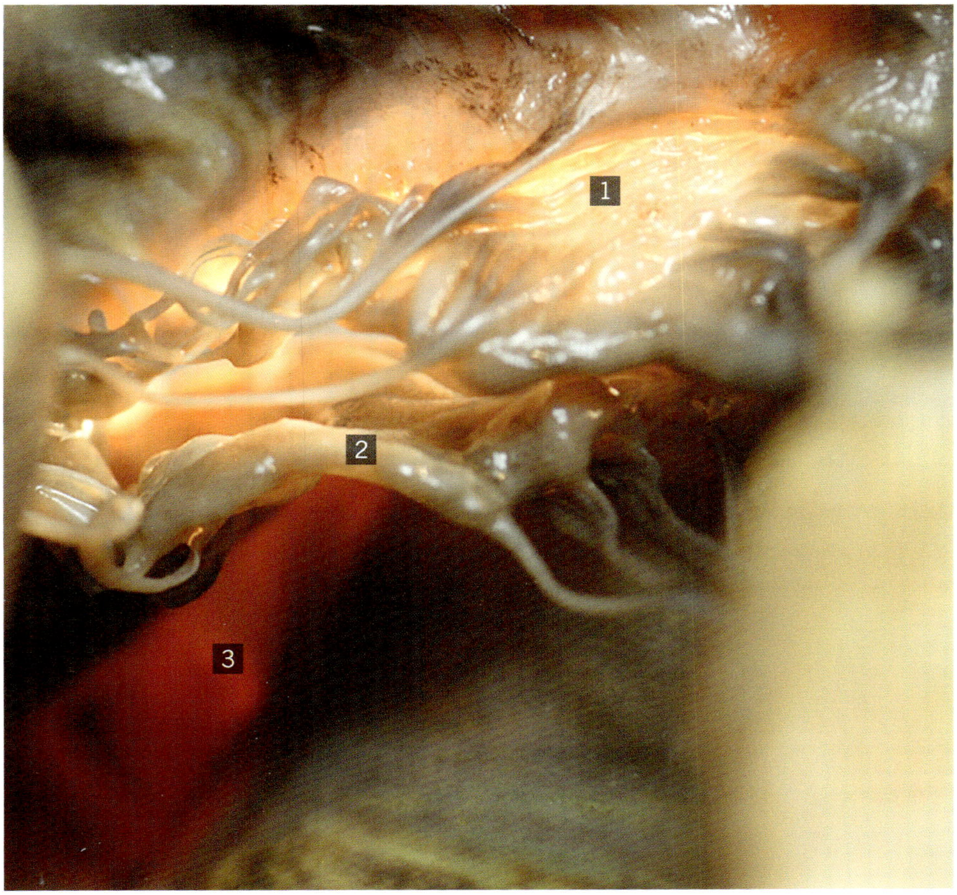

Figure 7.

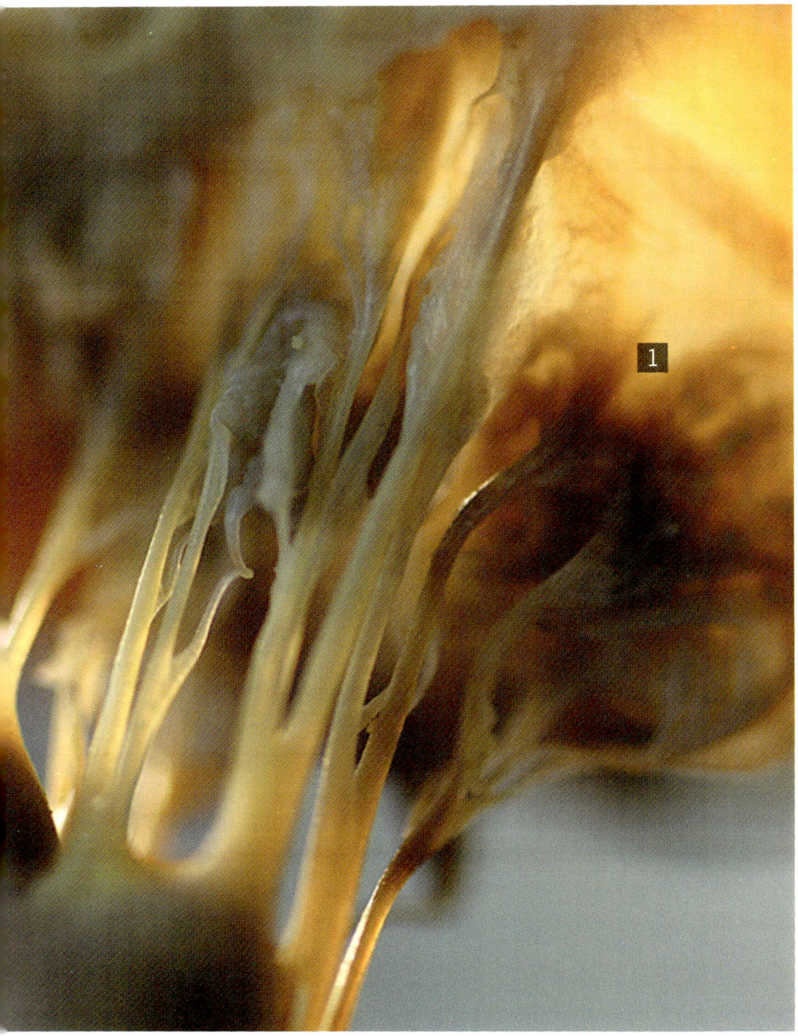

Figure 8. Chordae tendineae of the caudal leaflet.

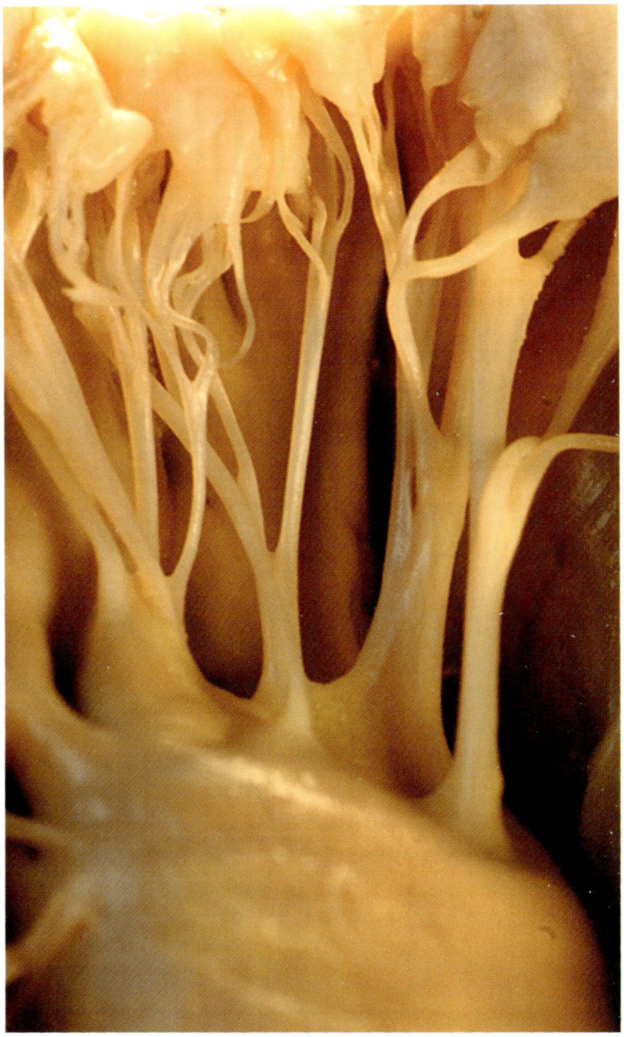

Figure 9. Chordae tendineae of the caudal leaflet.

CHORDAE TENDINEAE

[1 Rough zone]

They form the tensor apparatus of the valve and prevent the valve from prolapsing into the atrium during systole.

They run from the papillary muscles or, on some occasions, from the free ventricular wall to the ventricular surface of the leaflets or to their free edge. Most of them have branches.

A first classification distinguished three types of chordae:

- Primary chordae insert into the free edge.
- Secondary chordae, which are thicker than the previous ones, insert into the ventricular surface of the leaflets and then into their free edge, where they form the rough zone.
- Tertiary chordae are limited to the caudal leaflet. They arise from the ventricular wall or from small trabeculae and insert into the base of the leaflet.

[1 Primary chorda (strut)]

[2 Secondary chorda (rough)]

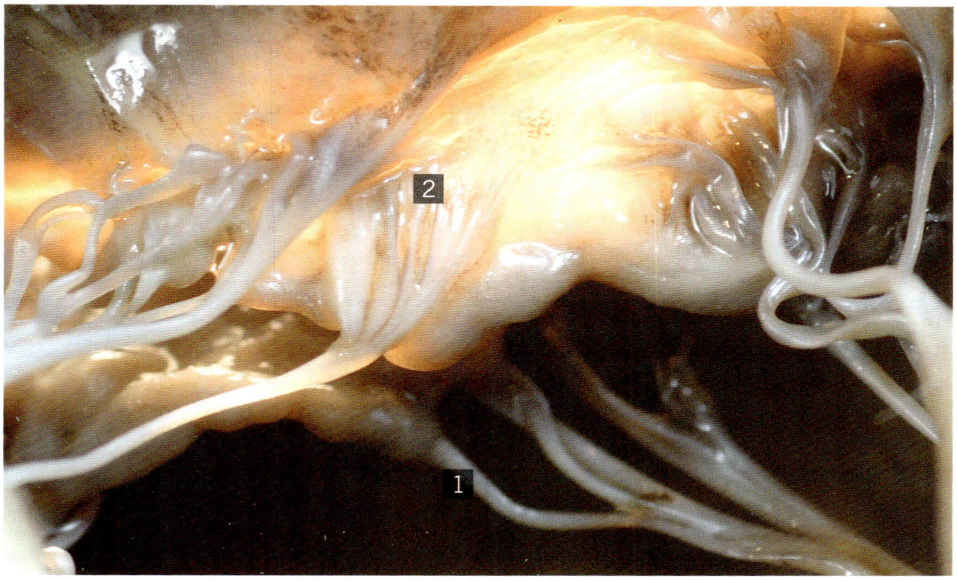

Figure 10.

[3 View of the area of insertion named rough zone]

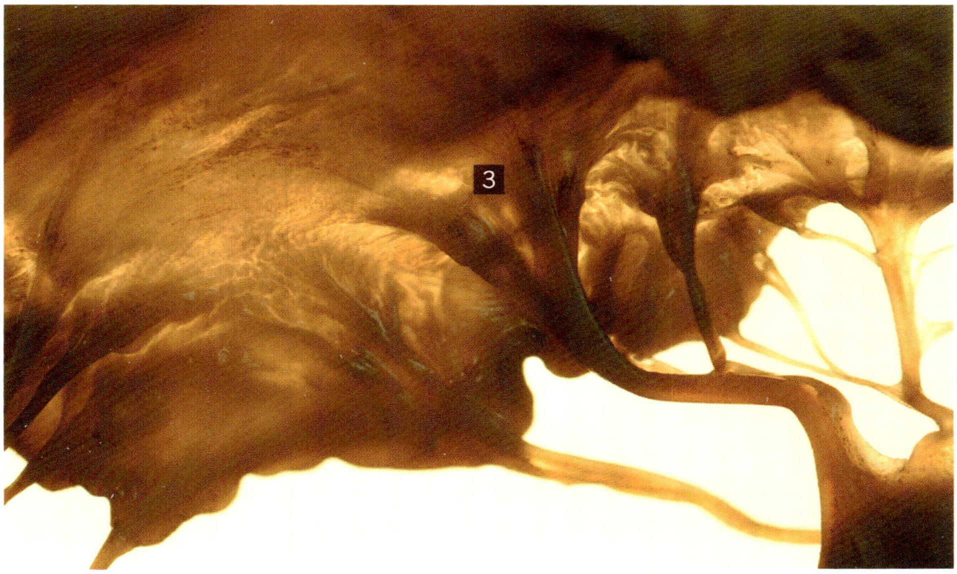

Figure 11. Rough zone.

A subsequent classification tells us about:

- **Commissural chordae**: they insert into the commissures of the leaflets.
- **Rough zone chordae**: they insert into the ventricular surface of both leaflets.
- **Strut chordae**: they insert into the free edge of the cranial leaflet.
- **Basal chordae**: they insert into the base of the caudal leaflet and arise from the ventricle or from small trabeculae.
- **Cleft chordae**: they insert into the free edge of the caudal leaflet.

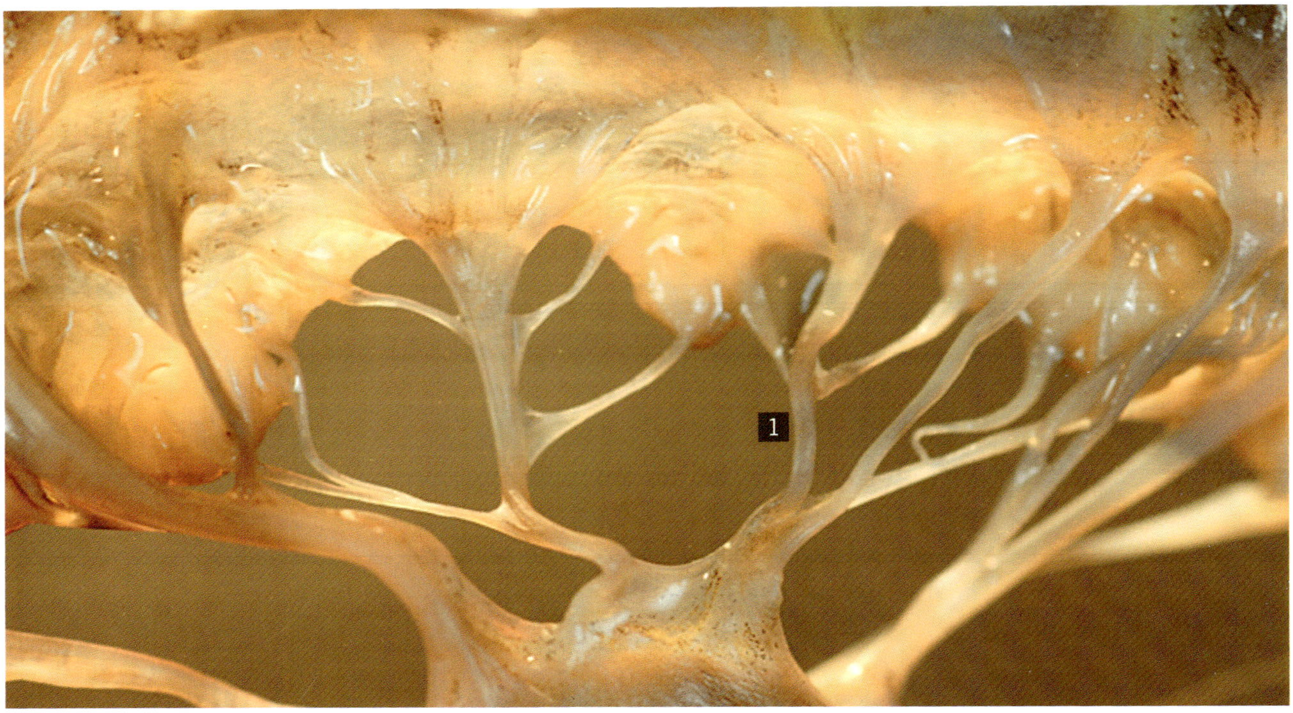

Figure 12.

[1 Commissural chordae (primary)]

[2 Cleft chorda (primary)]

[3 Rough zone chorda (secondary)]

[4 Basal chorda (tertiary)]

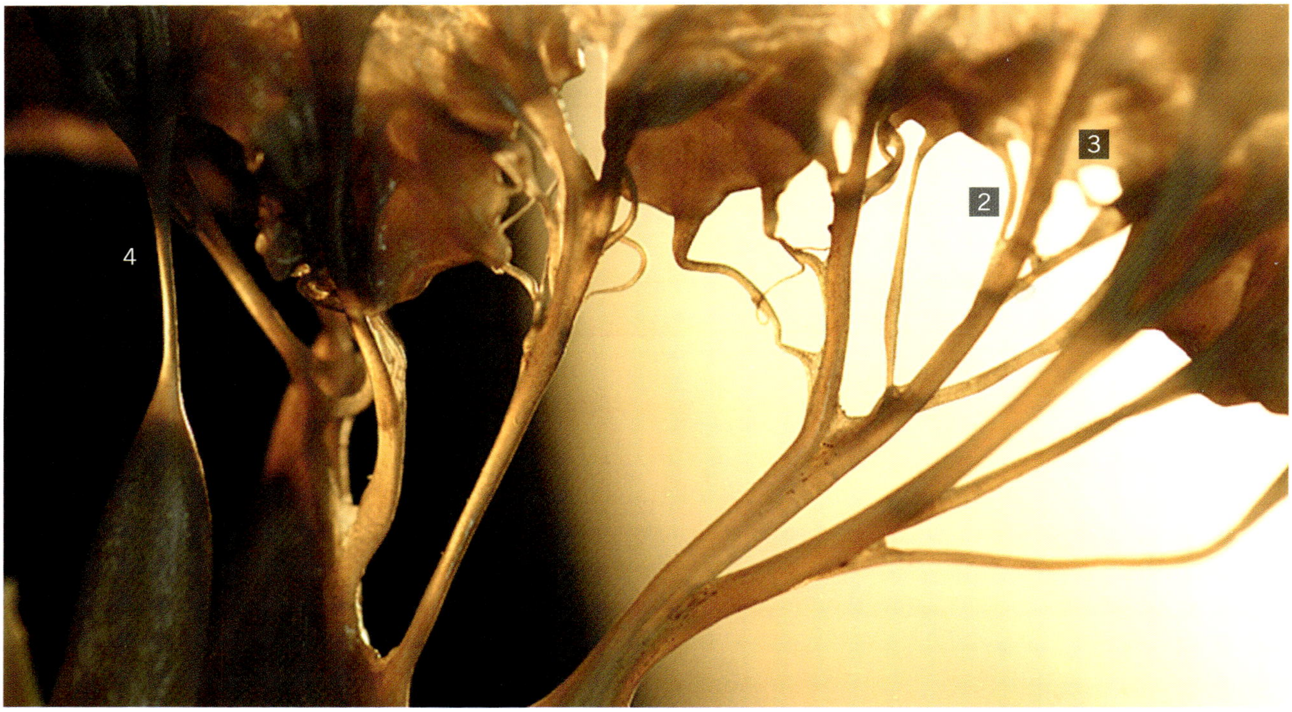

Figure 13.

[1 Basal chorda (tertiary)]

[2 Papillary muscle]

[3 Moderator bands]

[4 Origin of chordae tendineae]

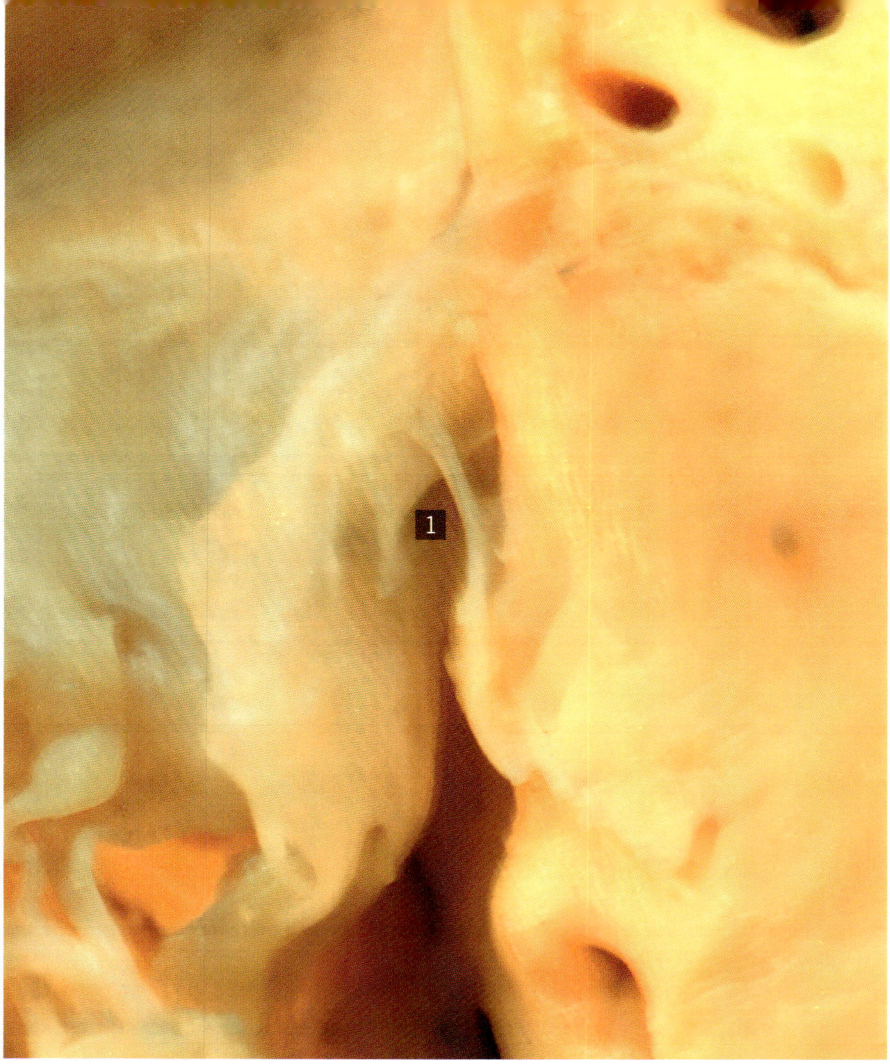

Figure 14.

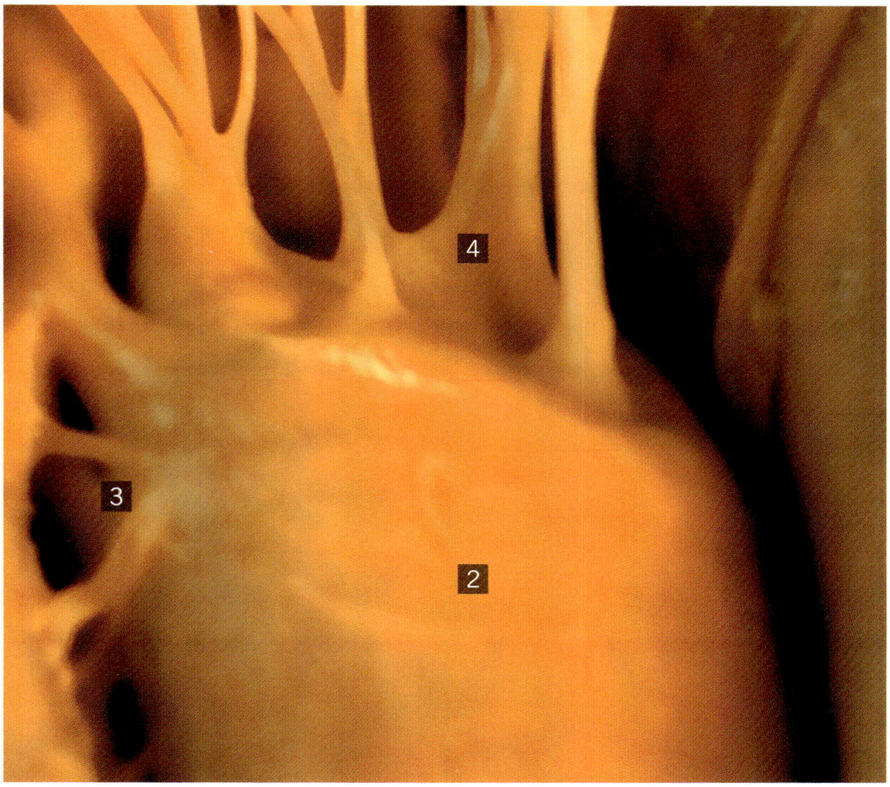

Figure 15.

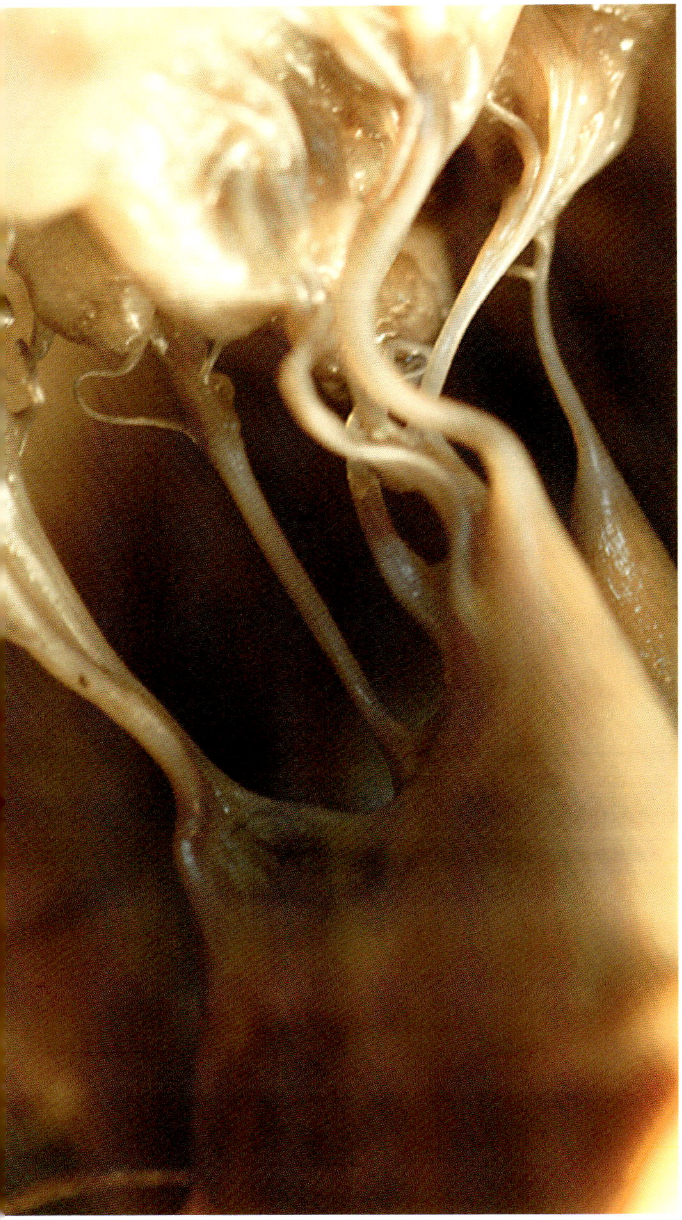

Figure 16. Papillary muscle.

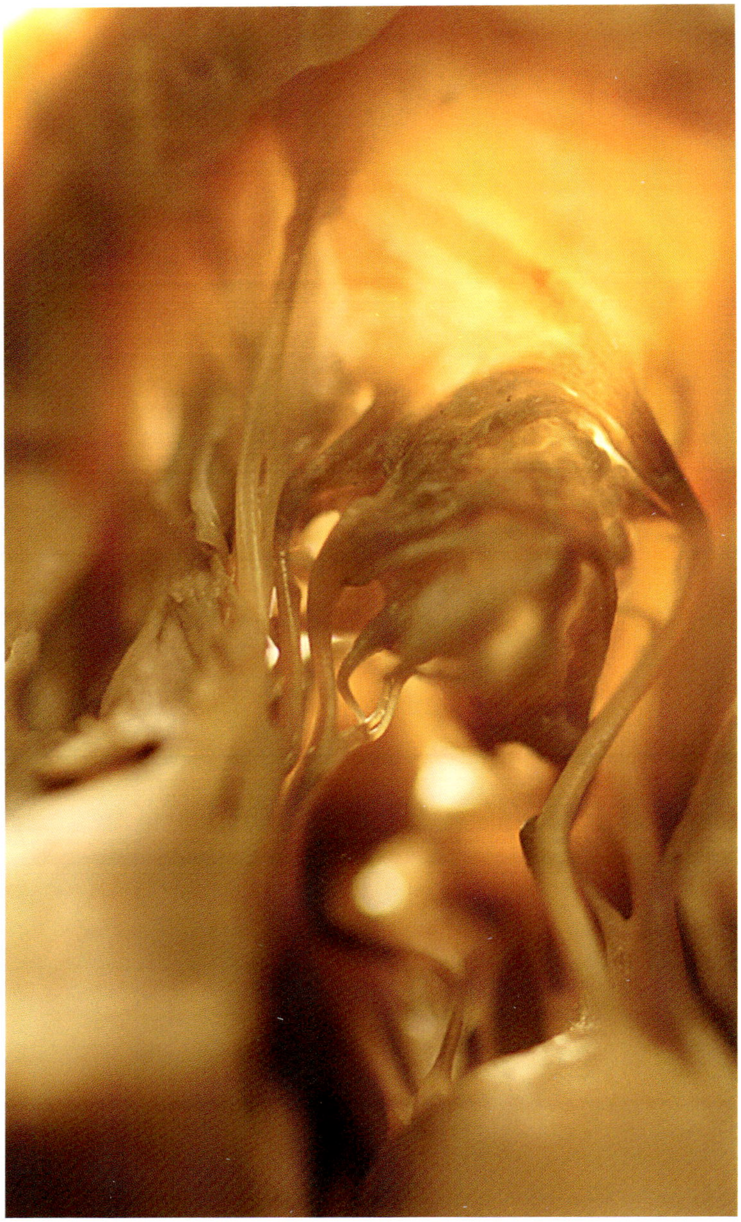

Figure 17. View of the two papillary muscles.

PAPILLARY MUSCLES

They are located between the apical and medial parts of the free wall of the ventricle and are the origin of the chordae tendineae, which attach to both leaflets. Their function is to hold the chordae in position and tighten them during ventricular systole, preventing the prolapse of the leaflets into the left atrium. They are sometimes divided at the end. Changes in the morphology of the left ventricle may affect their location and alter valvular function. The presence of moderator bands between them and the ventricular wall is common.

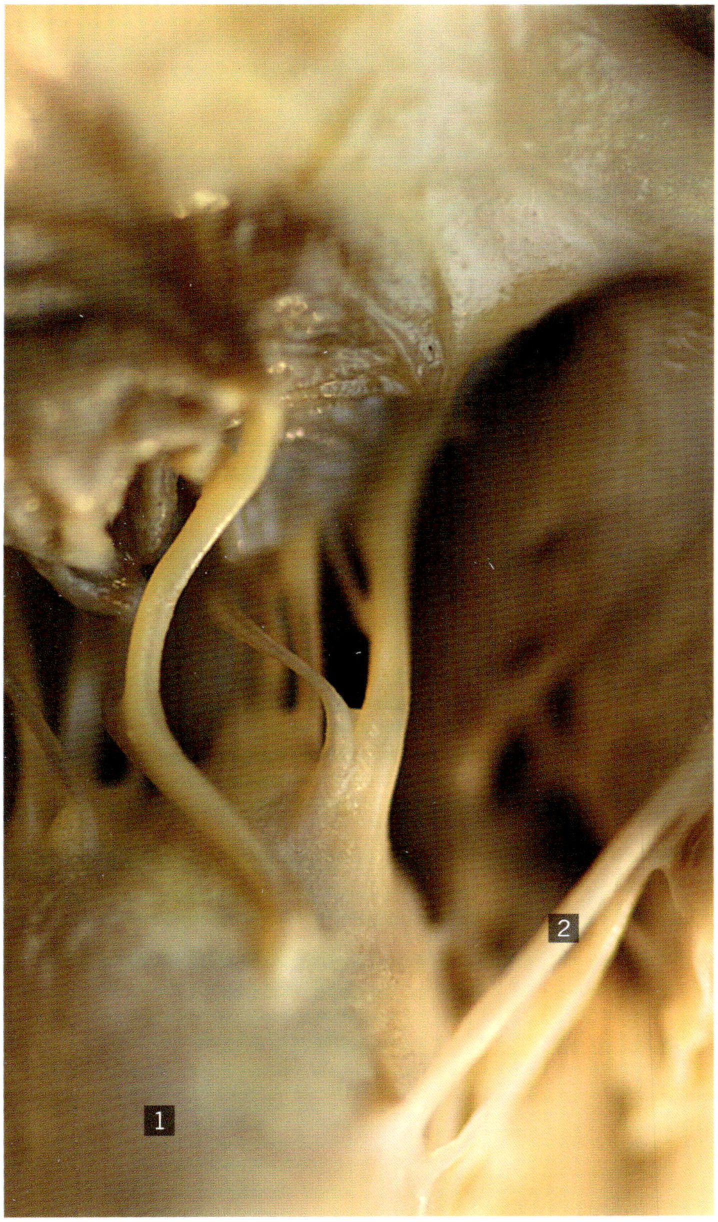

Figure 18.

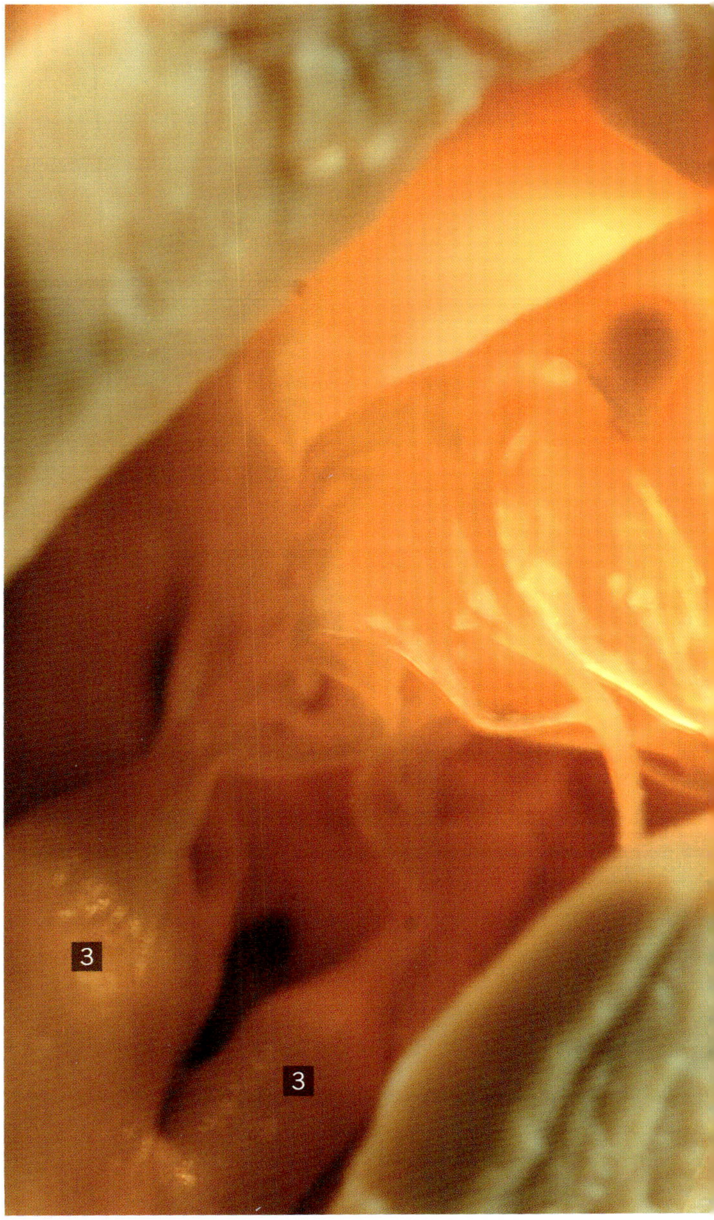

Figure 19.

[1 Papillary muscle] [2 Moderator bands] [3 Divided papillary muscle]

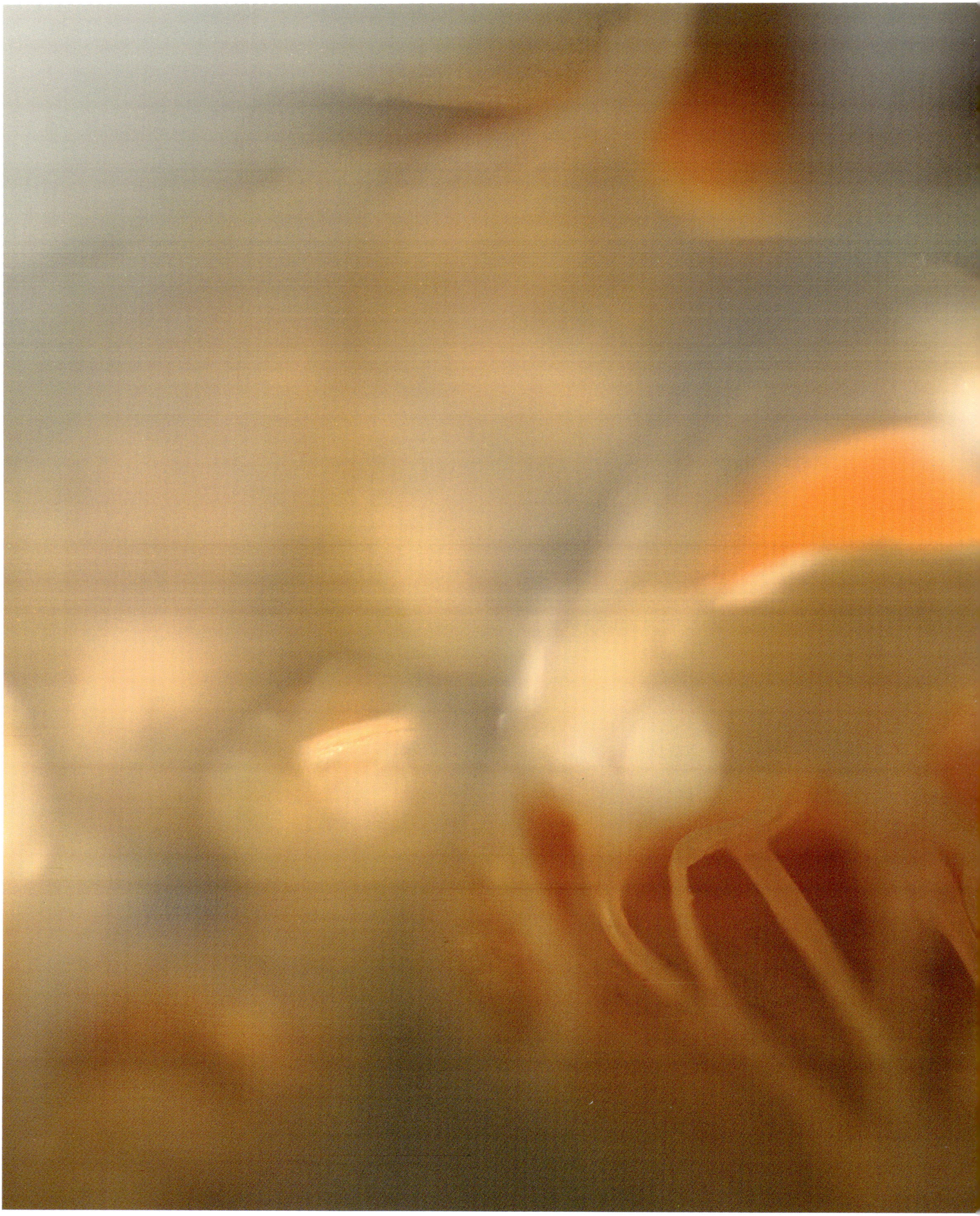

3

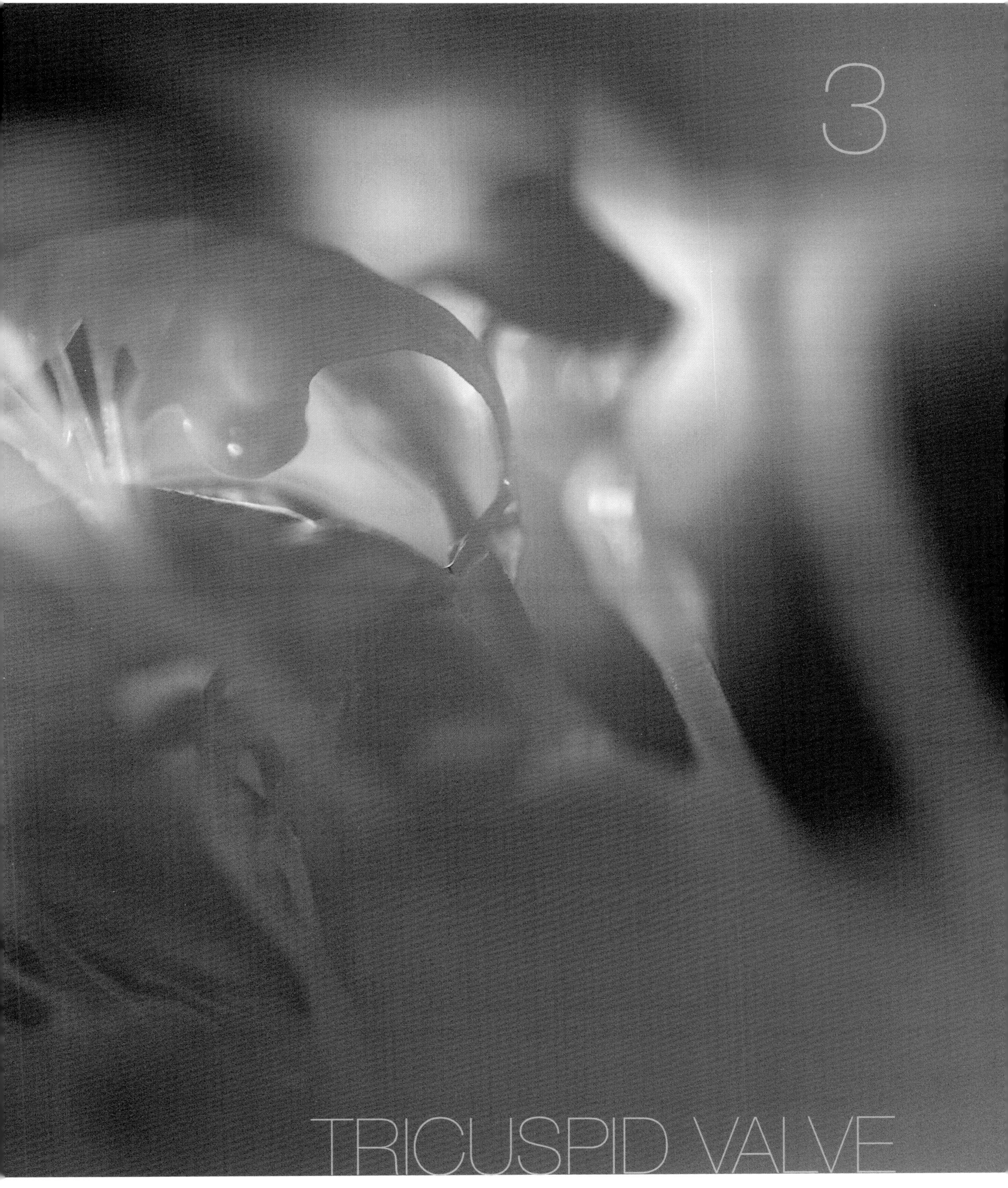

TRICUSPID VALVE

[1 Annulus]

[2 Leaflet]

[3 Chorda tendinea]

[4 Papillary muscle]

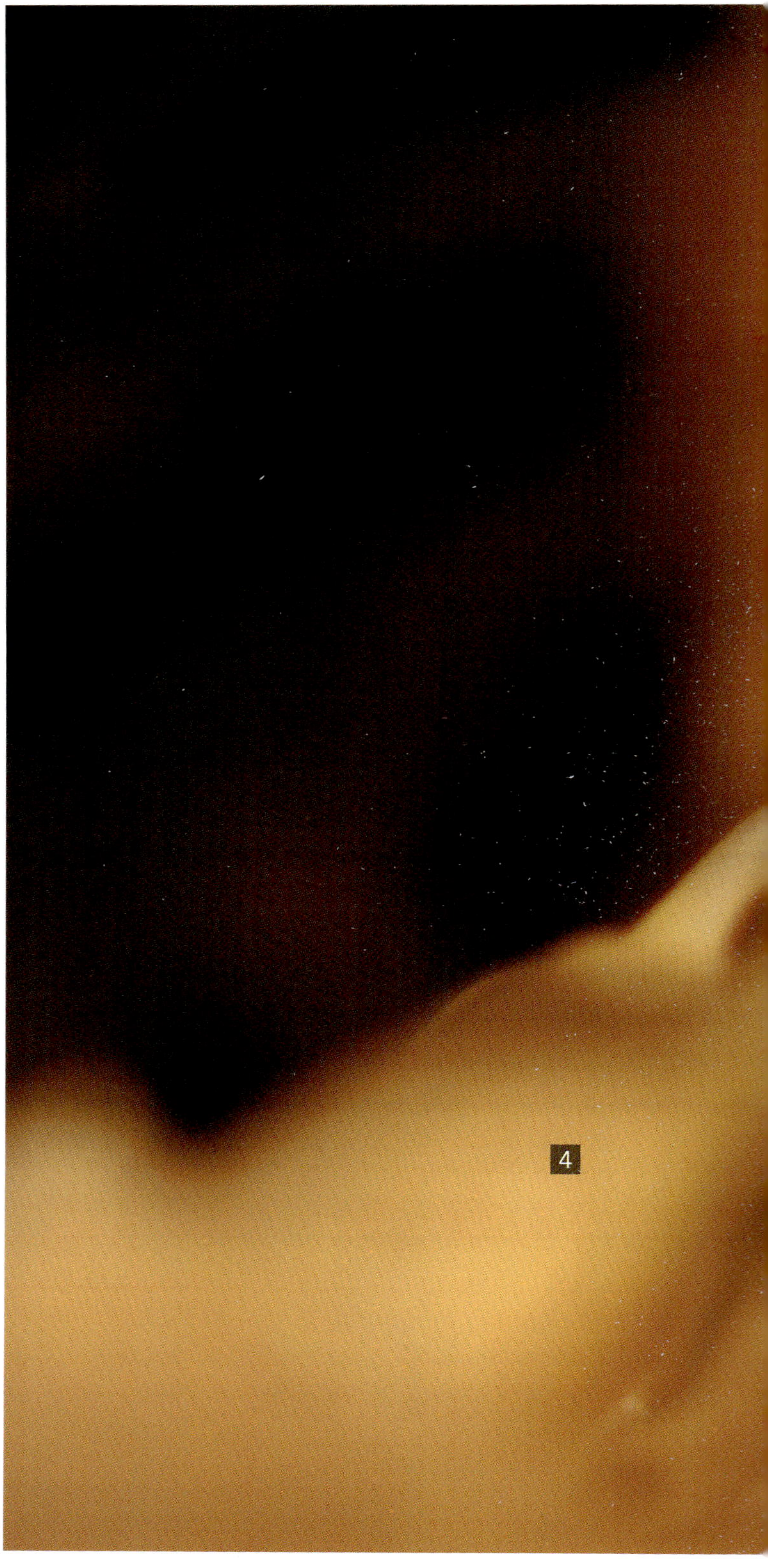

The tricuspid valve is located between the right atrium and ventricle. These cavities are adapted to lower pressures than those in the left side, which are due to the low vascular resistances of the pulmonary circuit. It is also important to know that, from the right atrium to the pulmonary artery, the blood flow forms an approximately right angle, as opposed to what occurs in the left side, where it forms a 180-degree angle.

The tricuspid valve apparatus is formed in a similar way to the mitral valve apparatus, but its structure is different due to the different conditions in which it works. It has:

- An annulus.
- Leaflets.
- Chordae tendineae.
- Papillary muscles.

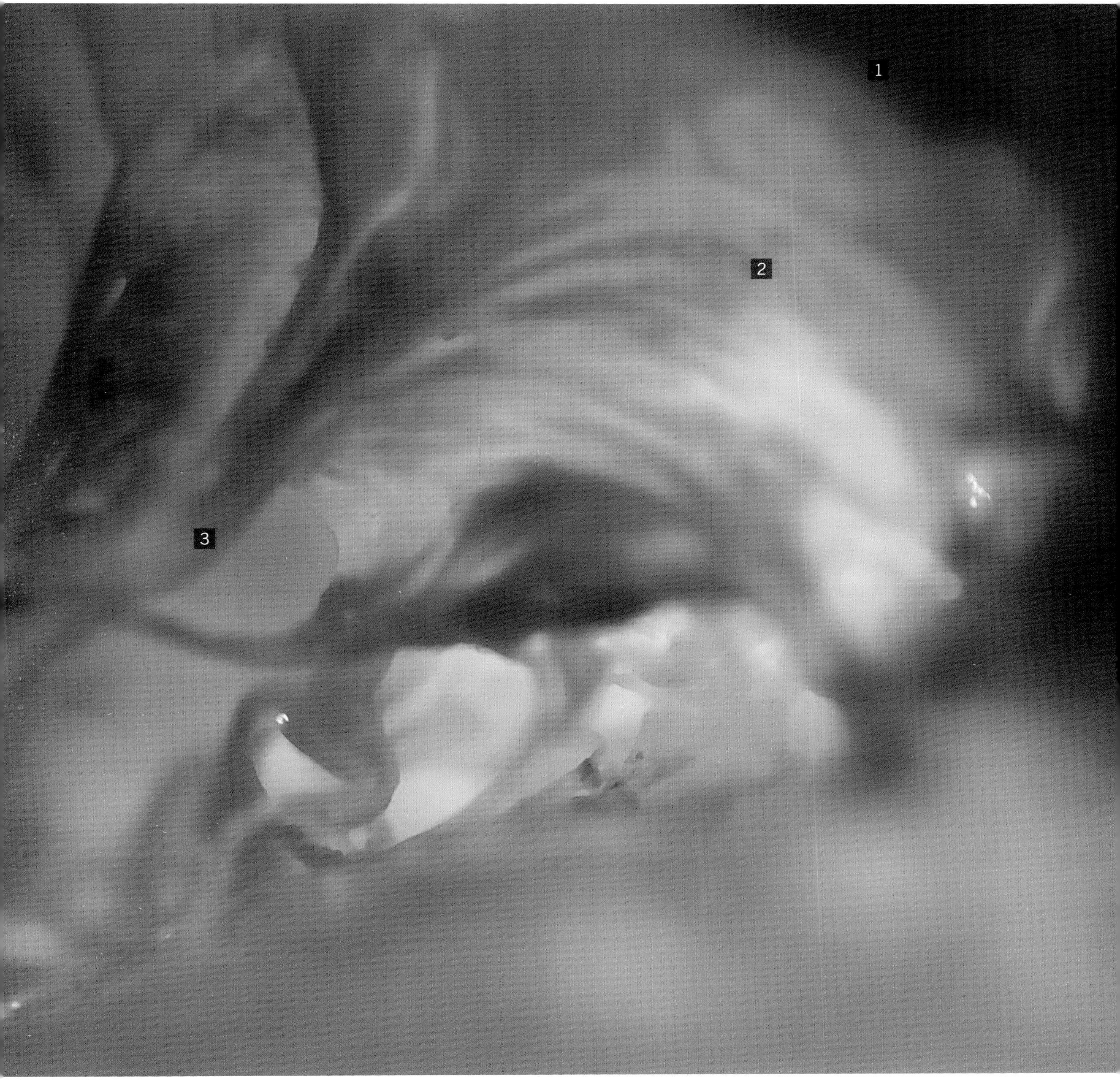

Figure 1. Tricuspid valve apparatus.

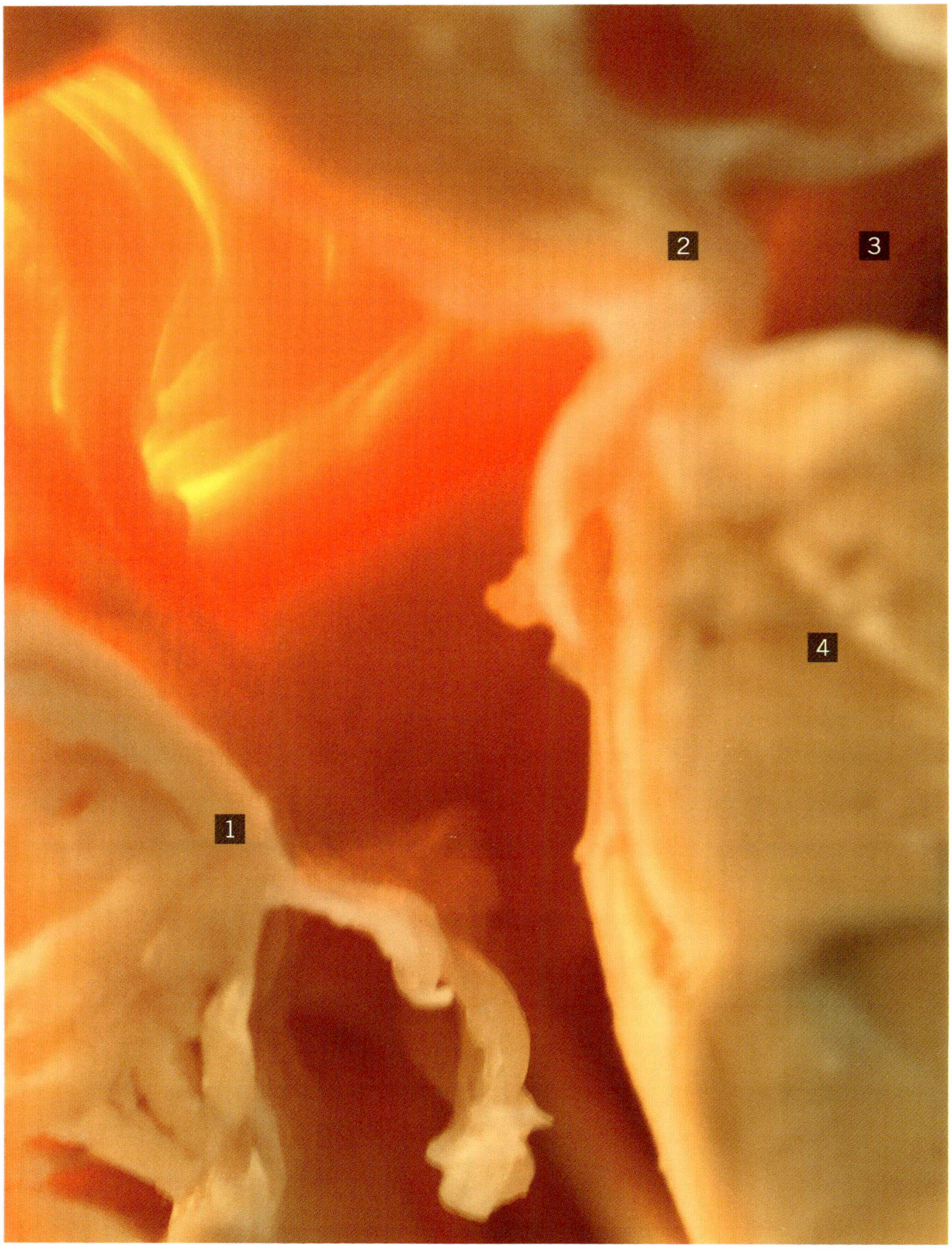

[1 Parietal area]

[2 Parietal area, corresponding to the membranous septum]

[3 Outflow tract of the left ventricle]

[4 Interventricular septum]

Figure 2. **Annulus.**

TRICUSPID VALVE ANNULUS

The leaflets are inserted into the annulus. This latter is less fibrous than that of the mitral valve, except in the area of the membranous septum, which forms part of the fibrous skeleton of the heart. The part that corresponds to the free wall is essentially muscular and is related to the right coronary artery.

[1 Parietal area, insertion of the mural leaflet]

[2 Right coronary artery]

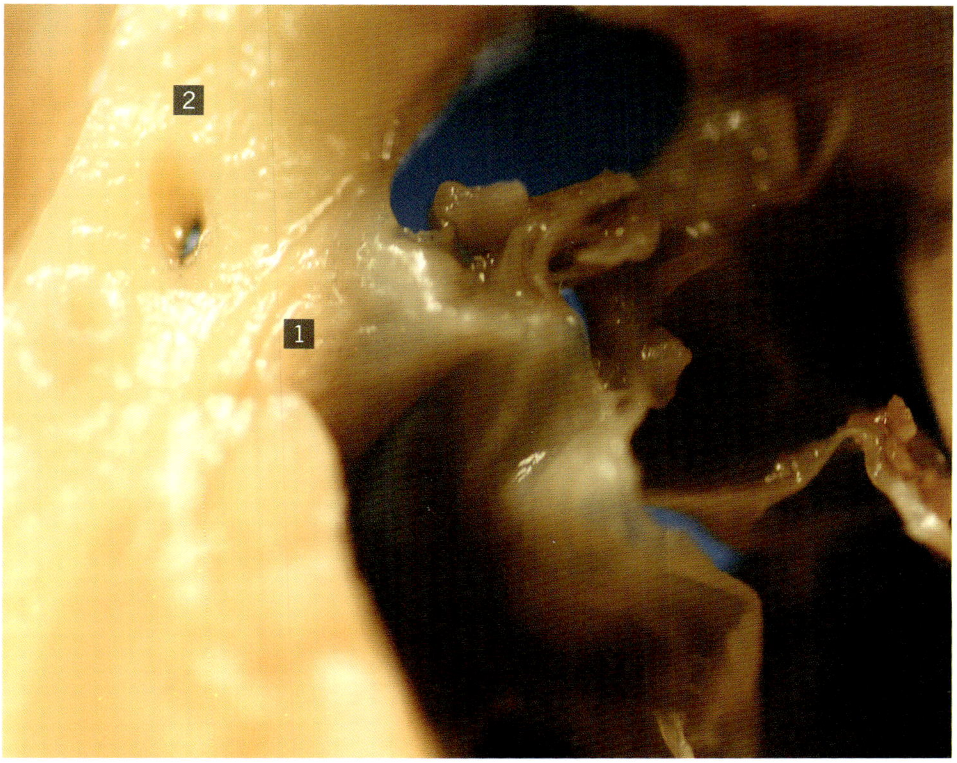

Figure 3. Annulus.

[1 Septal leaflet]

[2 Septum. Membranous septum]

[3 Free wall of the right ventricle]

[4 Right coronary artery]

[5 Aorta. Cross-section at leaflet level]

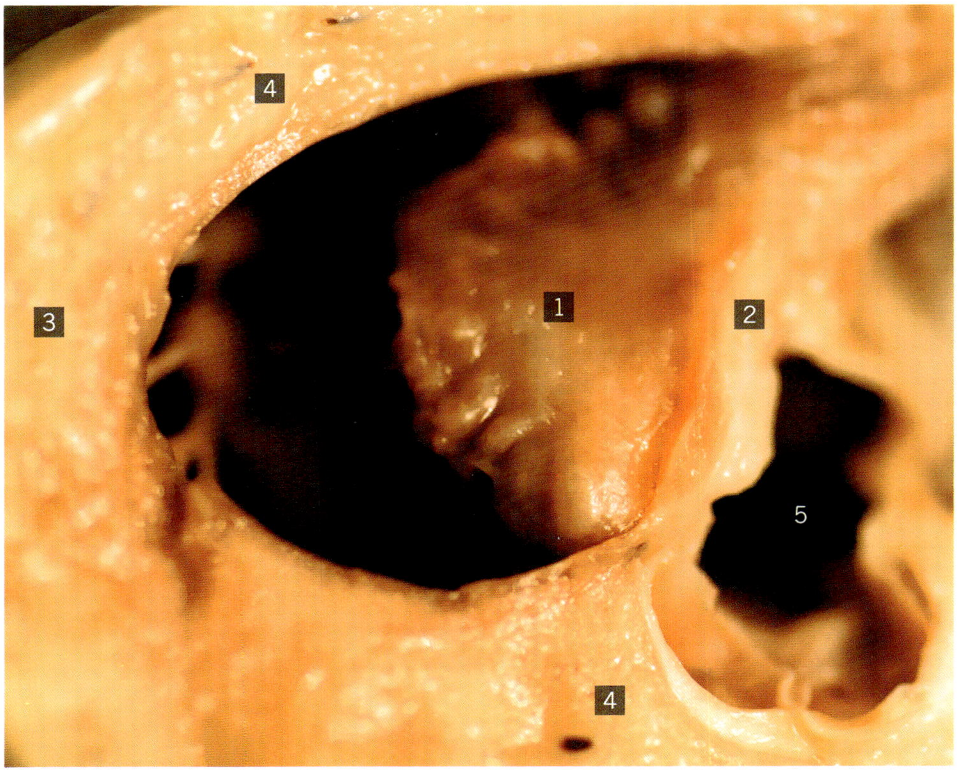

Figure 4. Triscupid valve annulus sectioned at the level of the membranous septum.

[1 Mural leaflet]

[2 Septal leaflet]

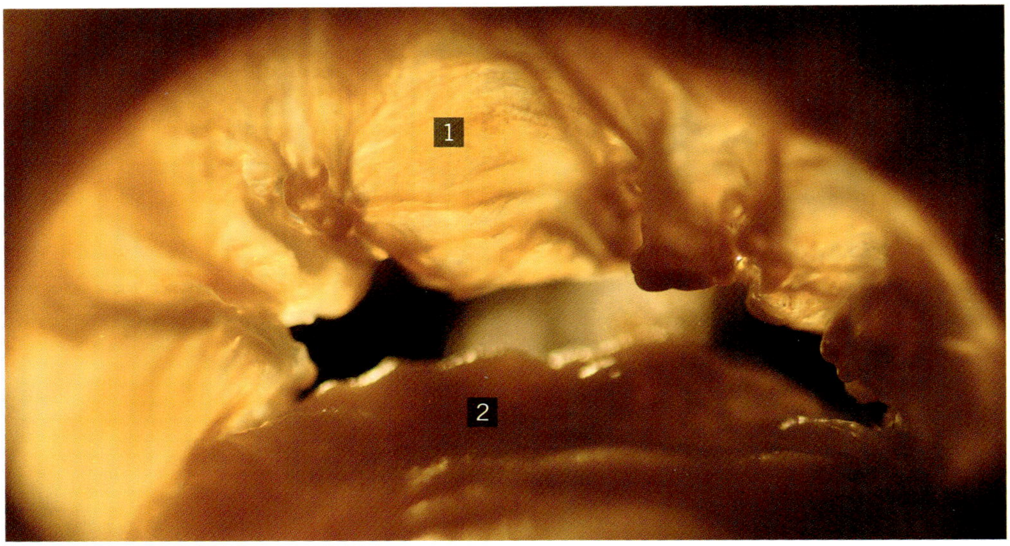

Figure 5. Leaflets, view from the right atrium. The outflow tract of the right ventricle would be on the left in the image.

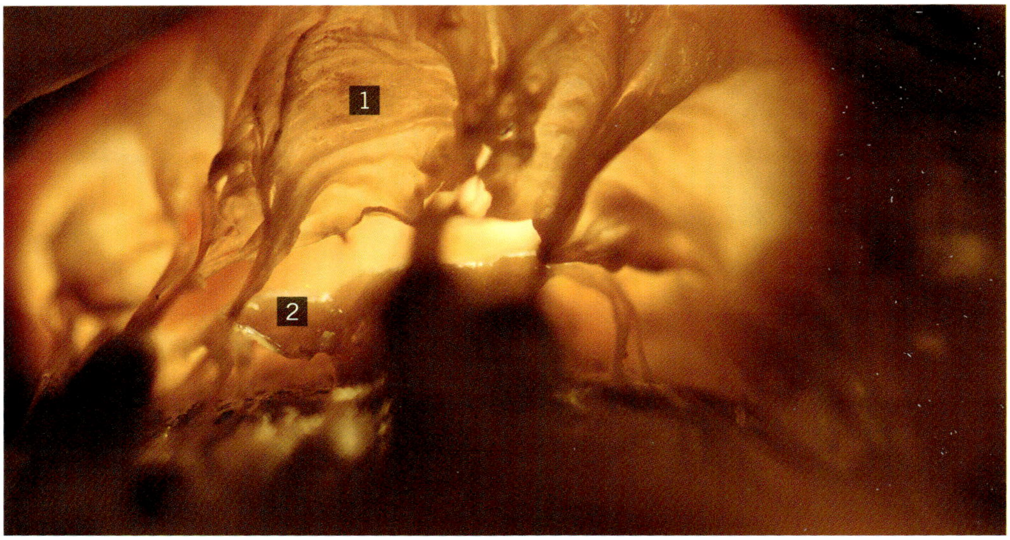

Figure 6. Leaflets, view from the right ventricle. The outflow tract of the right ventricle would be on the right in the image.

LEAFLETS

As opposed to what the name of the valve suggests, it only has two leaflets (bicuspid), a small one located on the interventricular septum –septal or dorsal leaflet– and a larger one located on the free wall –parietal, mural or ventral leaflet–. The atrial surface of the leaflets is smooth, while there are anchor sites for the chordae tendineae in their ventricular surface.

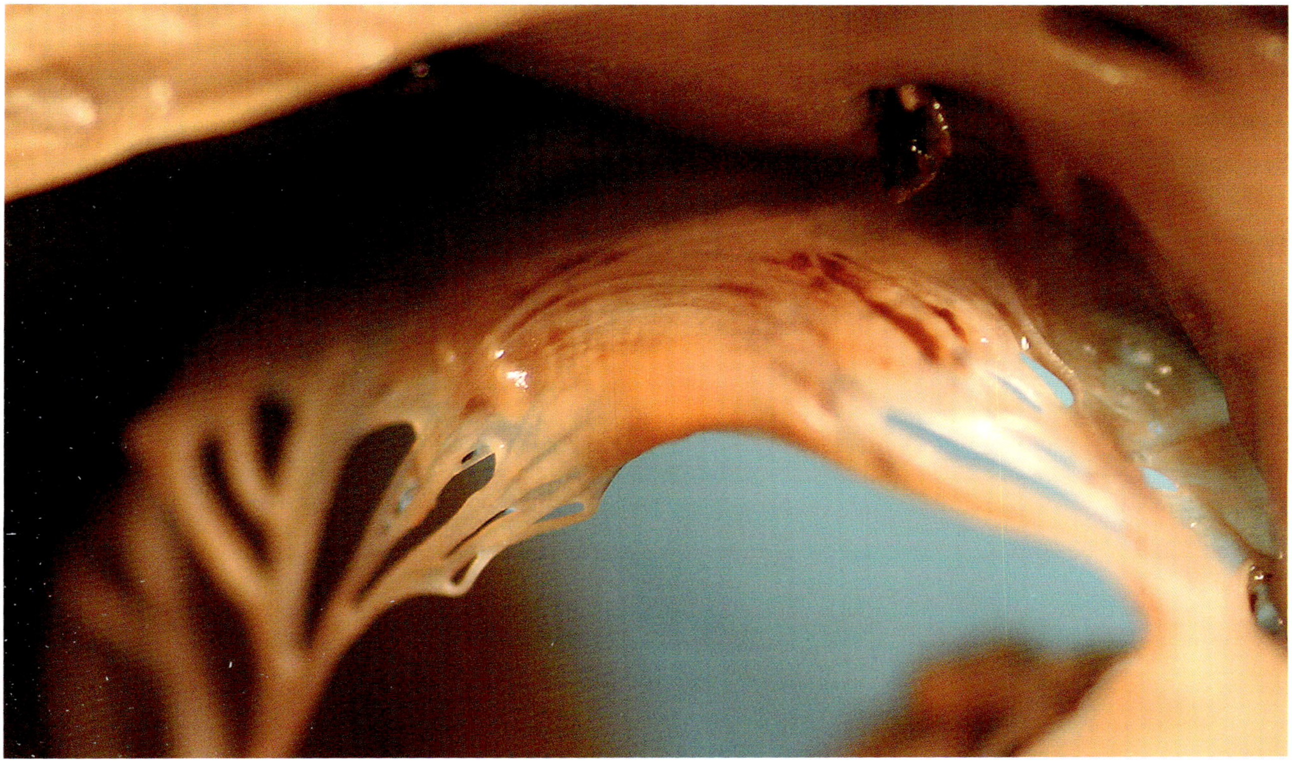

Figure 7. Segment of the mural leaflet. View from the right ventricle.

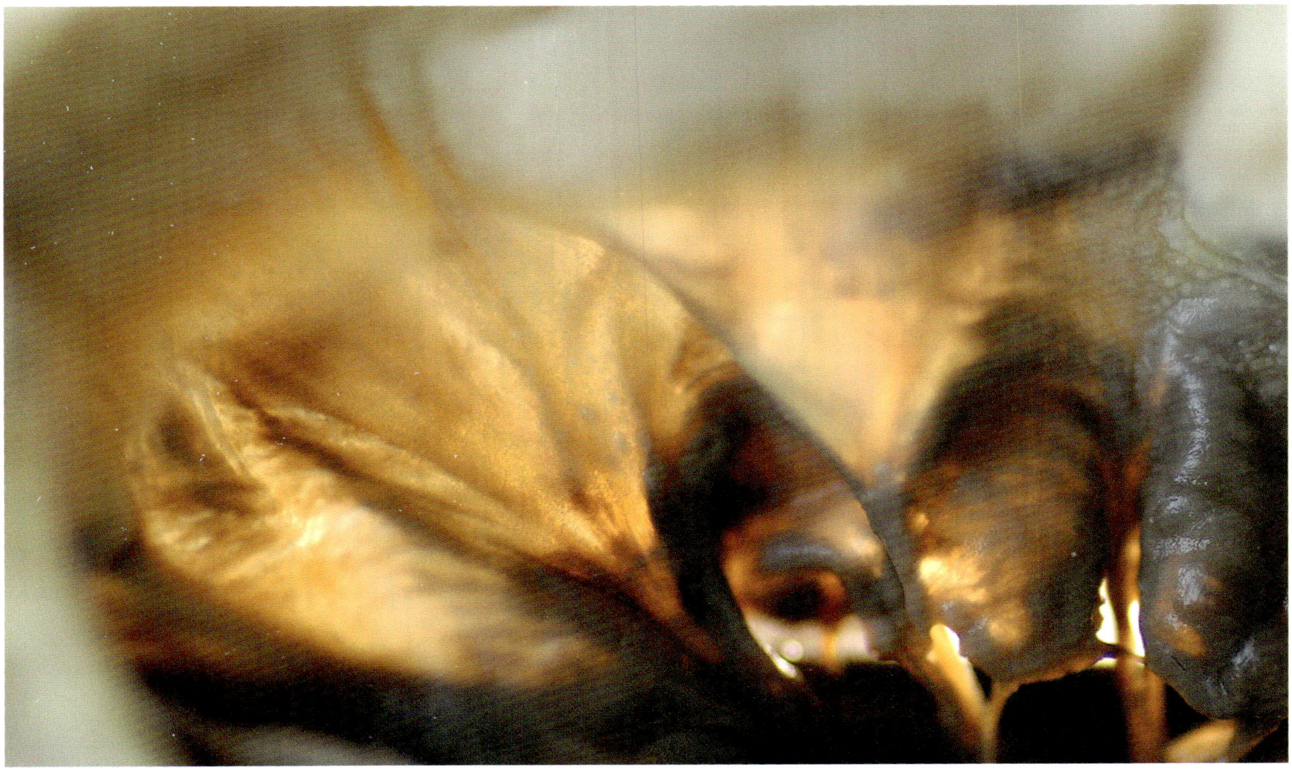

Figure 8. Cranial segment of the mural leaflet. View from the right atrium.

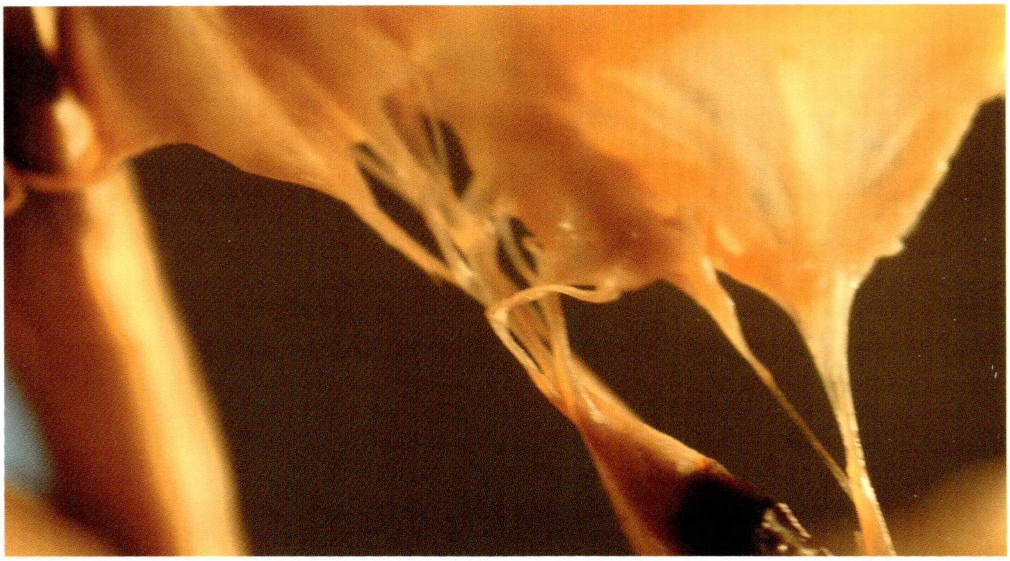

Figure 9. Chordae tendineae.

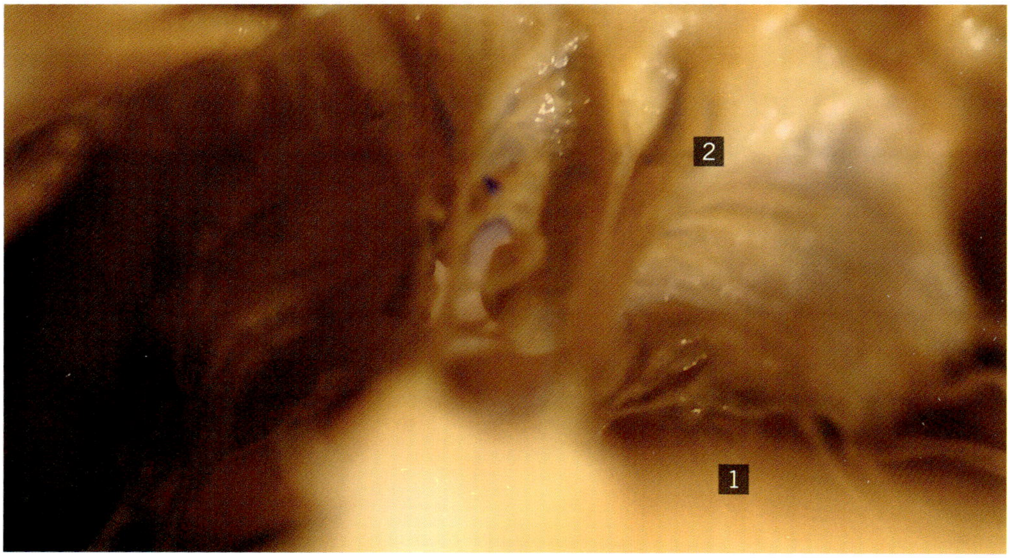

Figure 10. Chordae tendineae in the mural leaflet.

[1 Primary chordae tendineae]

[2 Secondary chordae tendineae]

CHORDAE TENDINEAE

Chordae tendineae are fibromuscular formations that originate from the papillary muscles and are attached to the edges of the leaflets and commissures –primary chordae tendineae– or to the ventricular surface of the leaflet –secondary chordae tendineae–. They usually have several branches and some of these may directly stretch to the free wall of the right ventricle. It is also common for them to split and then join again.

[1 Septum]

[2 Ventricular free wall]

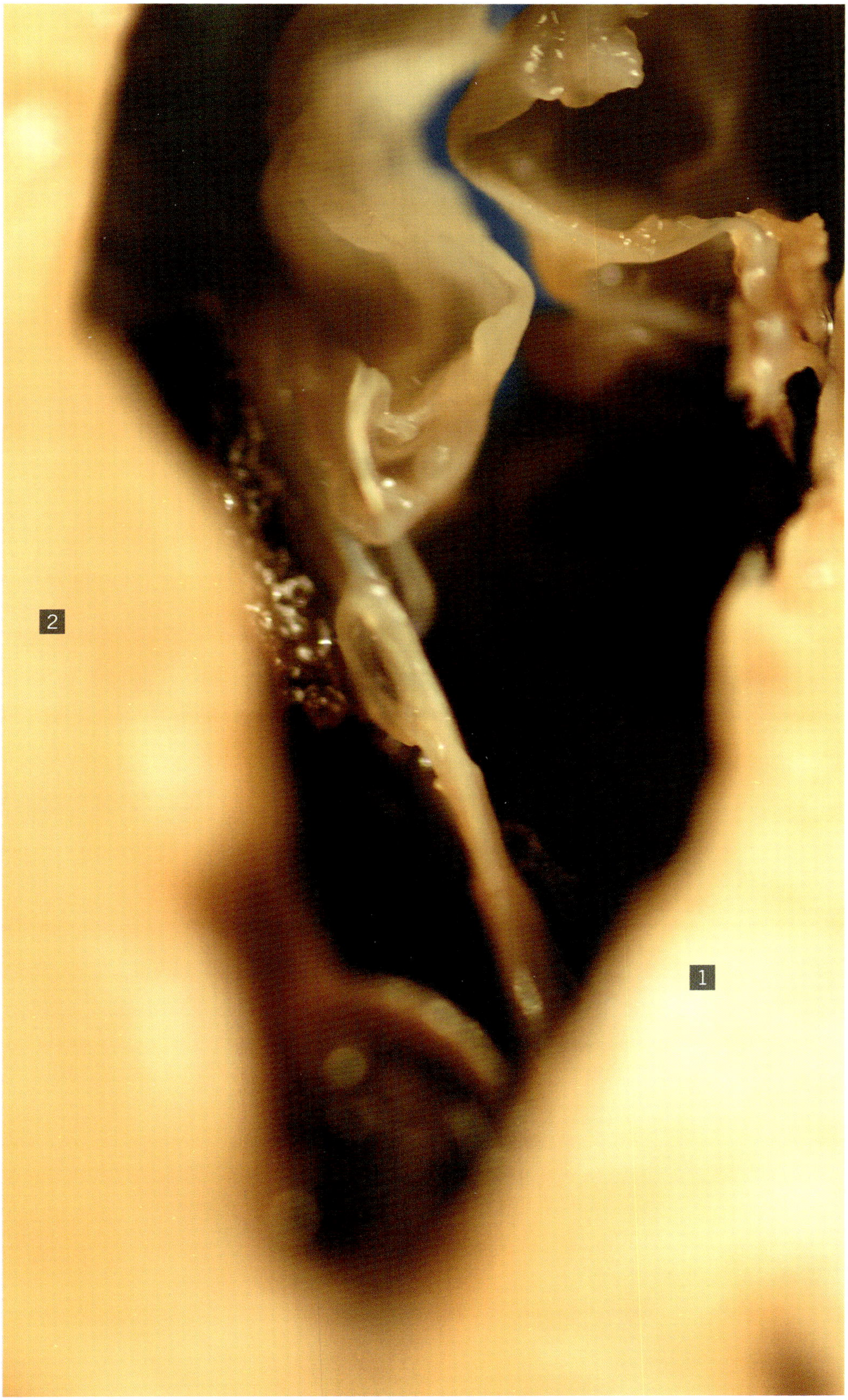

Figure 11. It is possible to observe how the chordae tendineae originate from the septum and run towards the mural leaflet.

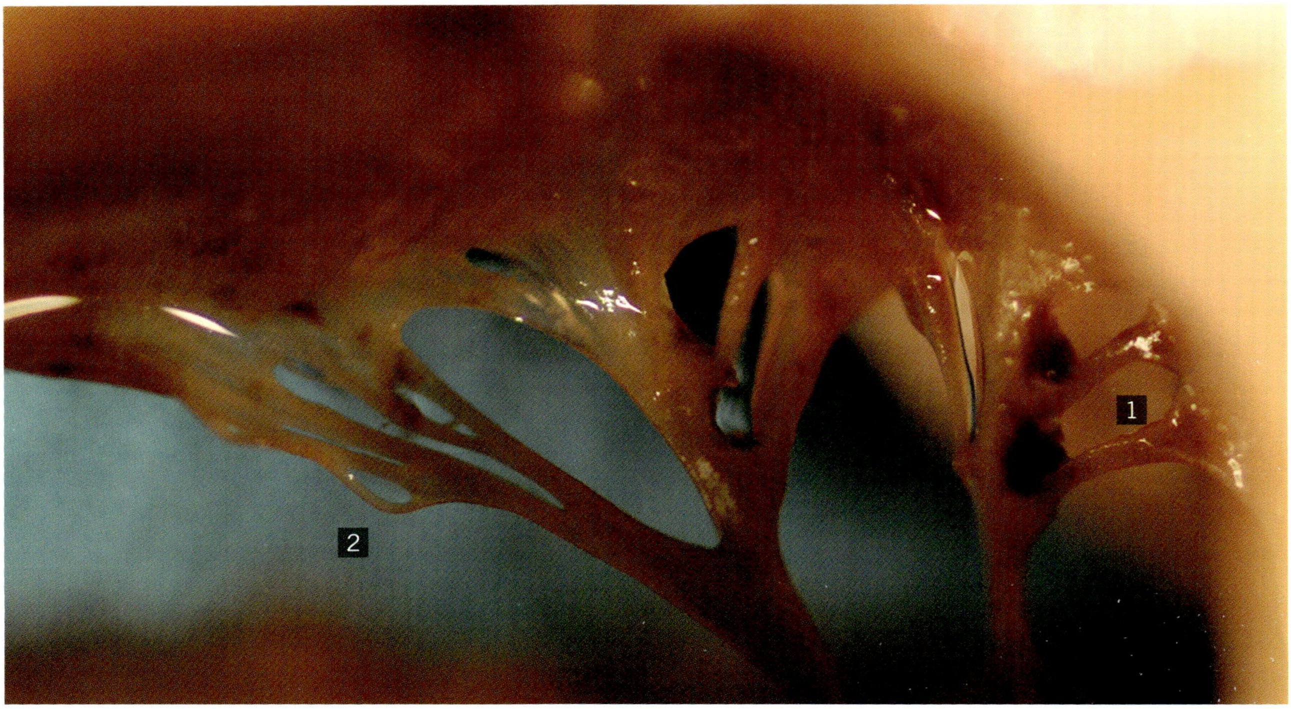

Figure 12. Chordae tendineae.

[1 Some branches may stretch directly to the free ventricular wall] [2 Splitting]

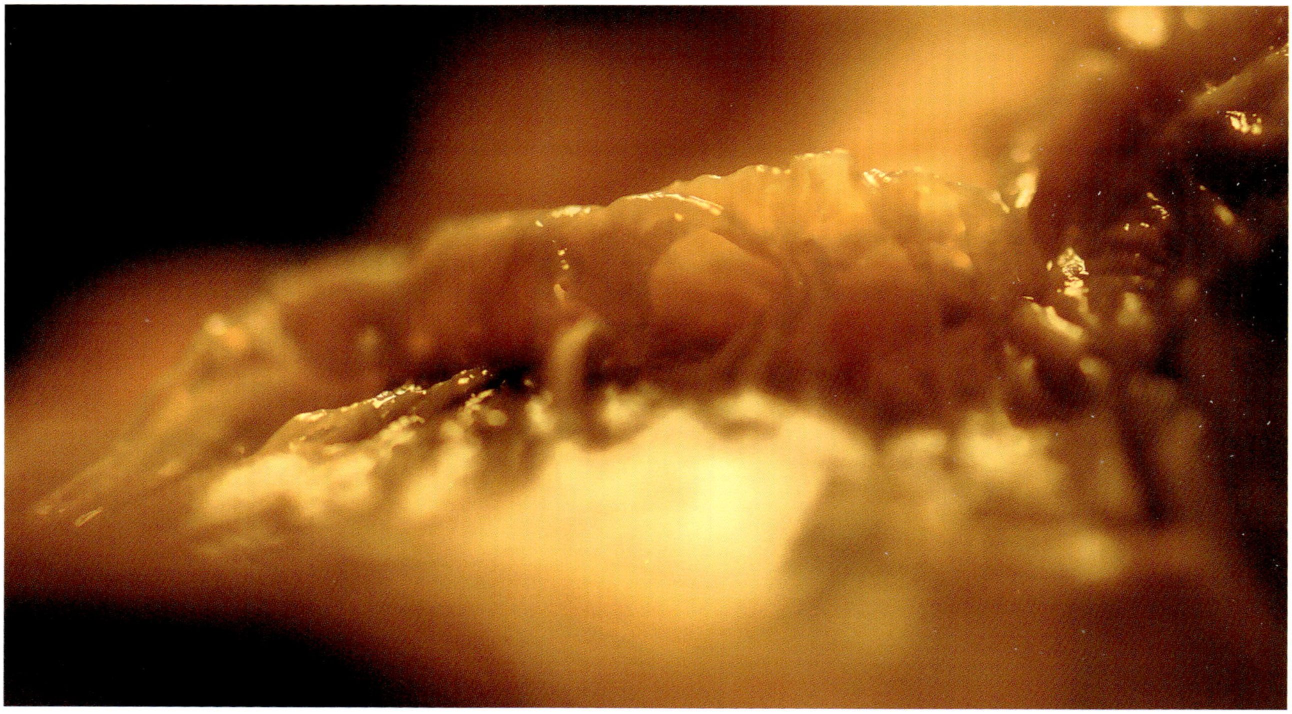

Figure 13. Chordae tendineae of the septal leaflet.

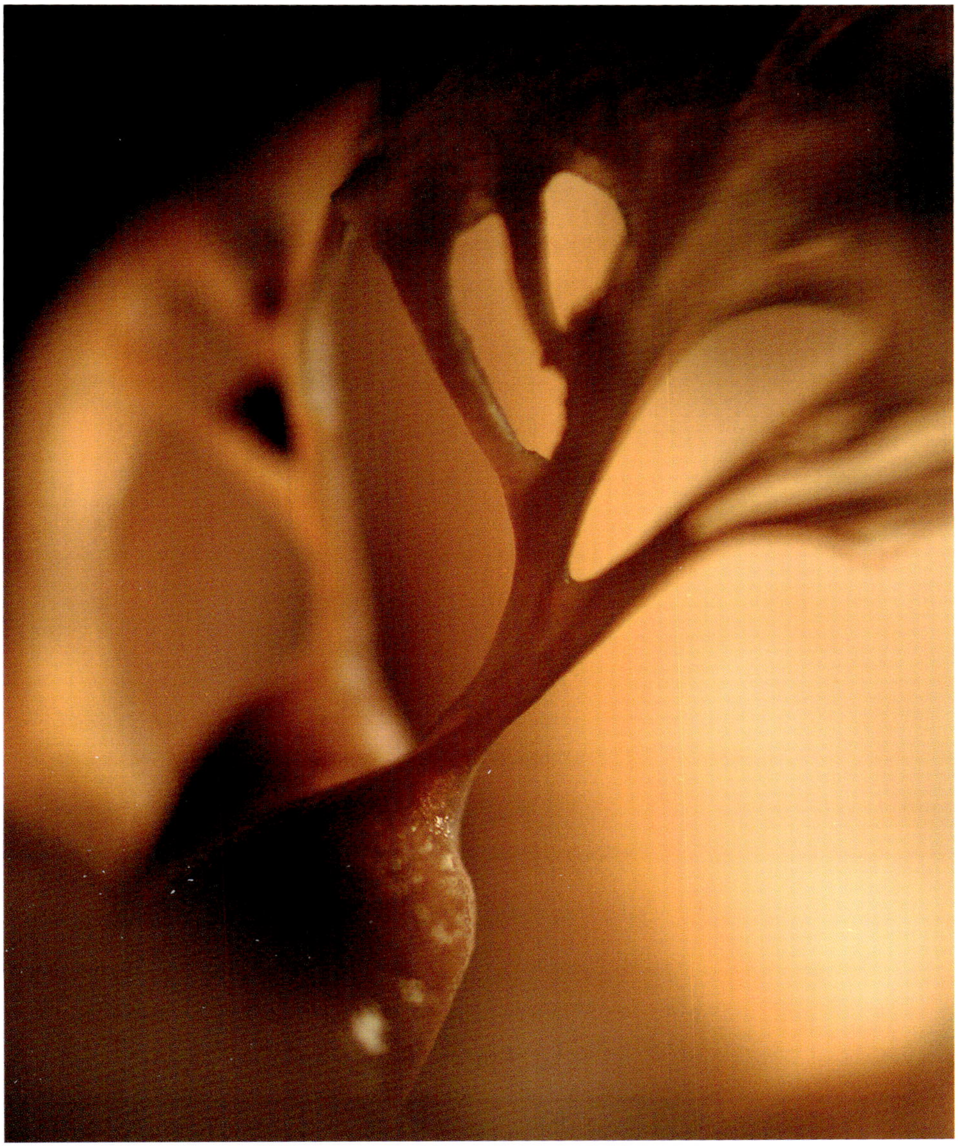

Figure 14. Papillary muscles.

PAPILLARY MUSCLES

In most cases we can find three main papillary muscles, although their number, shape and the points of origin of the chordae tendineae may vary. They originate from the apical third of the interventricular septum and their chordae tendineae only attach to the mural leaflet. Close to the angle formed by the septum and the free wall, and ventral to the supraventricular crest, we can find a small papillary muscle whose chorda tendinea is attached to the most caudodorsal part of the mural leaflet; it is the so-called papillary muscle of the conus.

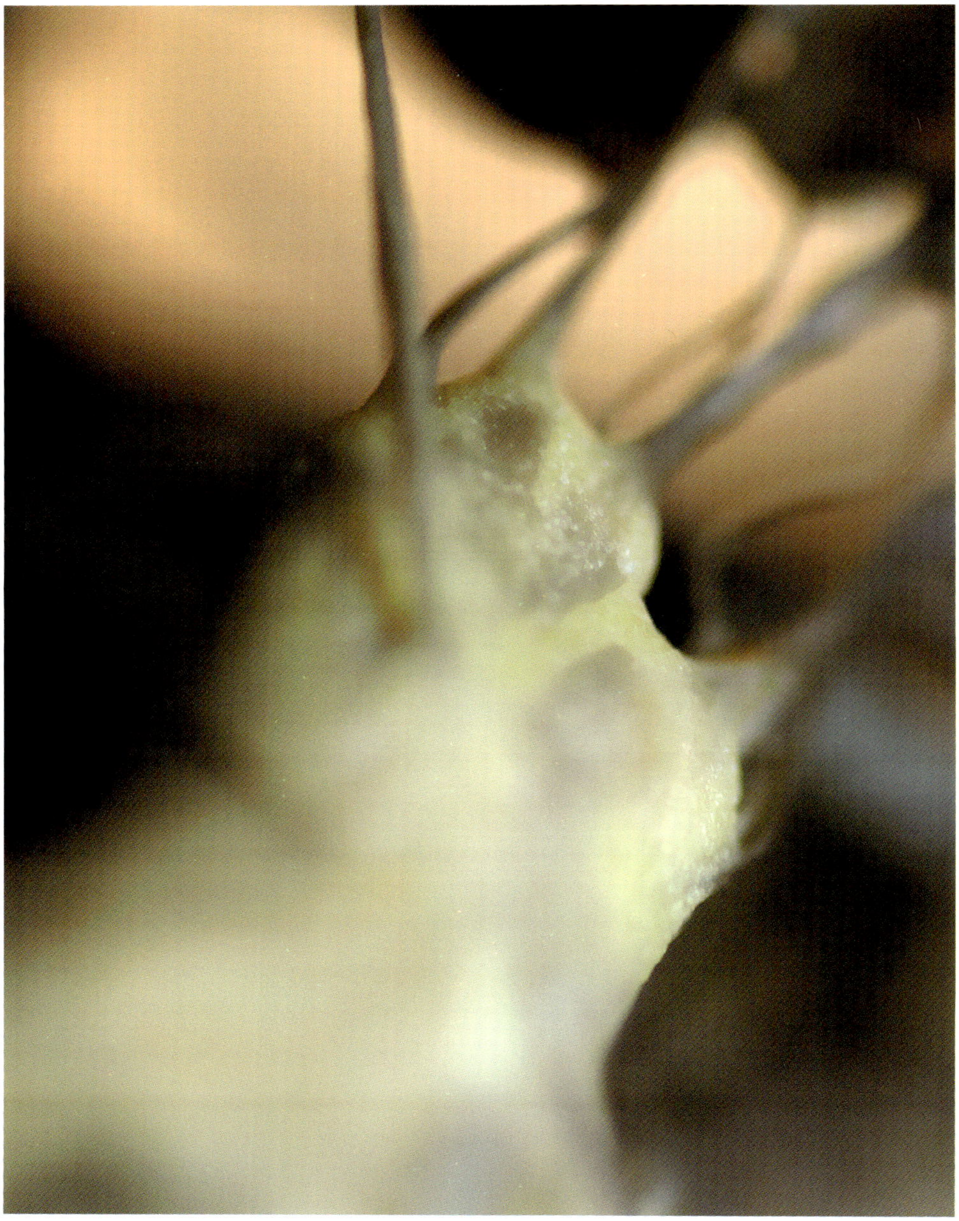

Figure 15. Papillary muscle, insertion of chordae tendineae at different levels and in different directions.

There are two other much smaller formations –muscular papillae– that also develop in the septum and are the origin of the chordae tendineae that run towards the septal leaflet. Their number greatly varies.

In addition to the supraventricular crest –a previously mentioned muscular ridge located between the cranial part of the annulus and the conus arteriosus, which connects the right ventricle with the pulmonary trunk–, there is another structure that should be known, although it is not directly related to the tricuspid valve apparatus; this structure is the septomarginal trabecula. It is a moderator band that originates close to the base of the major papillary muscle and runs to the free wall of the ventricle. It gives numerous branches and carries conducting fibres of the right branch of the bundle of His.

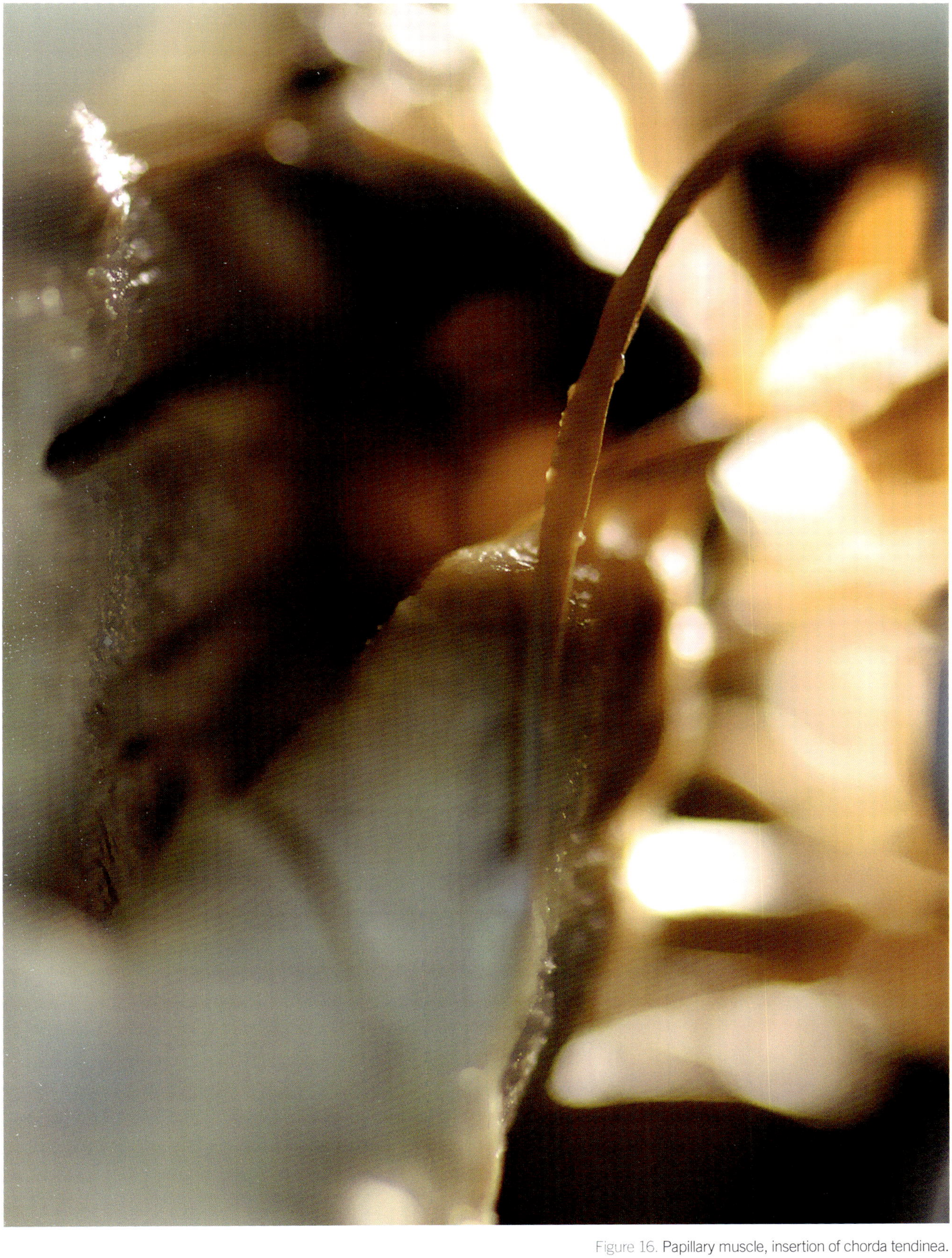

Figure 16. Papillary muscle, insertion of chorda tendinea.

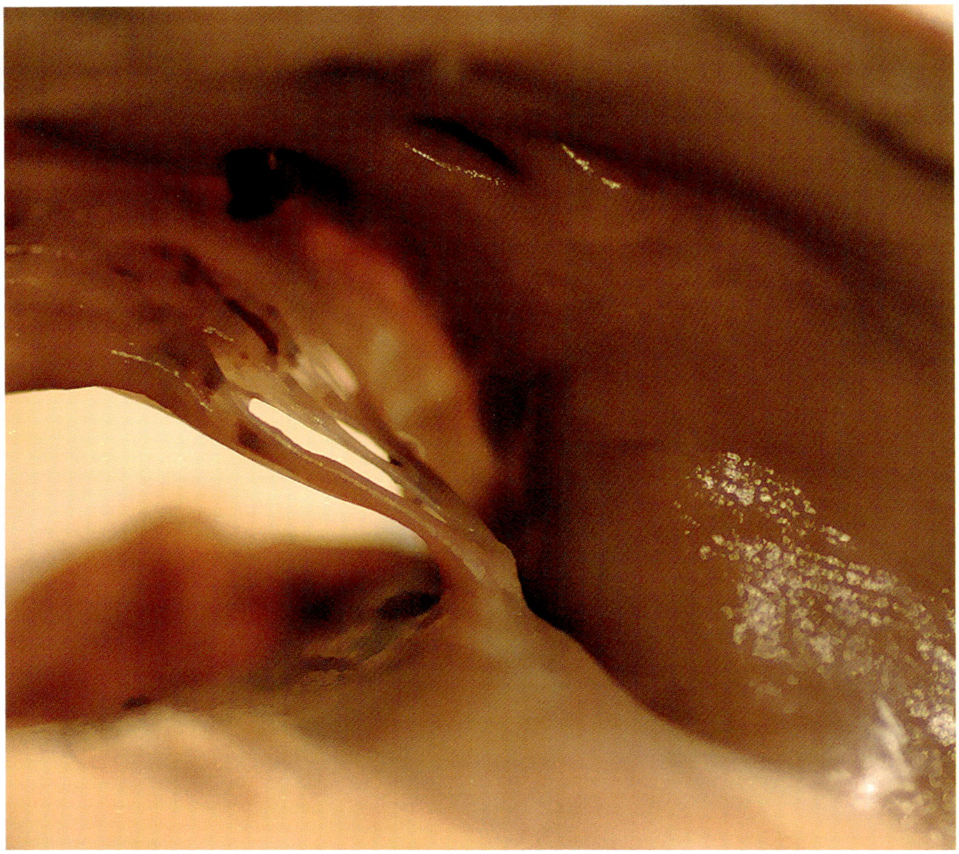

Figure 17. Papillary muscle of the conus.

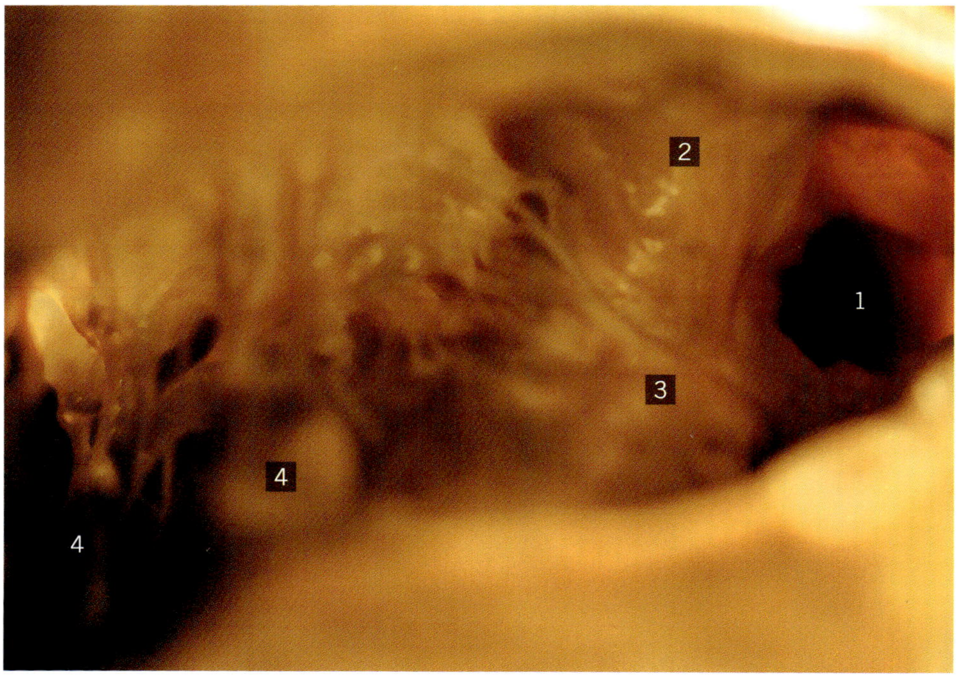

[1 Conus arteriosus]

[2 Supraventricular crest]

[3 Papillary muscle of the conus]

[4 Papillary muscles]

Figure 18. View of the tricuspid valve.

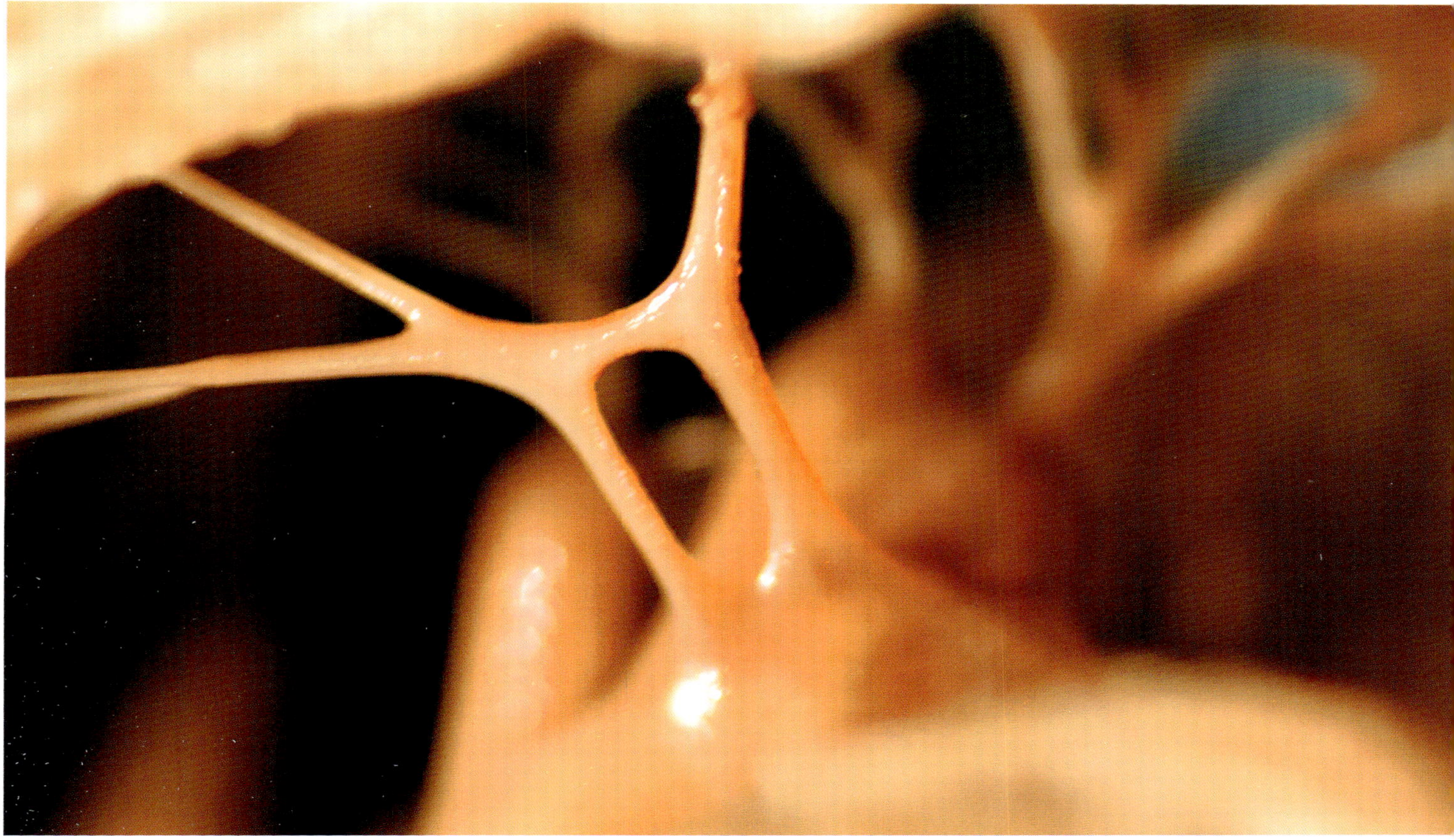

Figure 19. Septomarginal trabecula.

[1 Main papillary muscle]

[2 Septomarginal trabecula]

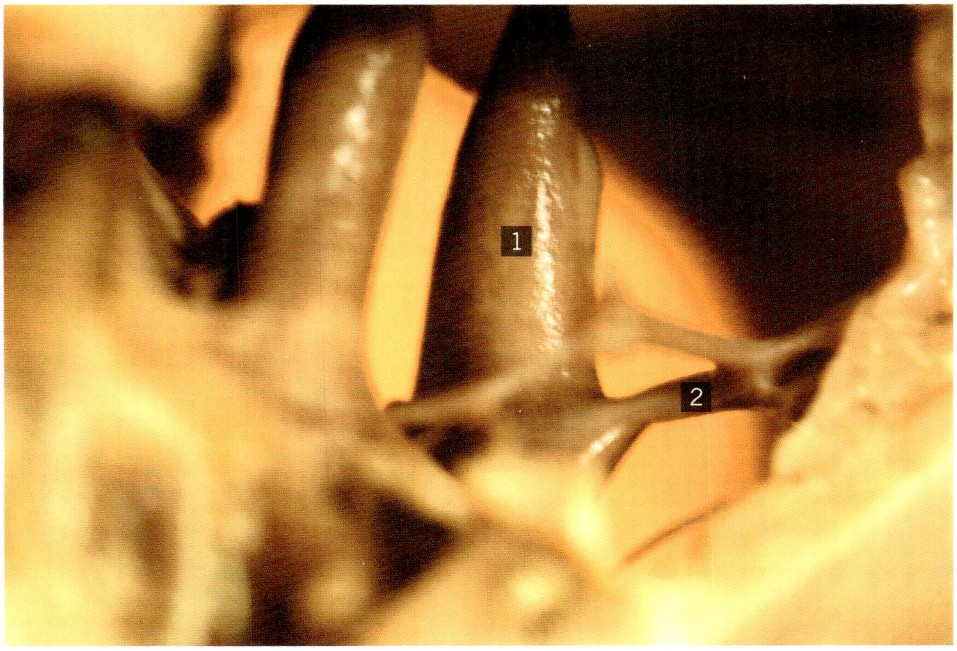

Figure 20. Papillary muscles. It is possible to observe the origin of the septomarginal trabecula from the main papillary muscle.

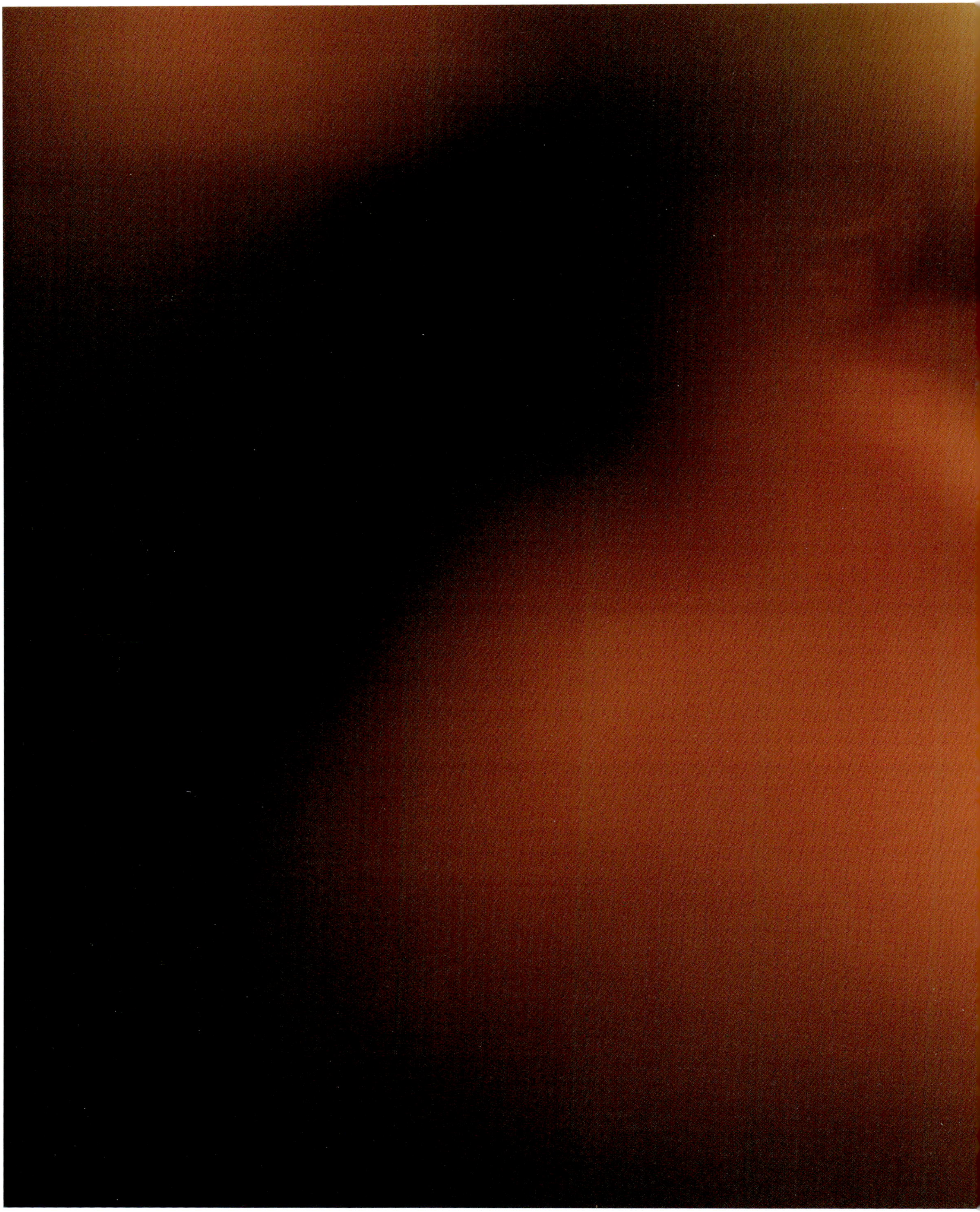

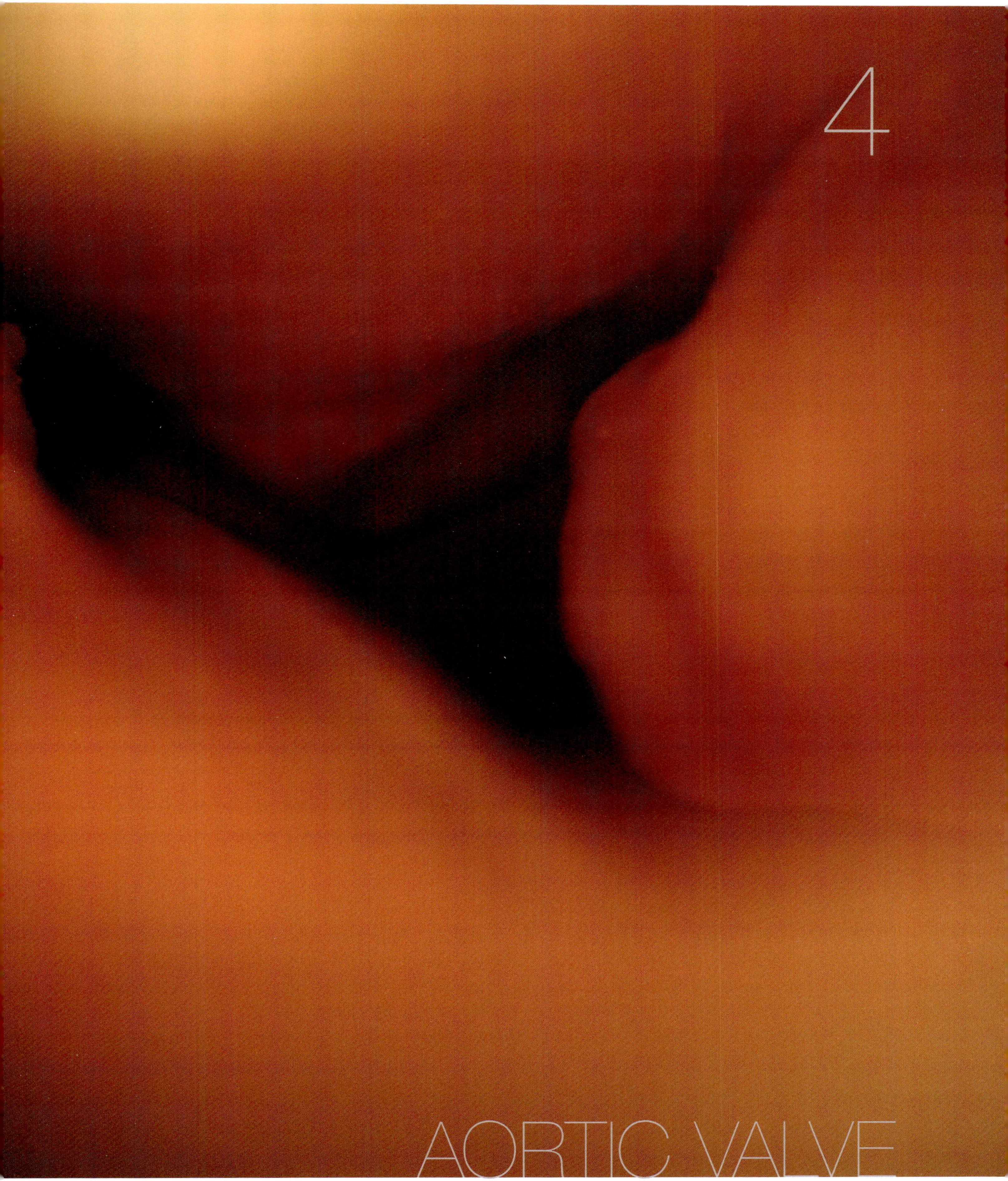

4 AORTIC VALVE

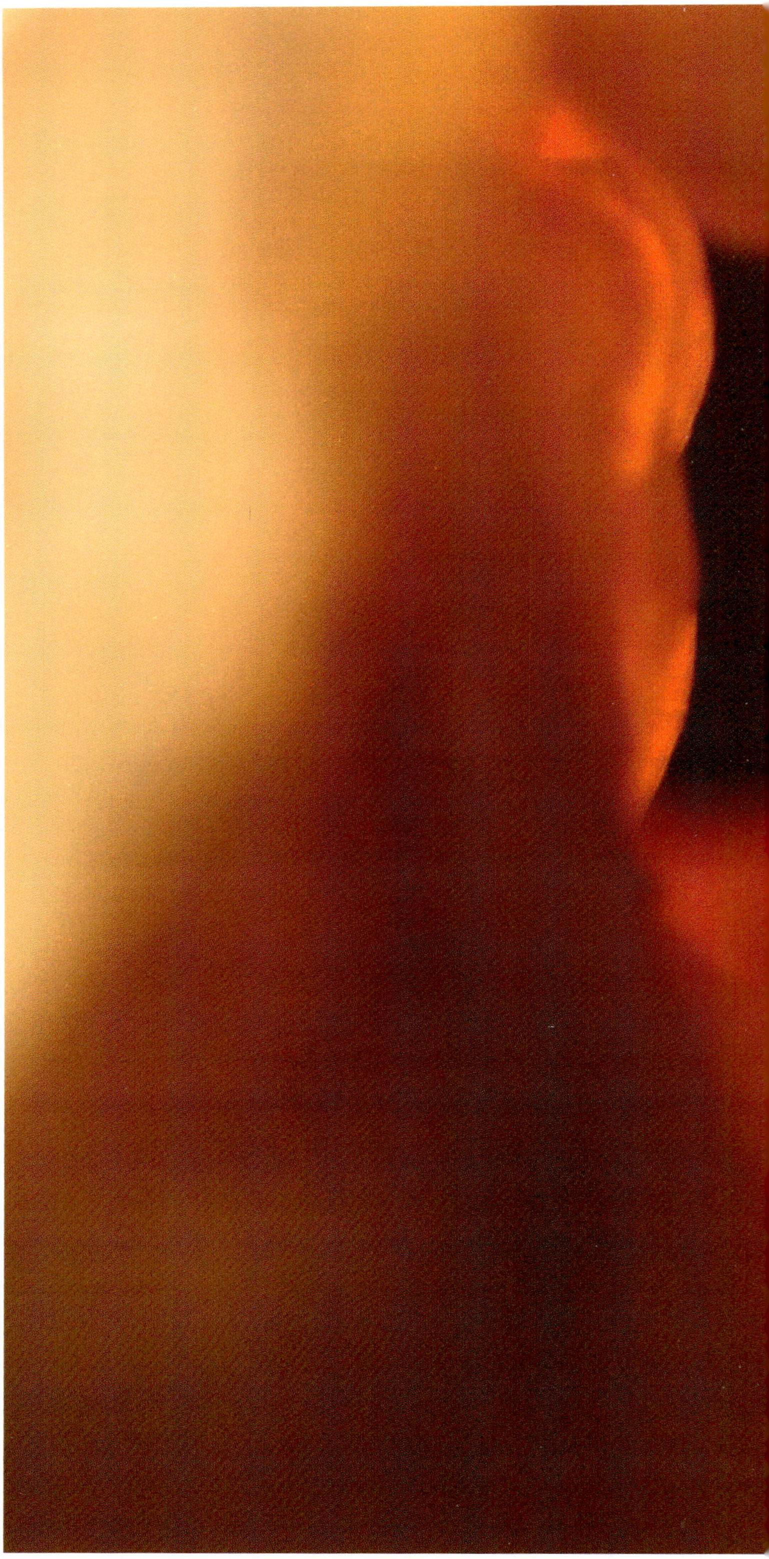

The aortic valve complex is formed by two defined parts, the outflow tract and the aortic root; both parts with their different components work to achieve the transmission of great volumes of blood and maintain a laminar flow with minimum resistance.

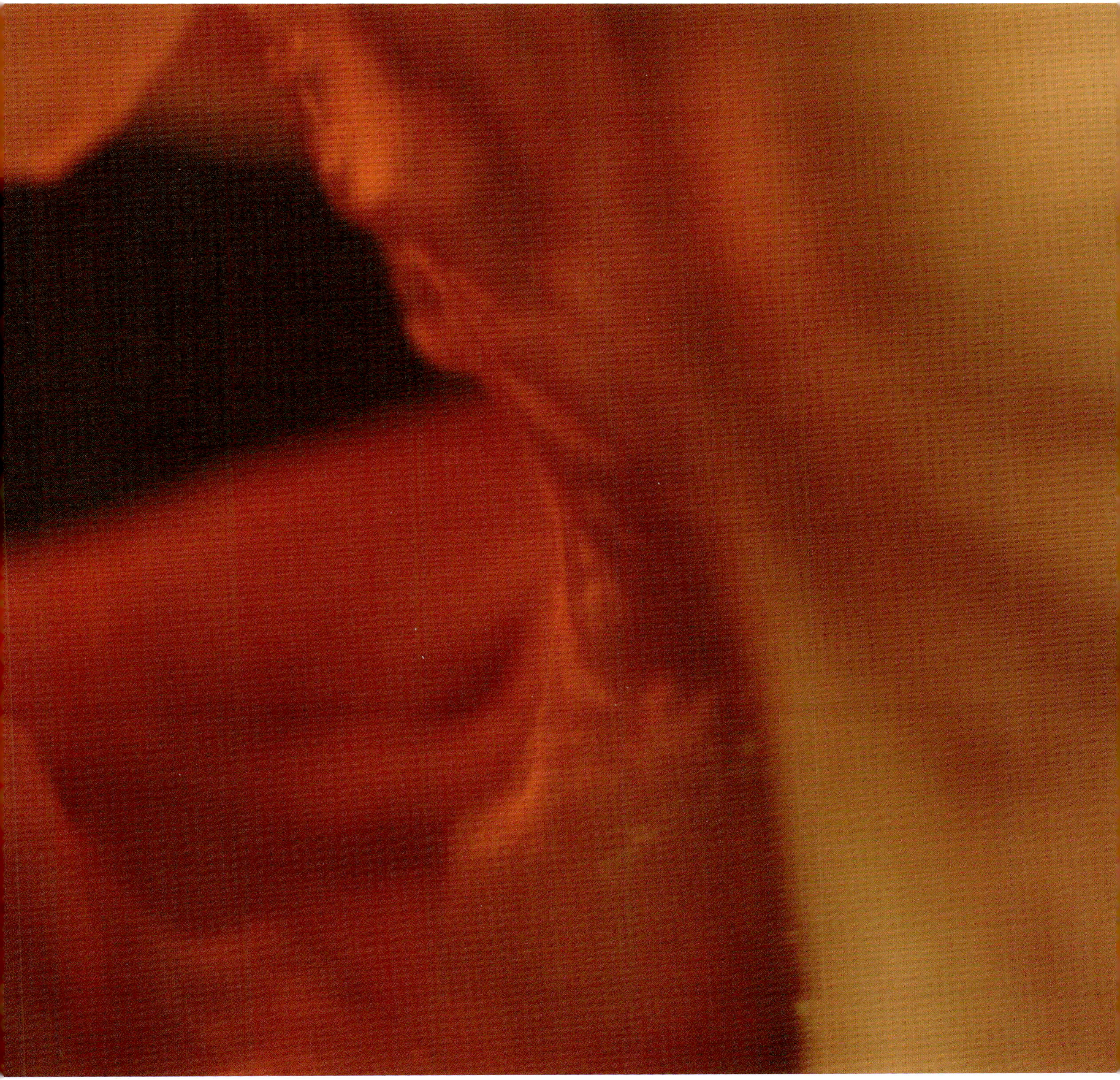

Figure 1. Outflow tract of the left ventricle.

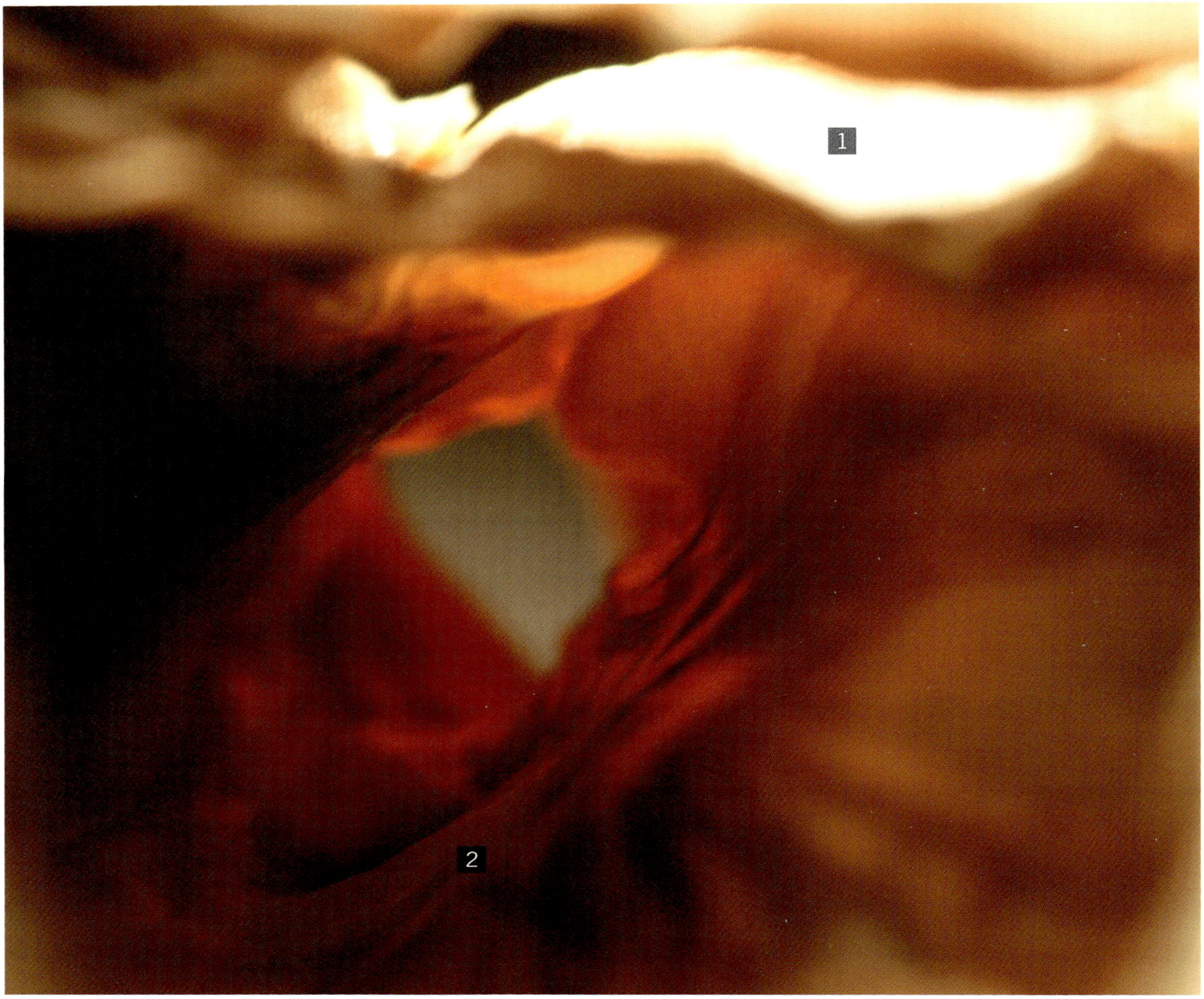

Figure 2. Outflow tract of the left ventricle. Cross-section.

[1 Cranial leaflet of the mitral valve]

[2 Interventricular septum]

OUTFLOW TRACT OF THE LEFT VENTRICLE

The outflow tract of the left ventricle is delimited by the interventricular septum, which forms the cranial wall, and the cranial leaflet of the mitral valve, which forms the caudal wall. The right and left trigones connect the two structures together.

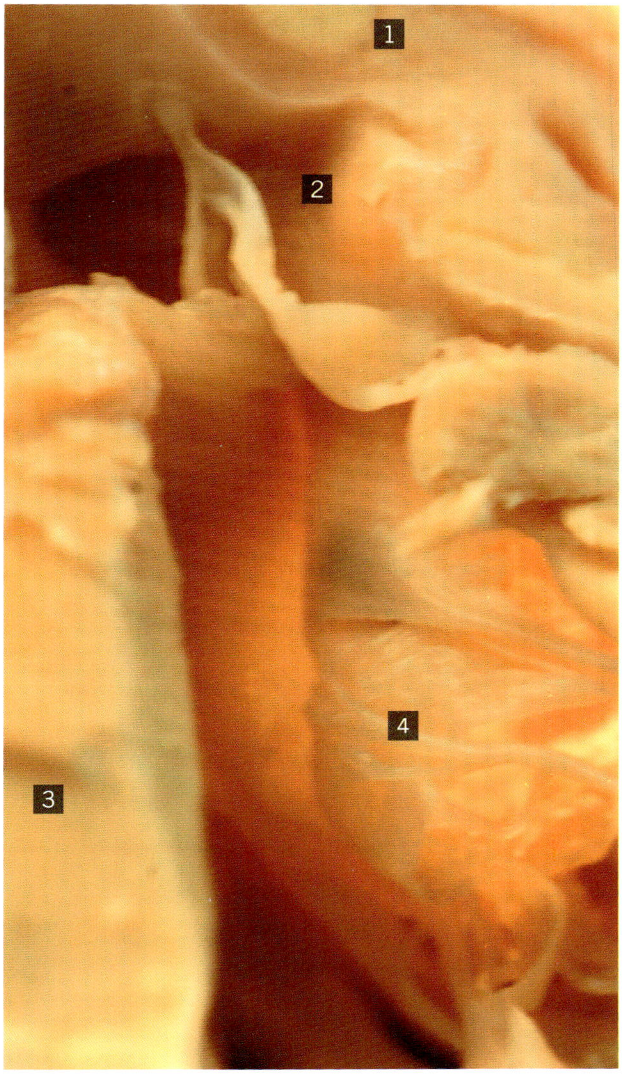

Figure 3. Outflow tract of the left ventricle. Longitudinal section.

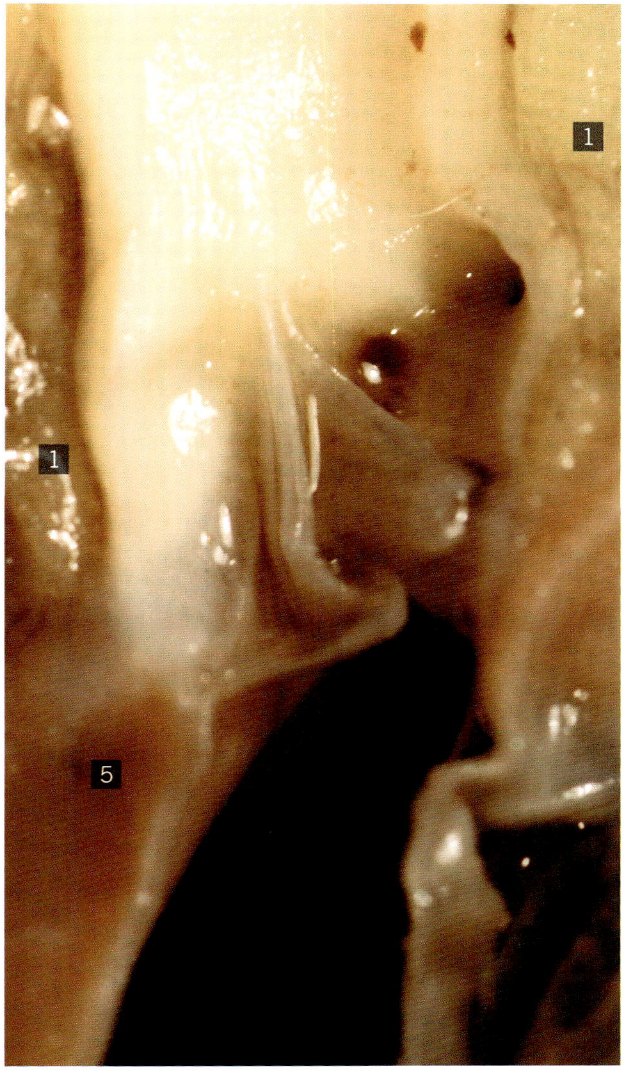

Figure 4. Outflow tract of the left ventricle in a cat. Longitudinal section.

[1 Aortic bulb]

[2 Sinus of Valsalva]

[3 Interventricular septum]

[4 Cranial leaflet of the mitral valve]

[5 Area of insertion of the aortic root in the septum, the more fibrous area on the left corresponds to the fibrous skeleton of the heart]

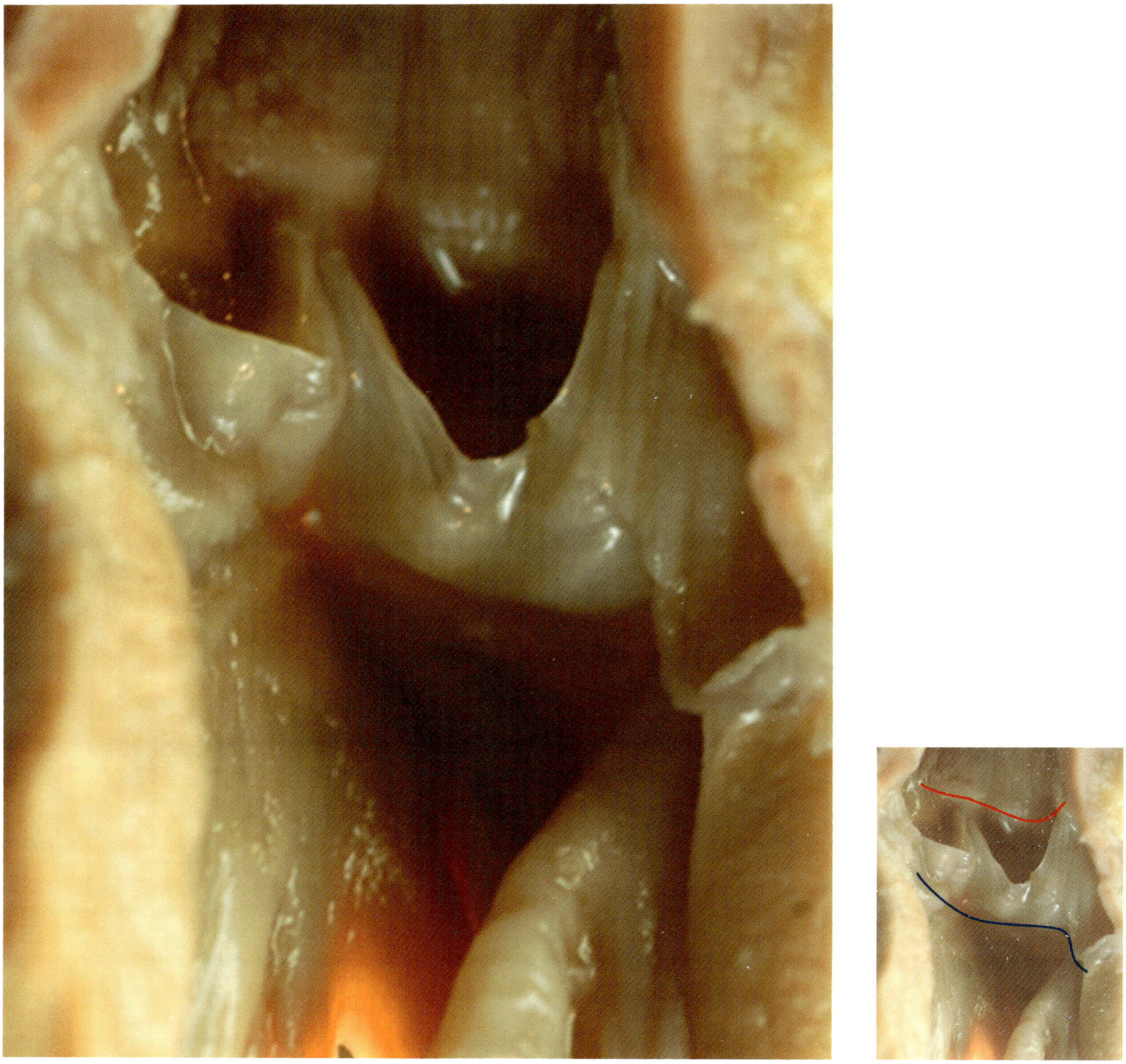

Figure 5. Aortic root, actually formed by three virtual rings: basal ring (blue line), superior ring (red line) and medial ring, which would be located between the two of them, where the cusps of the valve join.

AORTIC ROOT

The aortic root is an anatomical extension of the outflow tract. It is formed by:

- The aortic valve annulus.
- Semilunar leaflets or cusps.
- The sinuses of Valsalva.
- Coronary ostia.

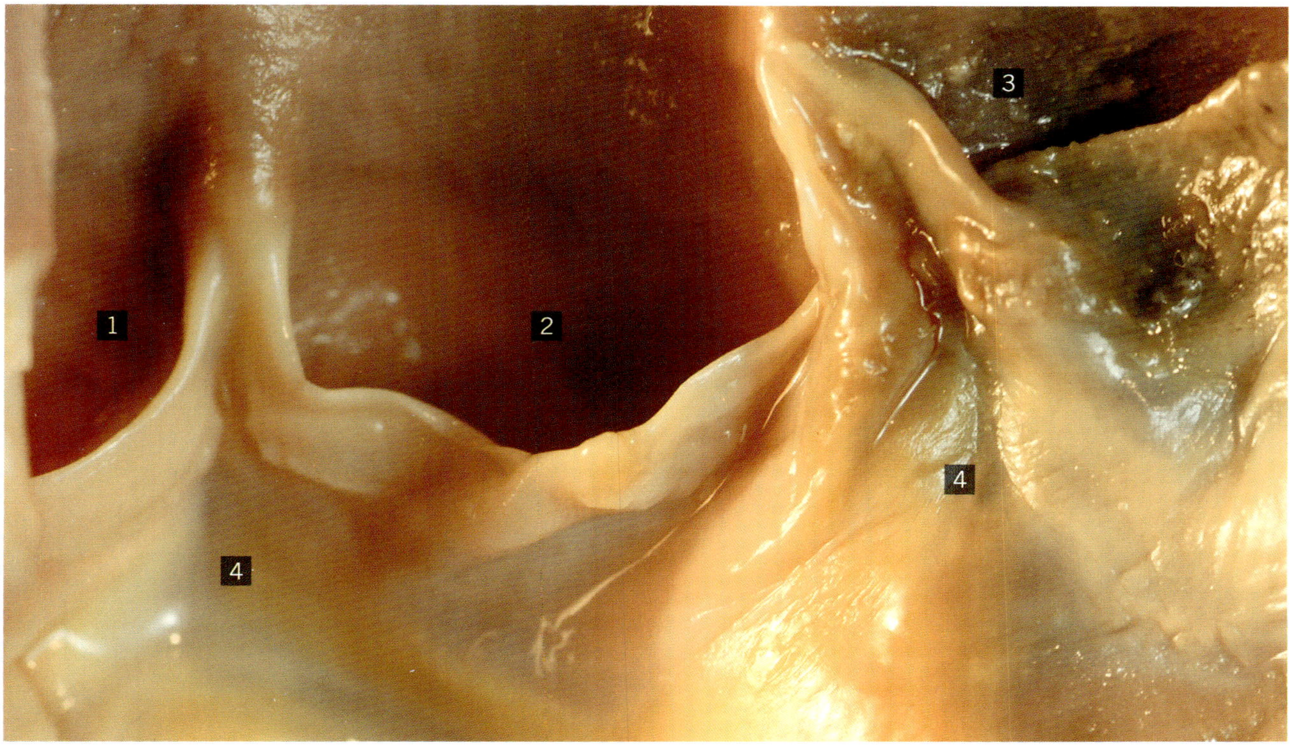

Figure 6. Aortic valve annulus. Medial ring, area of insertion of the three valve cusps.

[1 Right coronary cusp] [2 Non-coronary cusp] [3 Left coronary cusp] [4 Interleaflet triangles]

AORTIC VALVE ANNULUS

We can actually talk about three rings:

- A **basal ring**, which is formed by the virtual line of union of the lowest part of the areas of attachment of the cusps; strictly speaking, it is the union between the outflow tract and the aortic root.
- A **superior ring**, which corresponds to the union between the aortic root and the ascending aorta (sinotubular junction), and which is very rich in elastic fibres. In this area there are three points that correspond to the areas of union of two adjacent semilunar cusps and give the valve a crown-like shape.
- A **medial ring** located between the previous two rings, where the aortic valve cusps attach and form three semilunar areas (valve cusps), which are subject to aortic pressures, and three triangular areas (interleaflet triangles), which are subject to ventricular pressures. The triangle between the left coronary and non-coronary cusps is directly related to the membranous septum and, subendorcardially, to the bundle of His. In its lower part it corresponds to the insertion of the cranial leaflet of the mitral valve, this area being known as the aortic-mitral curtain.

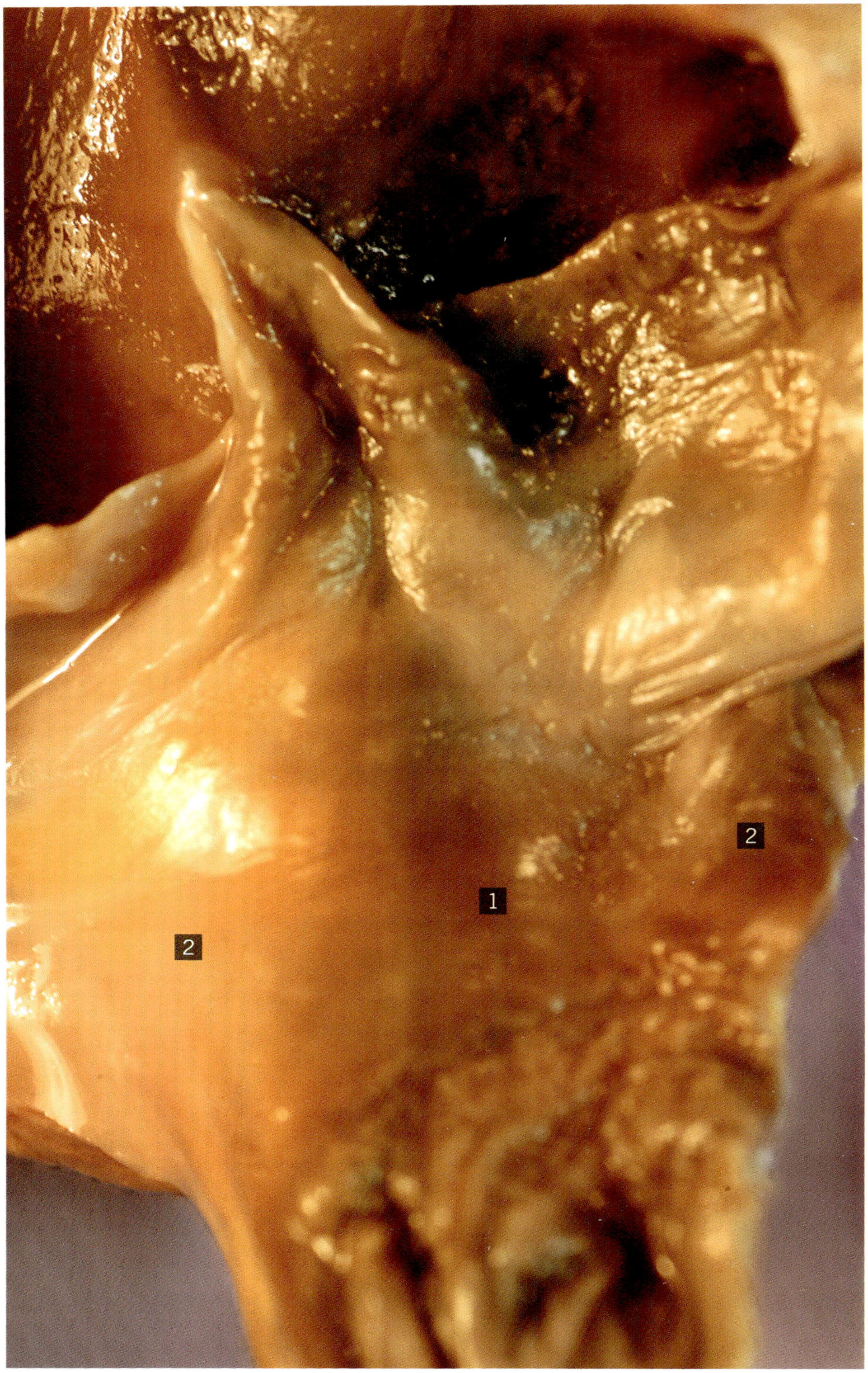

[1 Aortic-mitral curtain]

[2 Area corresponding to the insertion of the cranial mitral valve leaflet]

Figure 7. Interleaflet triangle located between the left coronary cusp and the non-coronary cusp.

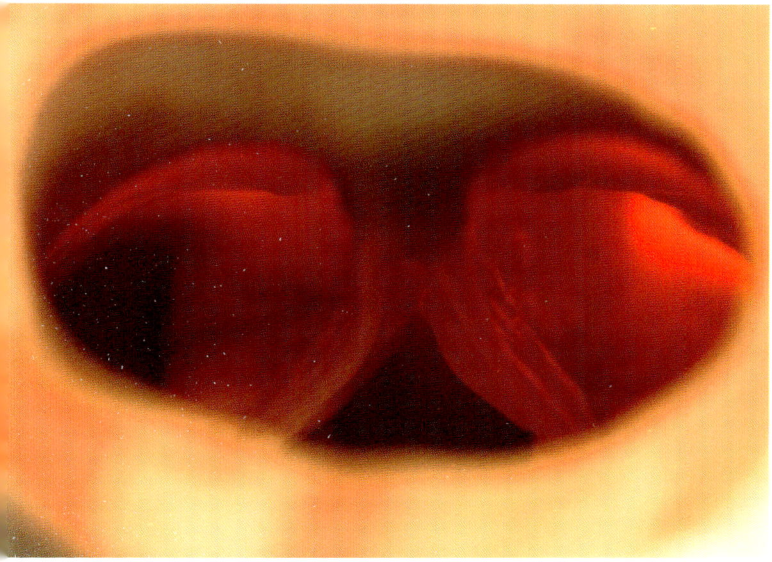

Figure 8. Sinotubular area. In the centre we can observe the area of union of the left and right coronary cusps. The three points corresponding to the unions of the three cusps give this area a crown-like shape.

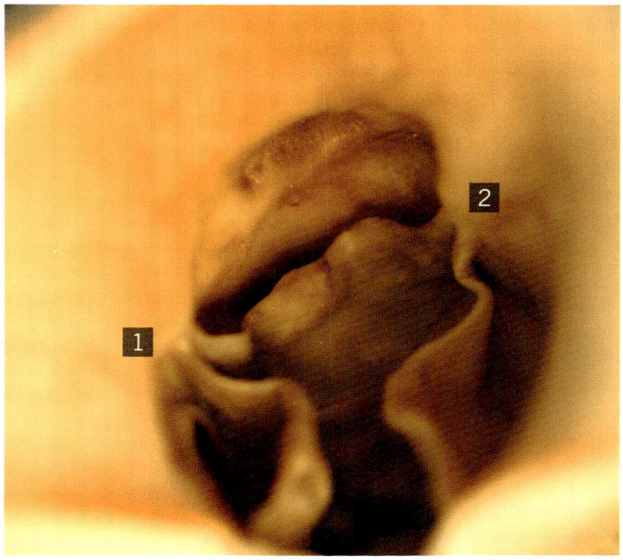

Figure 9. Sinotubular area. View of the three valve cusps from the ascending aorta.

[1 Area of union of the left and right coronary cusps]

[2 Area of union of the right coronary cusp with the non-coronary cusp]

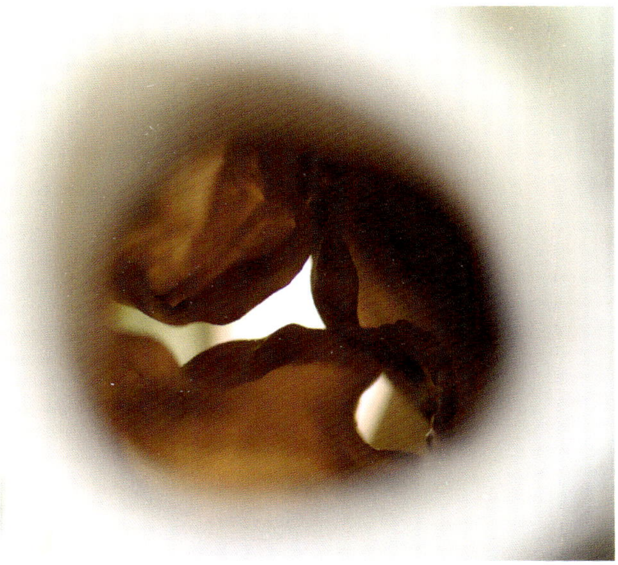

Figure 10. The three valve cusps seen from the ascending aorta.

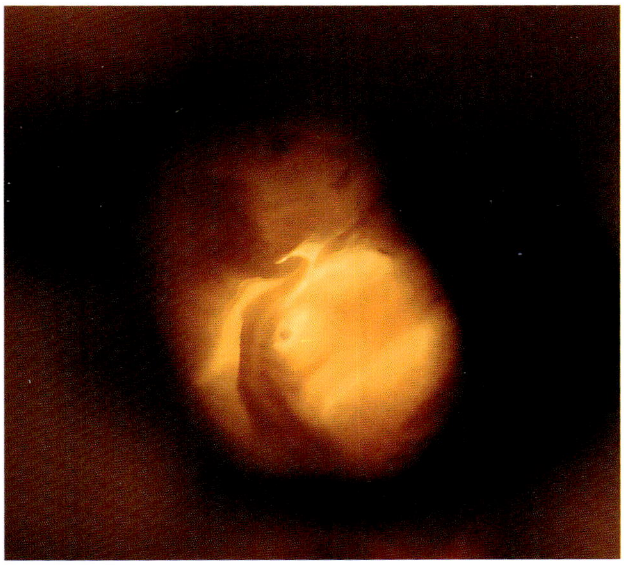

Figure 11. The three valve cusps seen from the outflow tract of the left ventricle.

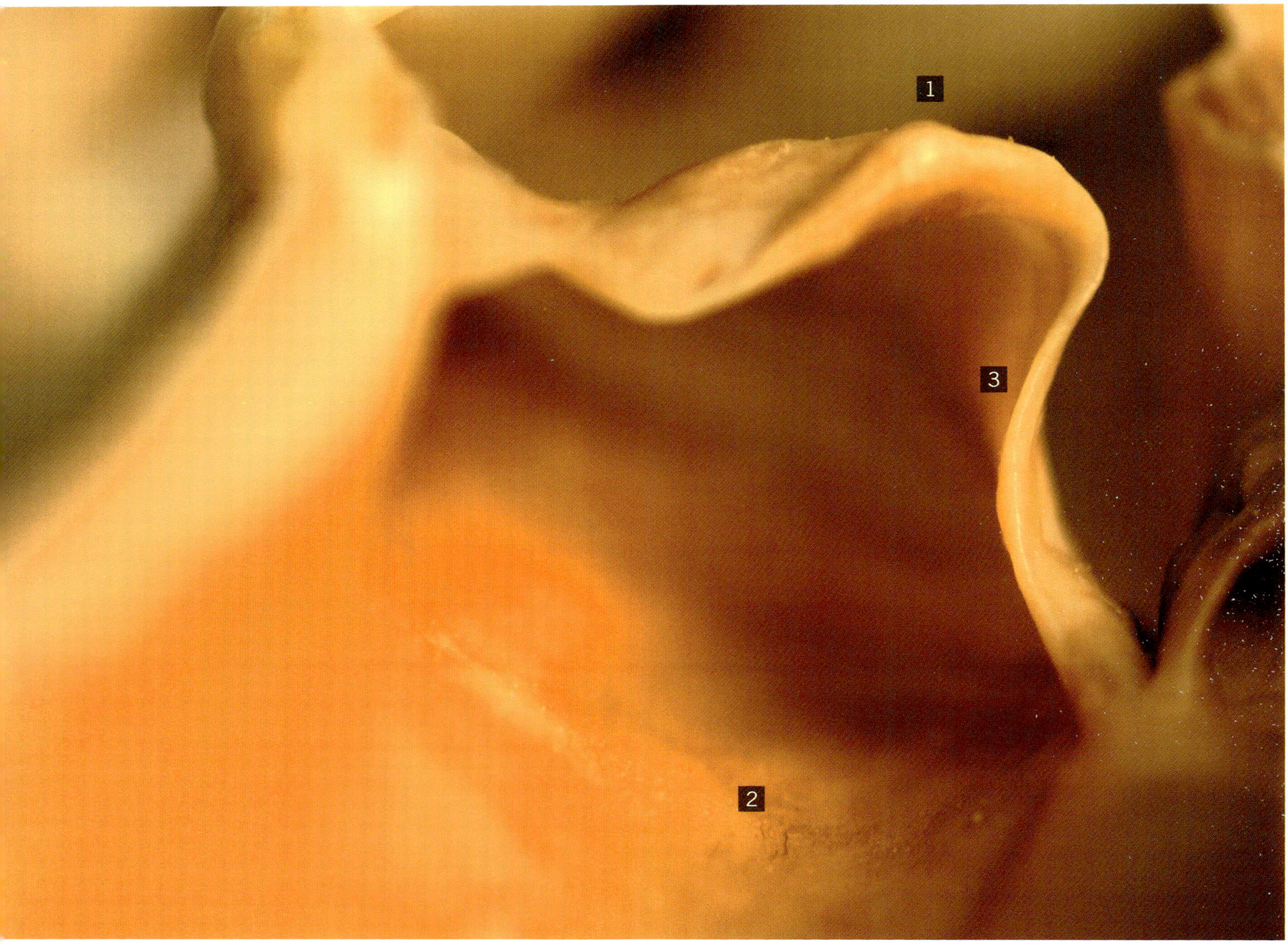

Figure 12. Non-coronary cusp.

[1 Nodule of Arantius]

[2 Sinotubular junction]

[3 Lunule]

SEMILUNAR CUSPS

There are three semilunar leaflets or aortic cusps –right, left and non-coronary– and they are formed by a stroma of fibrous tissue covered on both surfaces by endothelial tissue. A nodule, called nodule of the semilunar cusp or nodule of Arantius, can be found at the middle point of the free edge of each cusp. These nodules close the central space, which would otherwise be open due to the union of three adjacent arches. The thinner and more translucent areas are called lunules.

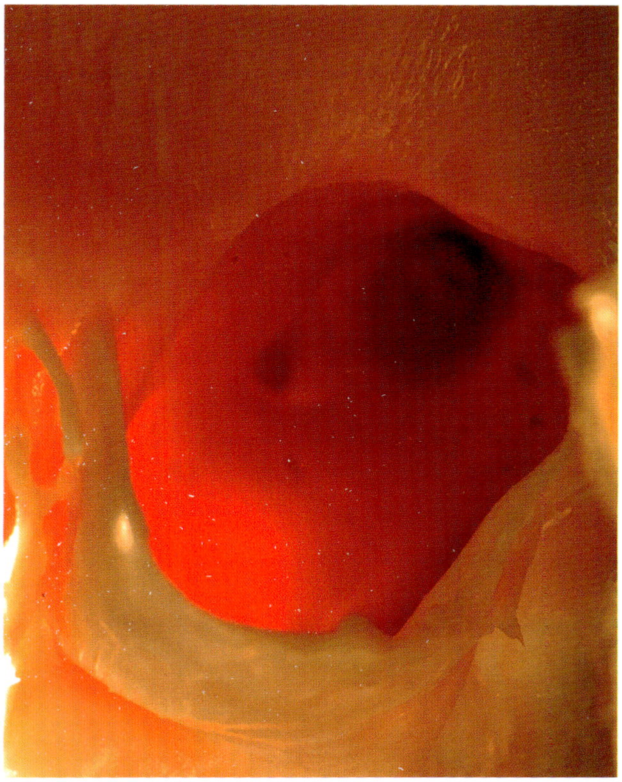

Figure 13. Coronary cusp.

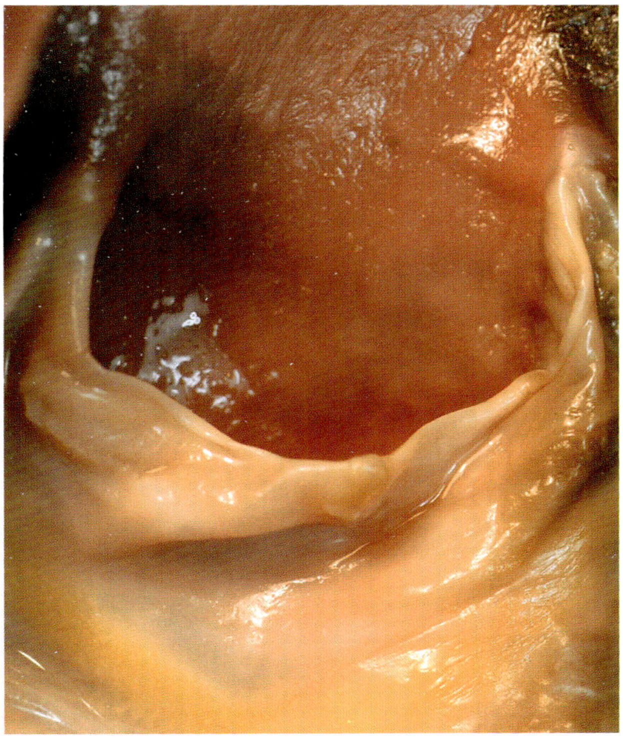

Figure 14. Non-coronary cusp. The basal ring can be made out in the area of attachment of the cusp; union between the outflow tract and the aortic root.

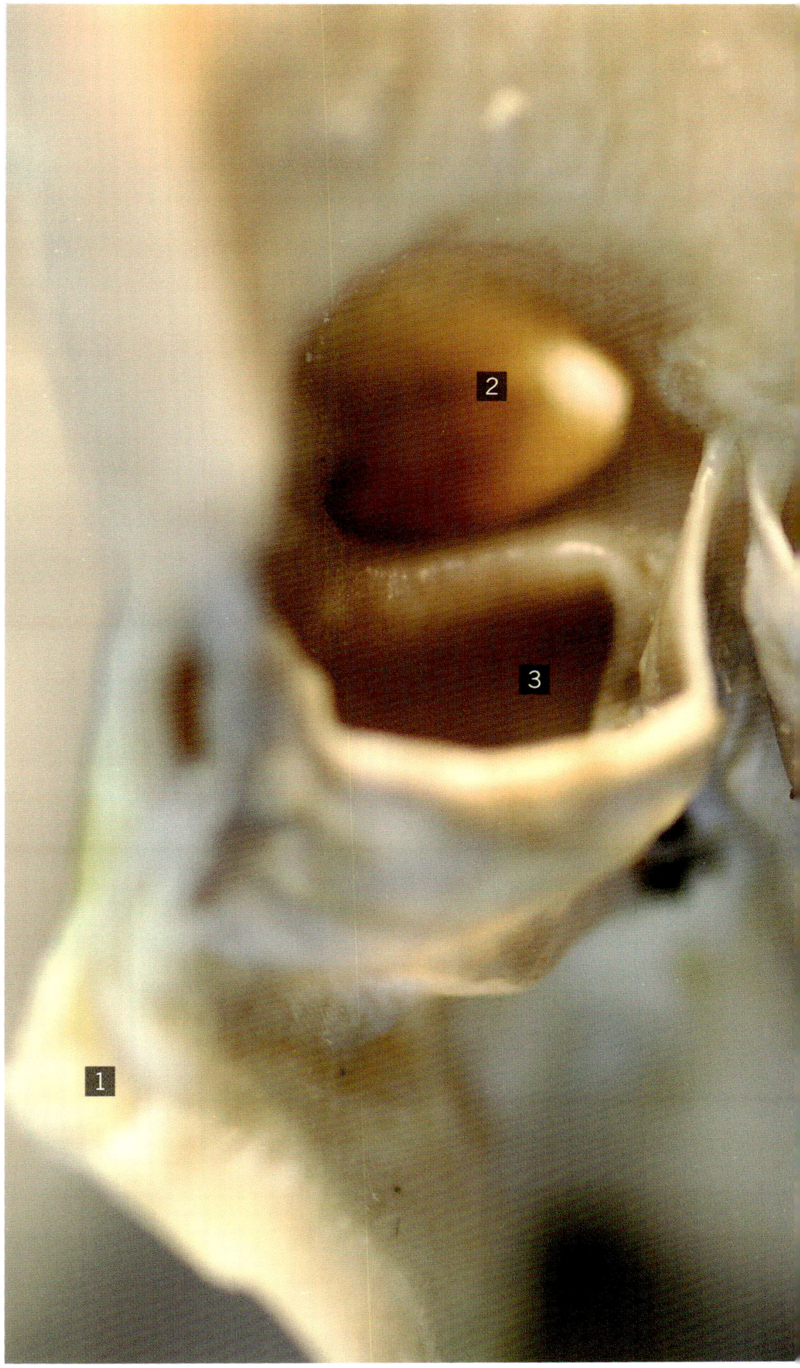

Figure 15. Right coronary cusp.

[1 Aortic bulb]

[2 Origin of the right coronary artery]

[3 Sinus of Valsalva]

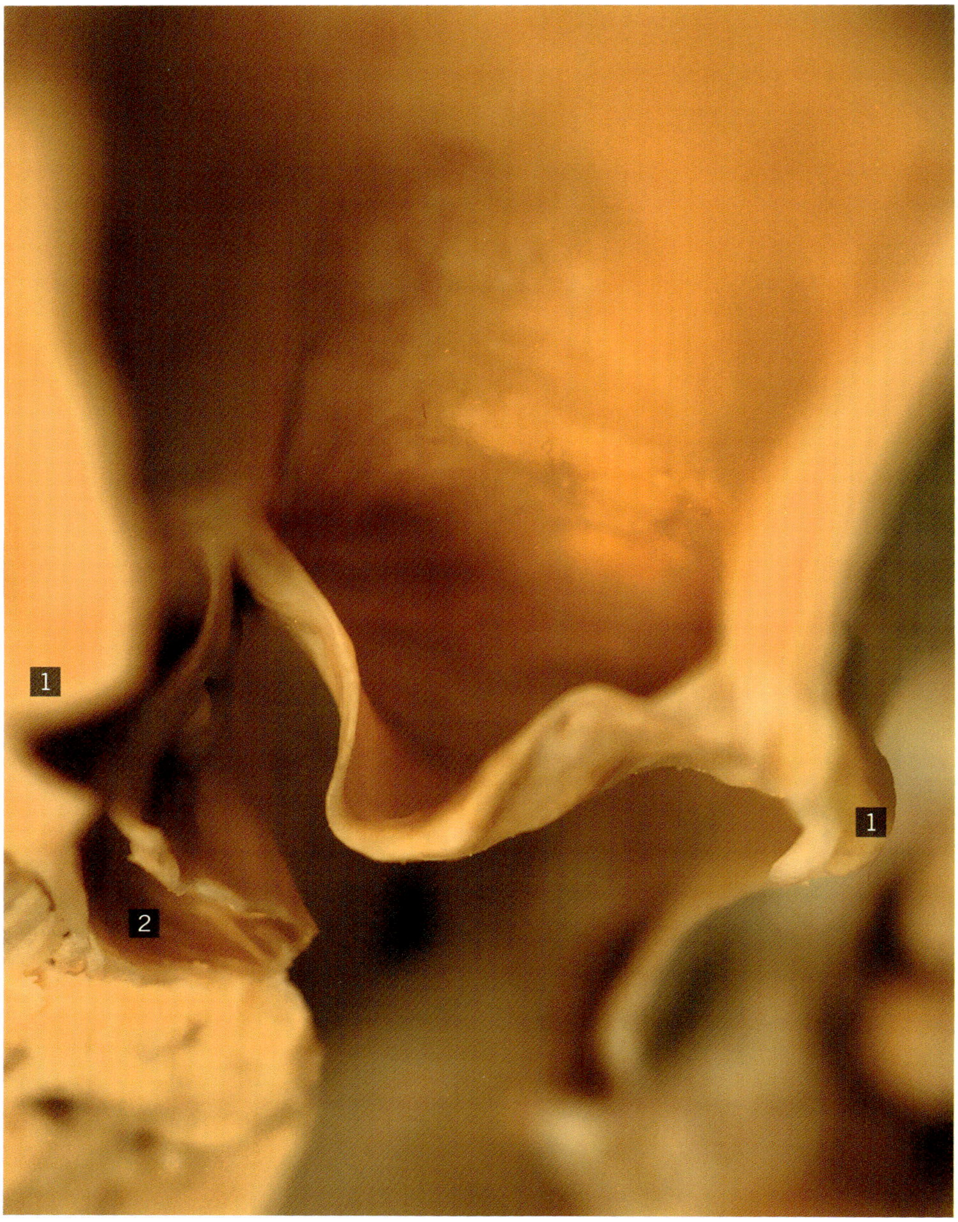

[1 Aortic bulb]

[2 Sinus of Valsalva]

Figure 16.

SINUSES OF VALSALVA

The sinuses of Valsalva or aortic sinuses are located in the aortic root and opposite each of the semilunar cusps; they are dilations of the aortic wall. This creates a swelling at the base of the ascending aorta that is named the aortic bulb.

The orifice of origin of the left and right coronary arteries is located in the sinuses of Valsalva of the respective cusps.

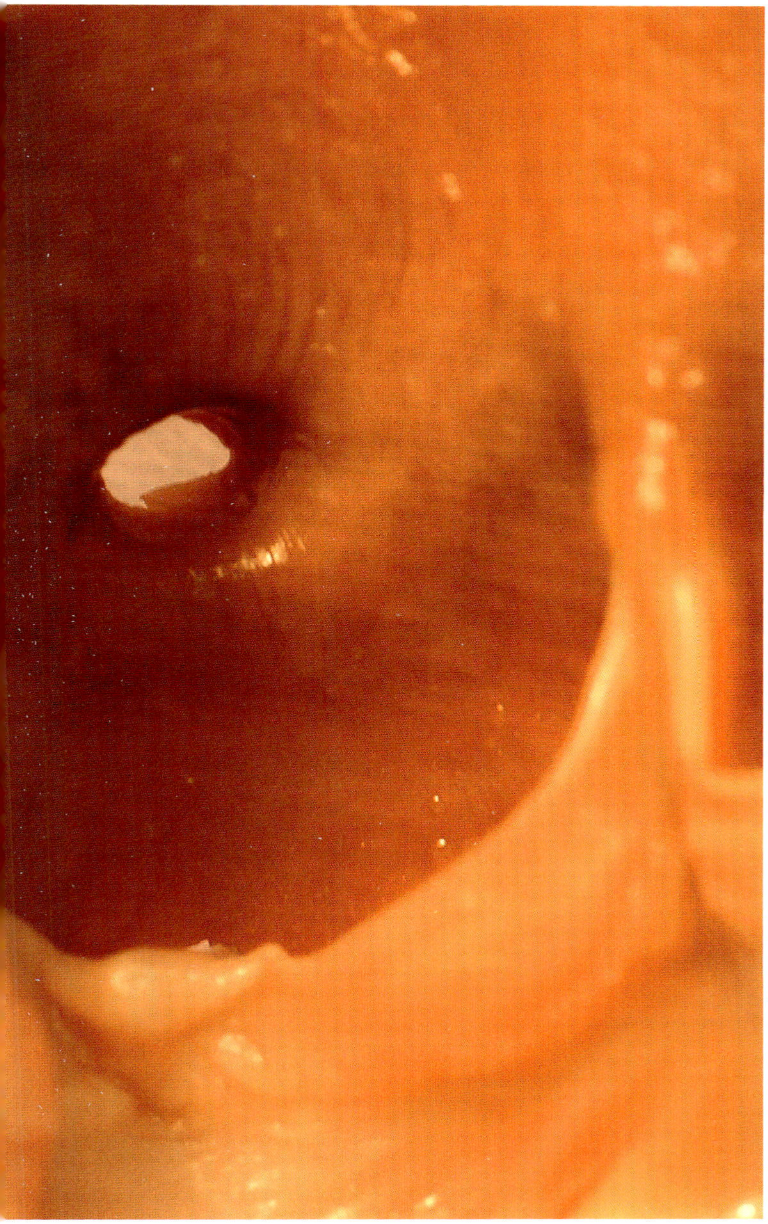

Figure 17. Origin of the right coronary artery.

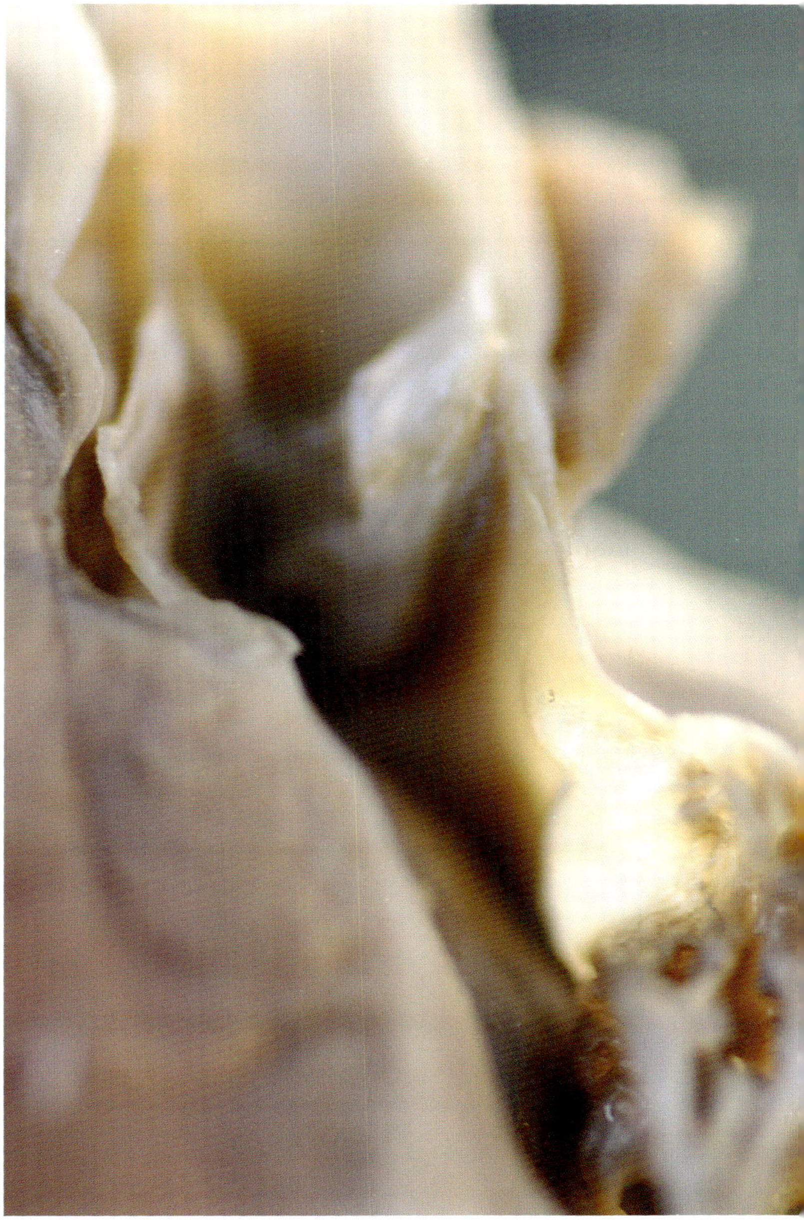

Figure 18. Outflow tract and aortic root.

CORONARY OSTIA

The coronary ostia are located, as previously mentioned, in the right and left sinuses of Valsalva, usually just below the sinotubular junction.

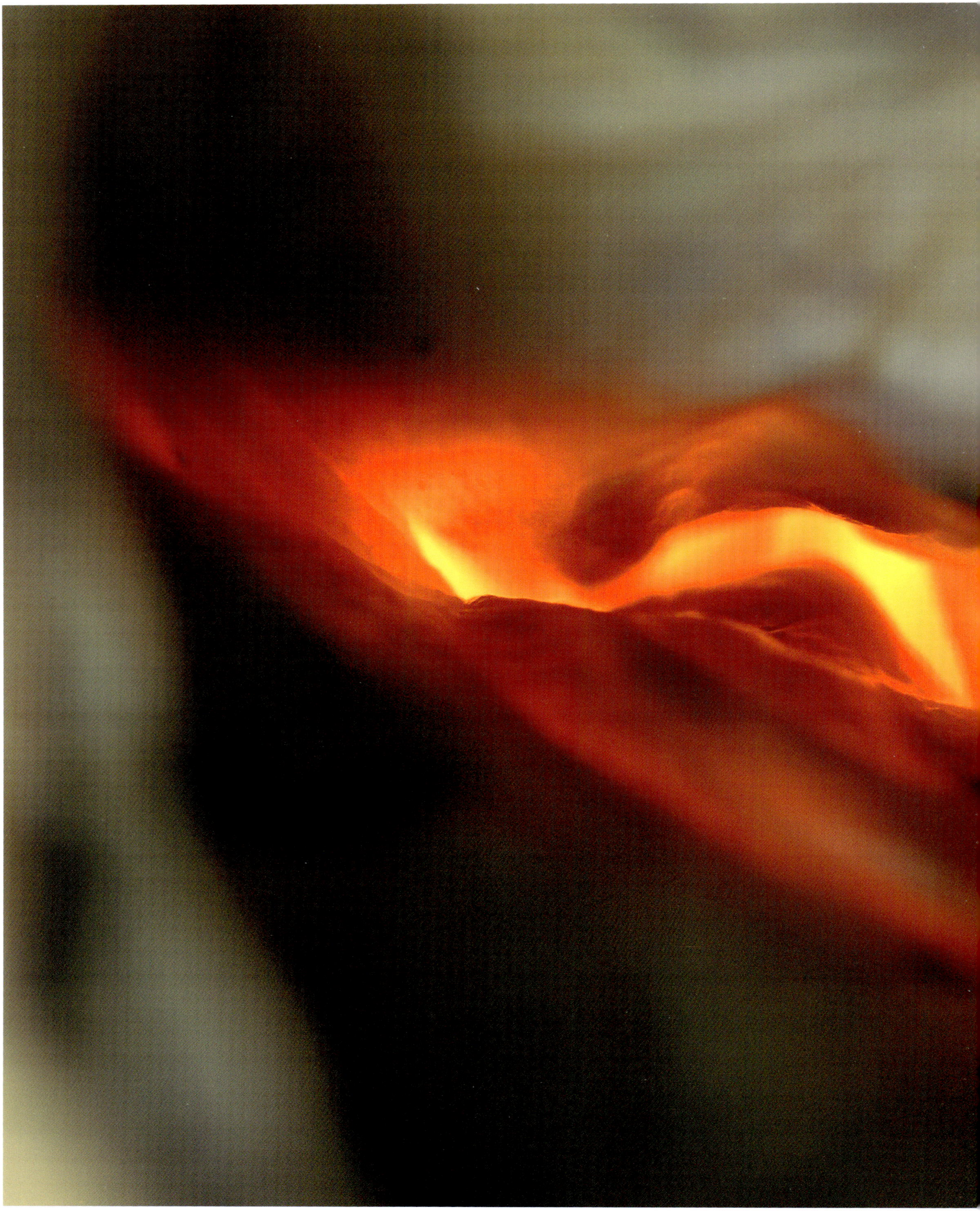

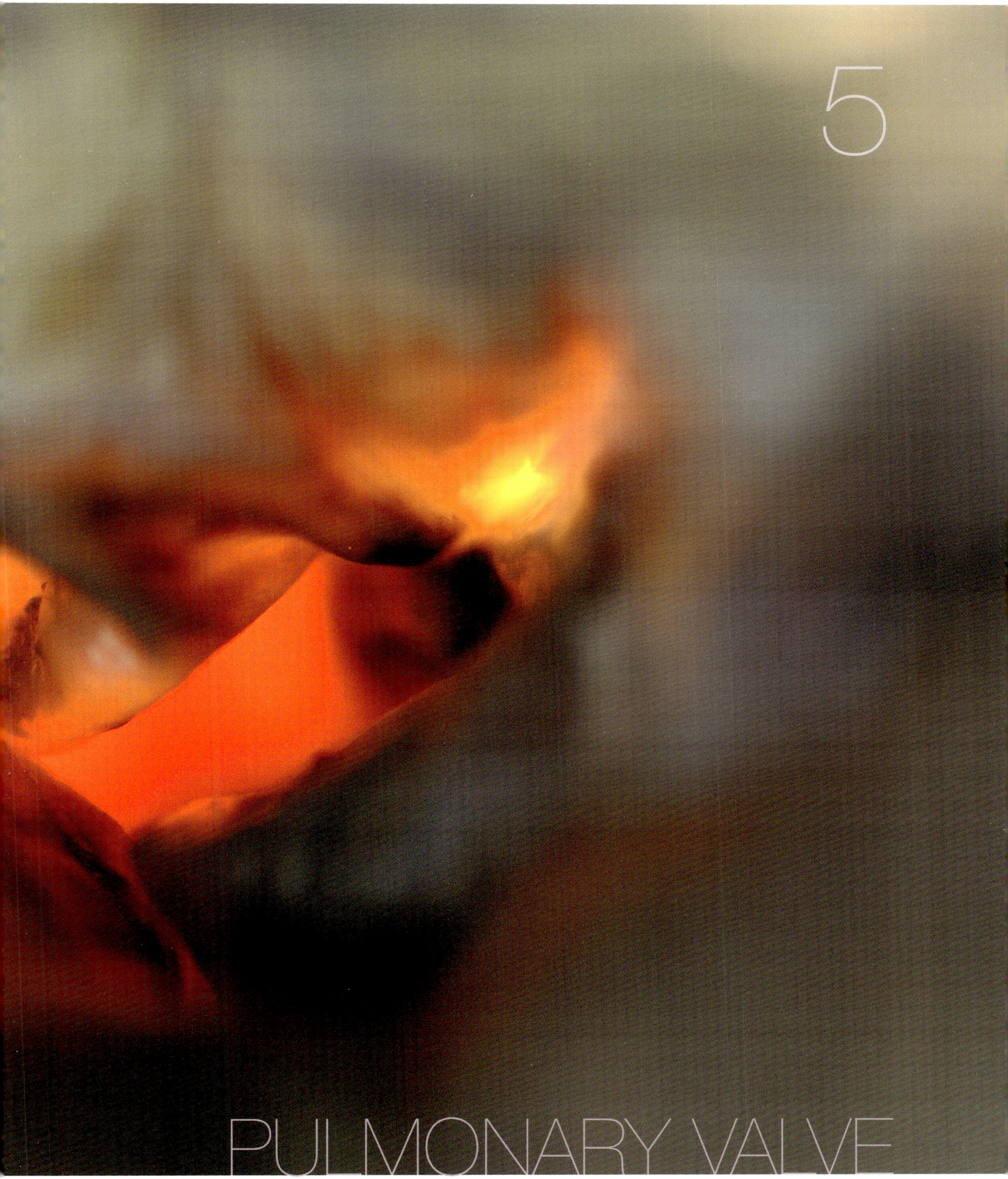

5

PULMONARY VALVE

[1 Intermediate cusp of the pulmonary valve]

[2 Left cusp]

[3 Right cusp]

[4 Septal or non-coronary cusp]

[5 Left coronary cusp]

[6 Right coronary cusp]

[7 Conus ligament]

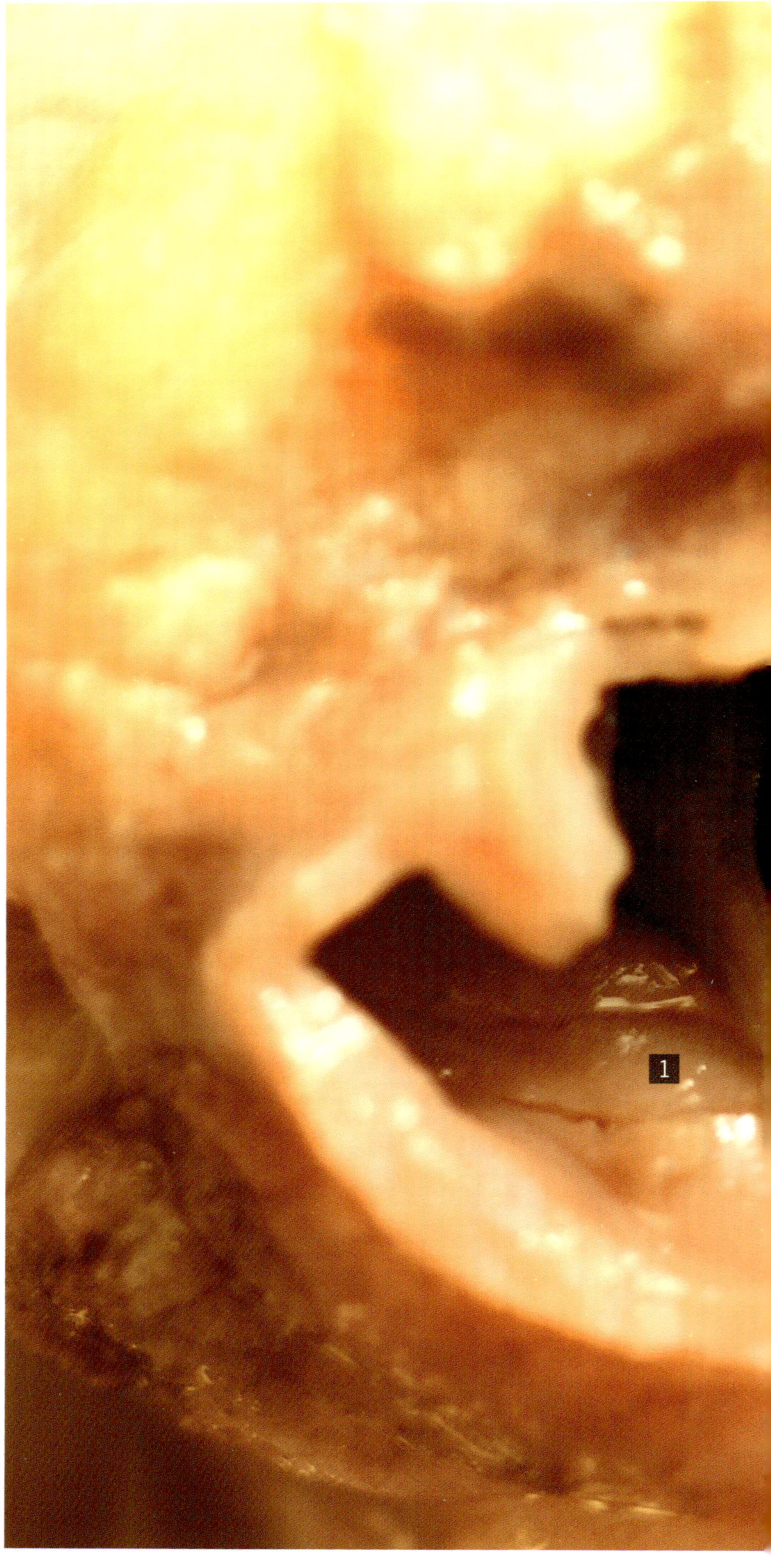

The pulmonary valve is located cranial to the aortic valve and craniodorsal and to the left of the tricuspid valve. As opposed to what occurs with those of the aortic and mitral valves, the annuli of the pulmonary and tricuspid valves are separated.

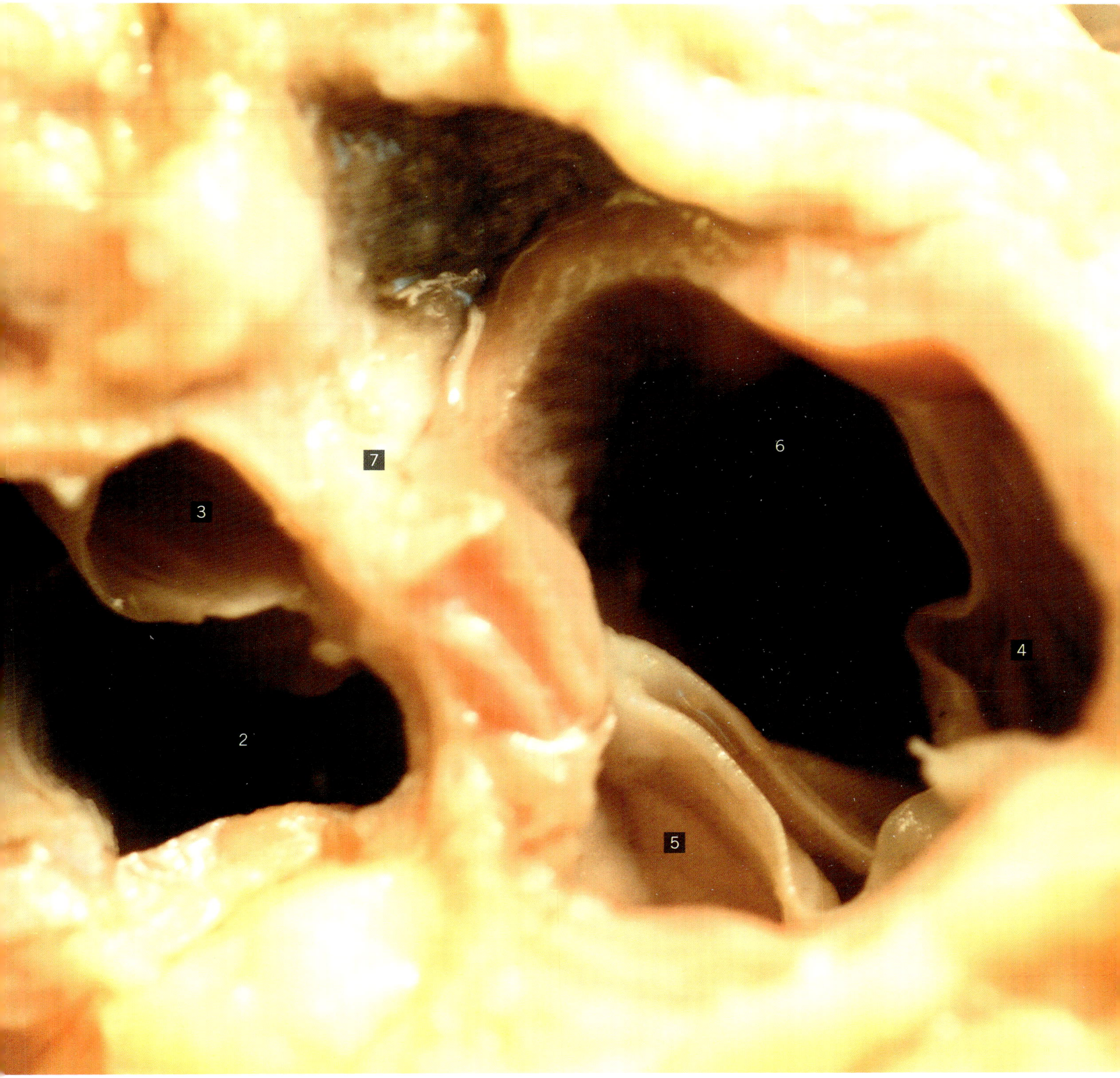

Figure 1. Pulmonary valve and its relation with the aortic valve.

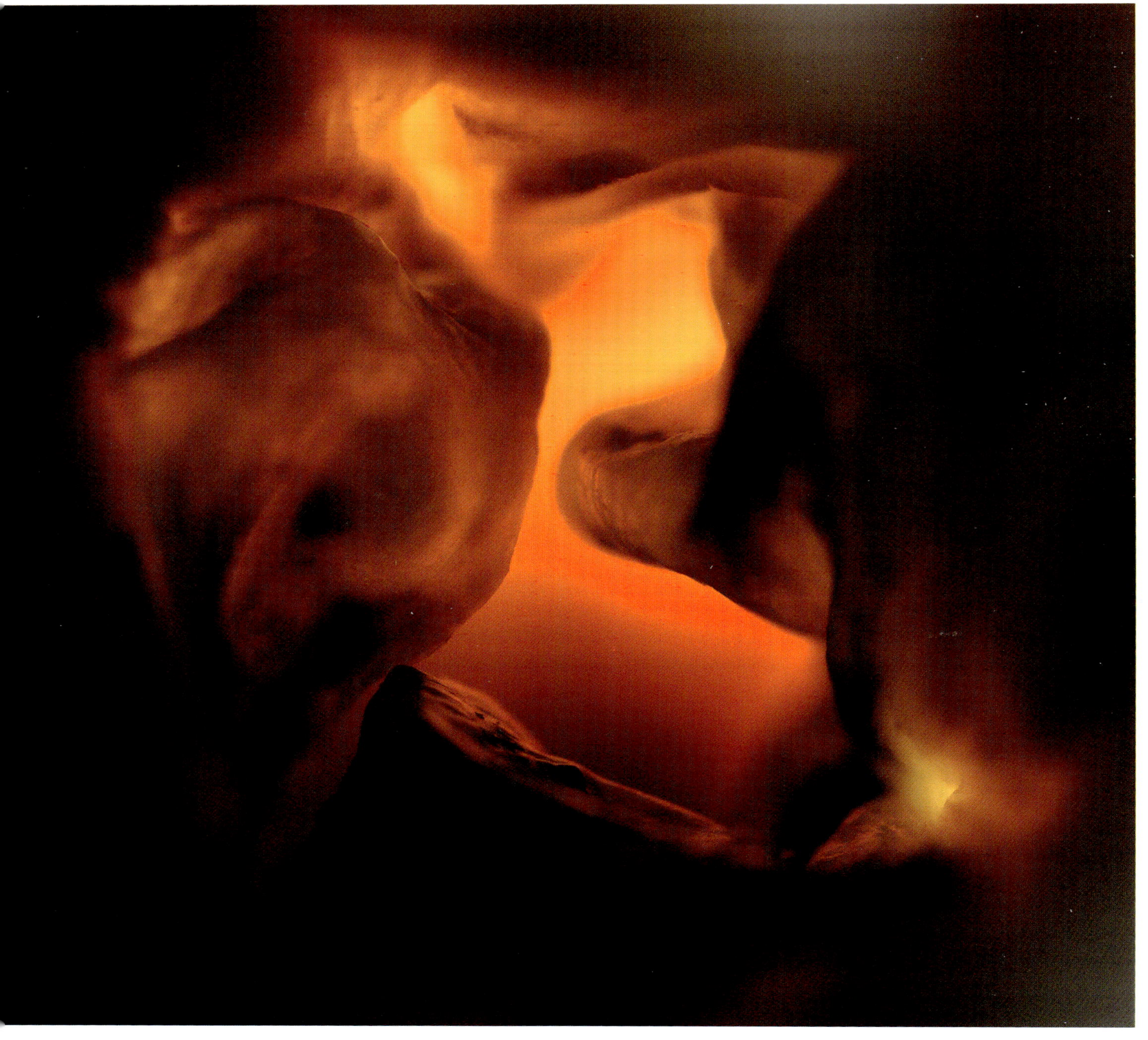

Figure 2. View of the pulmonary valve from the infundibulum.

The outflow tract of the right ventricle, which leads to the pulmonary valve and trunk of the pulmonary artery, is a long and rounded muscular structure named conus arteriosus or infundibulum.

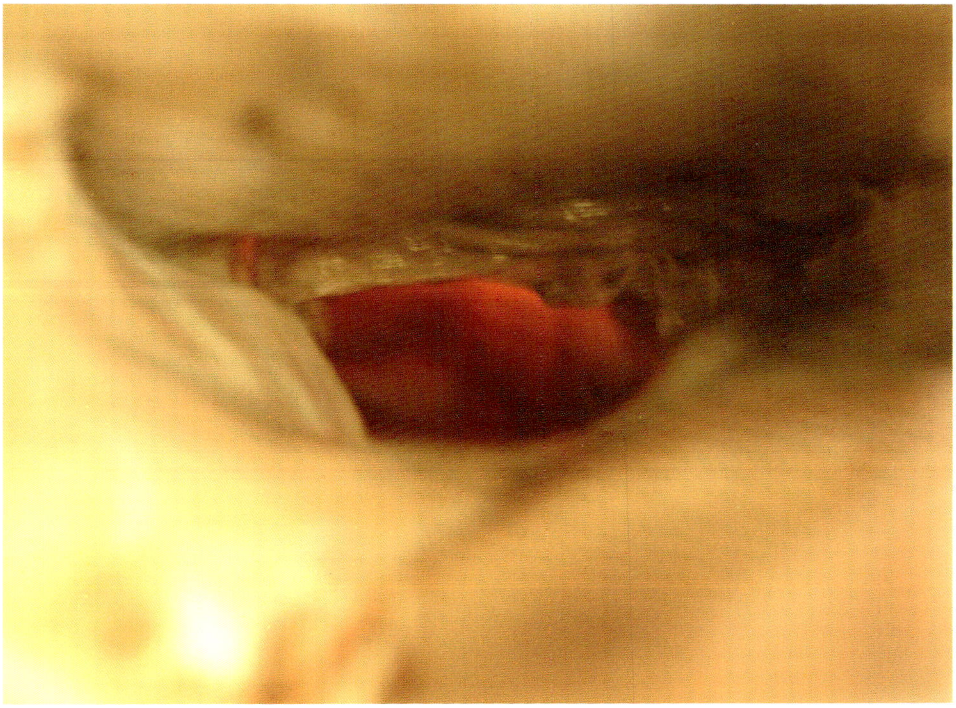

Figure 3. Infundibulum. Outflow tract of the right ventricle.

[1 Tricuspid valve]

[2 Papillary muscle of the conus]

[3 Supraventricular crest]

[4 Pulmonary valve]

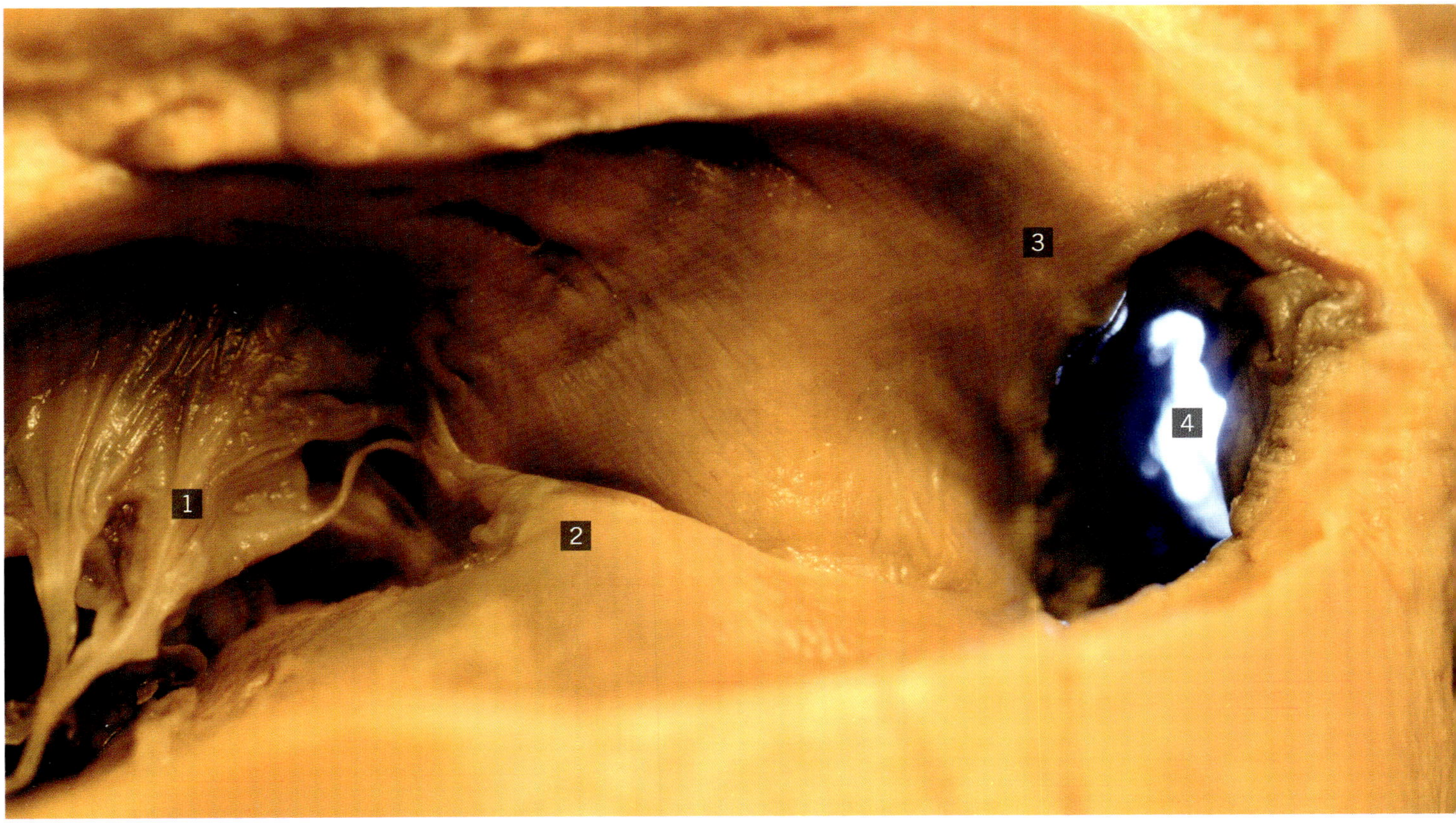

Figure 4. General view of the conus arteriosus or infundibulum, which includes the area from the atrioventricular orifice to the pulmonary valve.

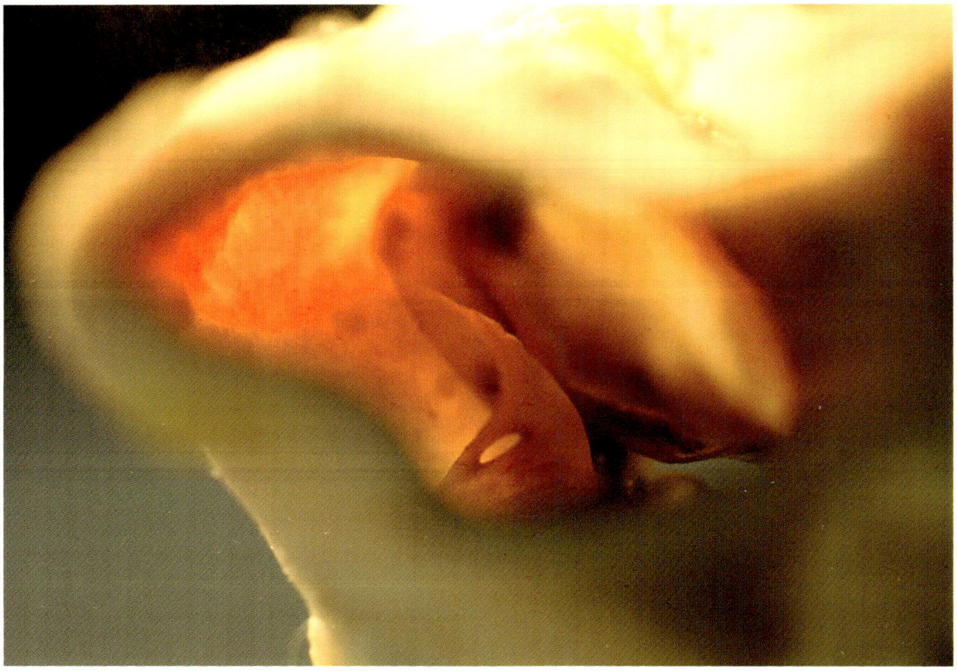

Figure 5. Pulmonary valve. Intermediate cusp seen from the pulmonary trunk.

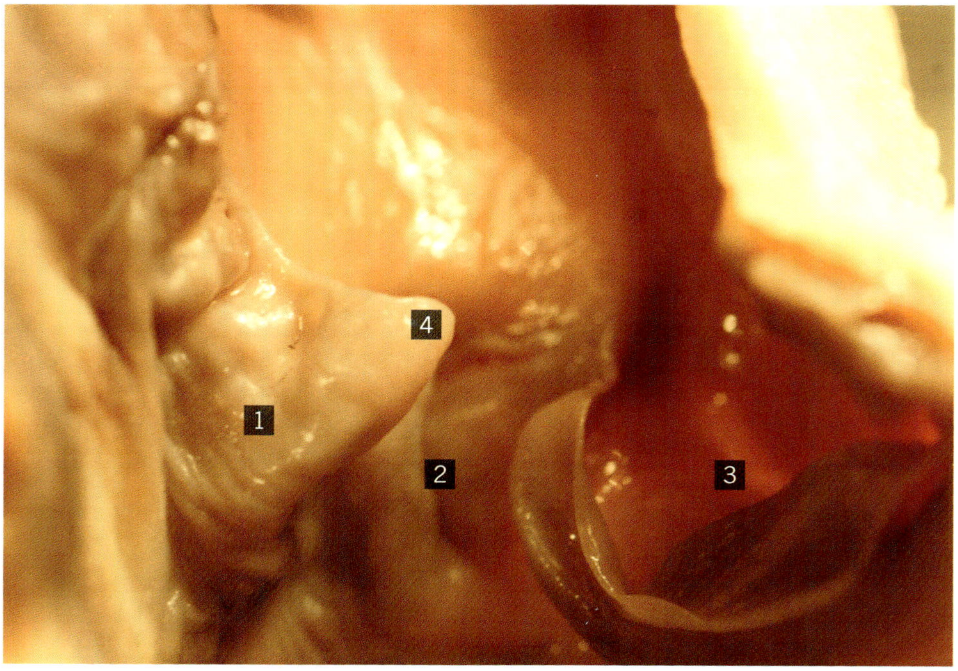

[1 Left cusp]

[2 Right cusp]

[3 Intermediate cusp]

[4 Fibrous nodule]

Figure 6. Valve cusps.

The pulmonary valve has a similar structure to that of the aortic valve; however, as the arterial pressure in the pulmonary trunk is considerably lower than in the aorta, the cusps and other related structures are not as developed.

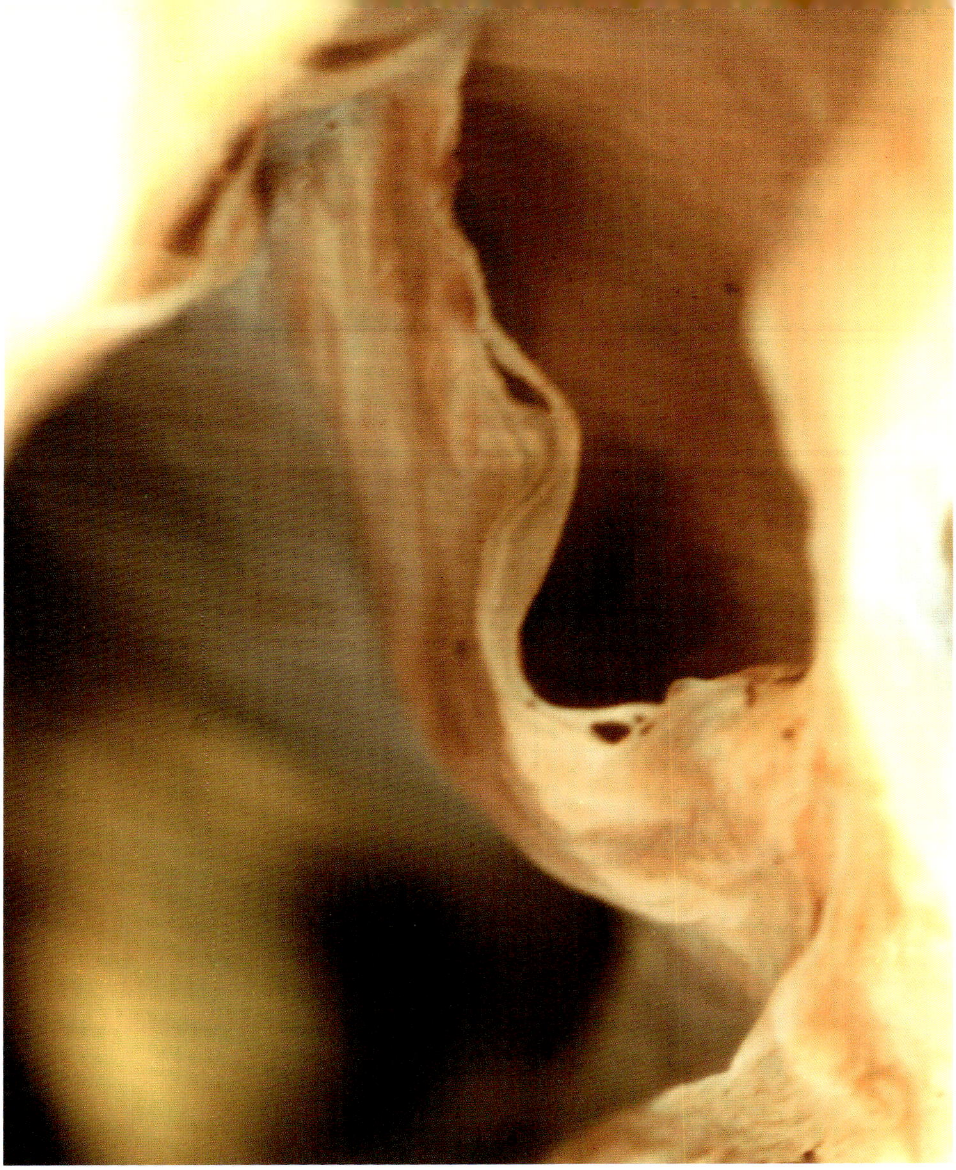

Figure 7. Intermediate cusp.

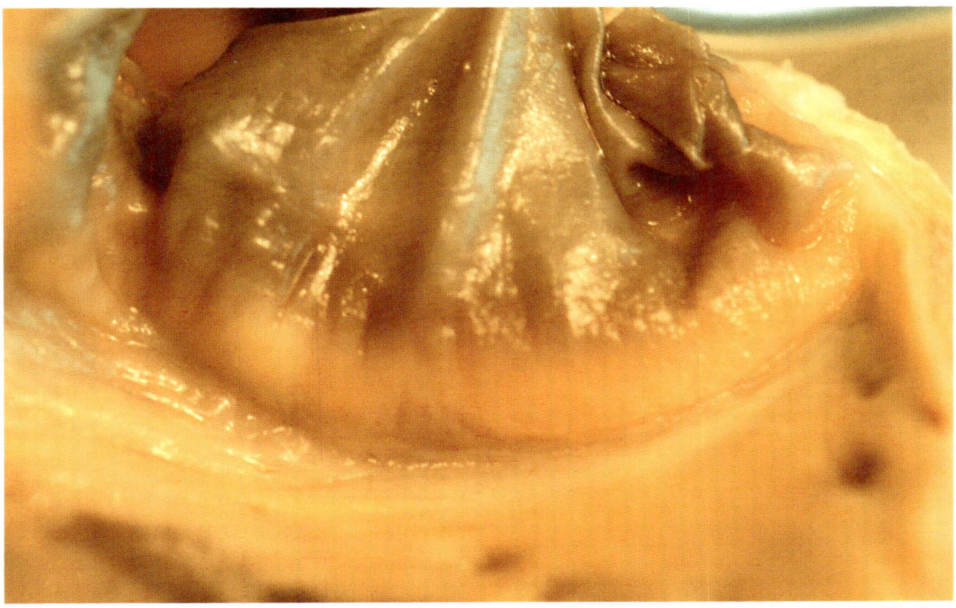

Figure 8. Cusp. Attachment to the valve annulus.

[1 Valve annulus]

[2 Semilunar leaflet or cusp]

[3 Commissure]

[4 Sinotubular junction]

[5 Subcommissural trigones]

[6 Sinus of Valsalva]

[7 Ventriculopulmonary junction]

The valve apparatus is therefore formed by:

- An annulus.
- Cusps.
- Commissures.
- A sinotubular junction.
- Subcommissural trigones.
- Sinuses of Valsalva.

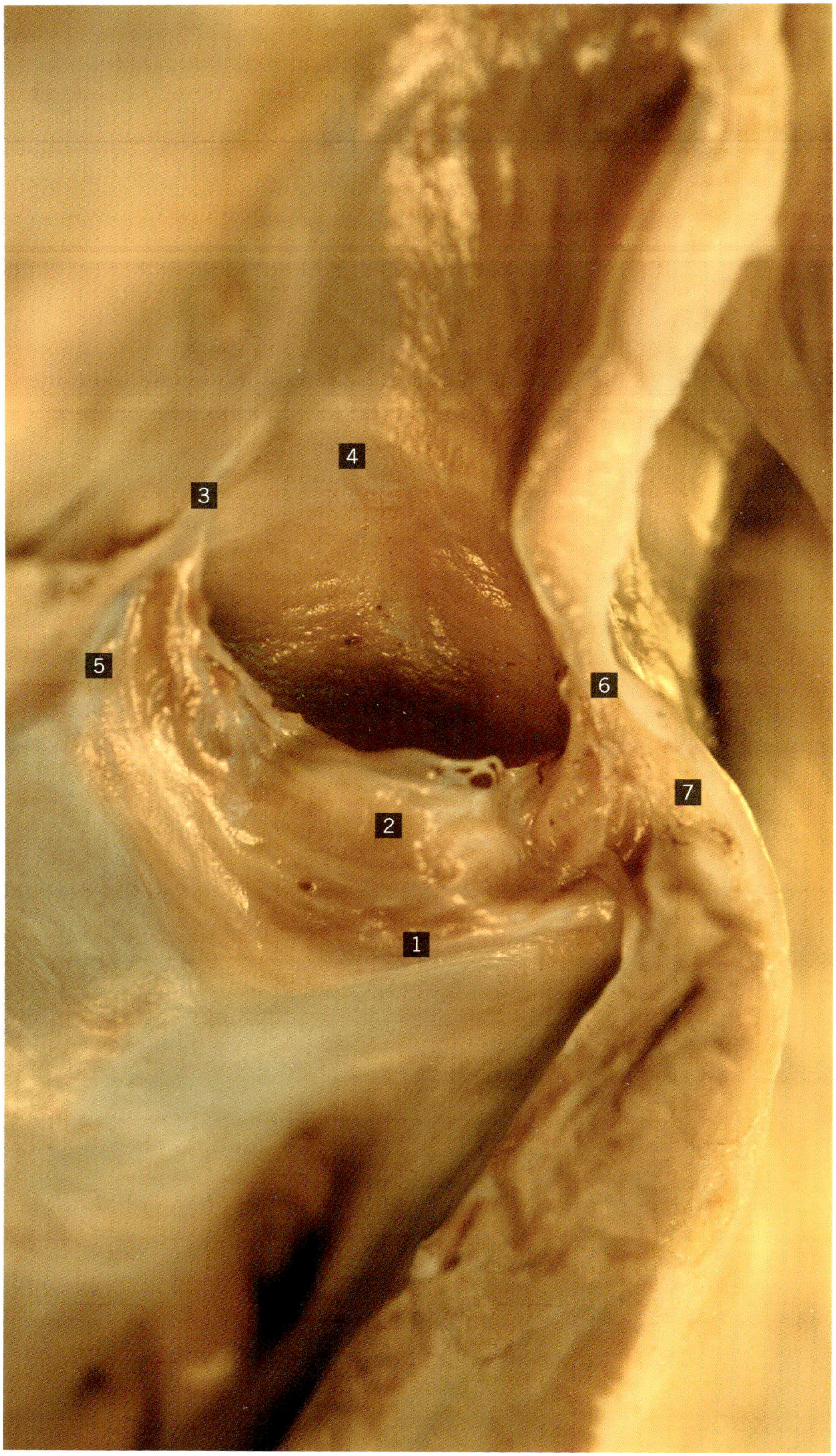

Figure 9. Sagittal section of the pulmonary valve apparatus.

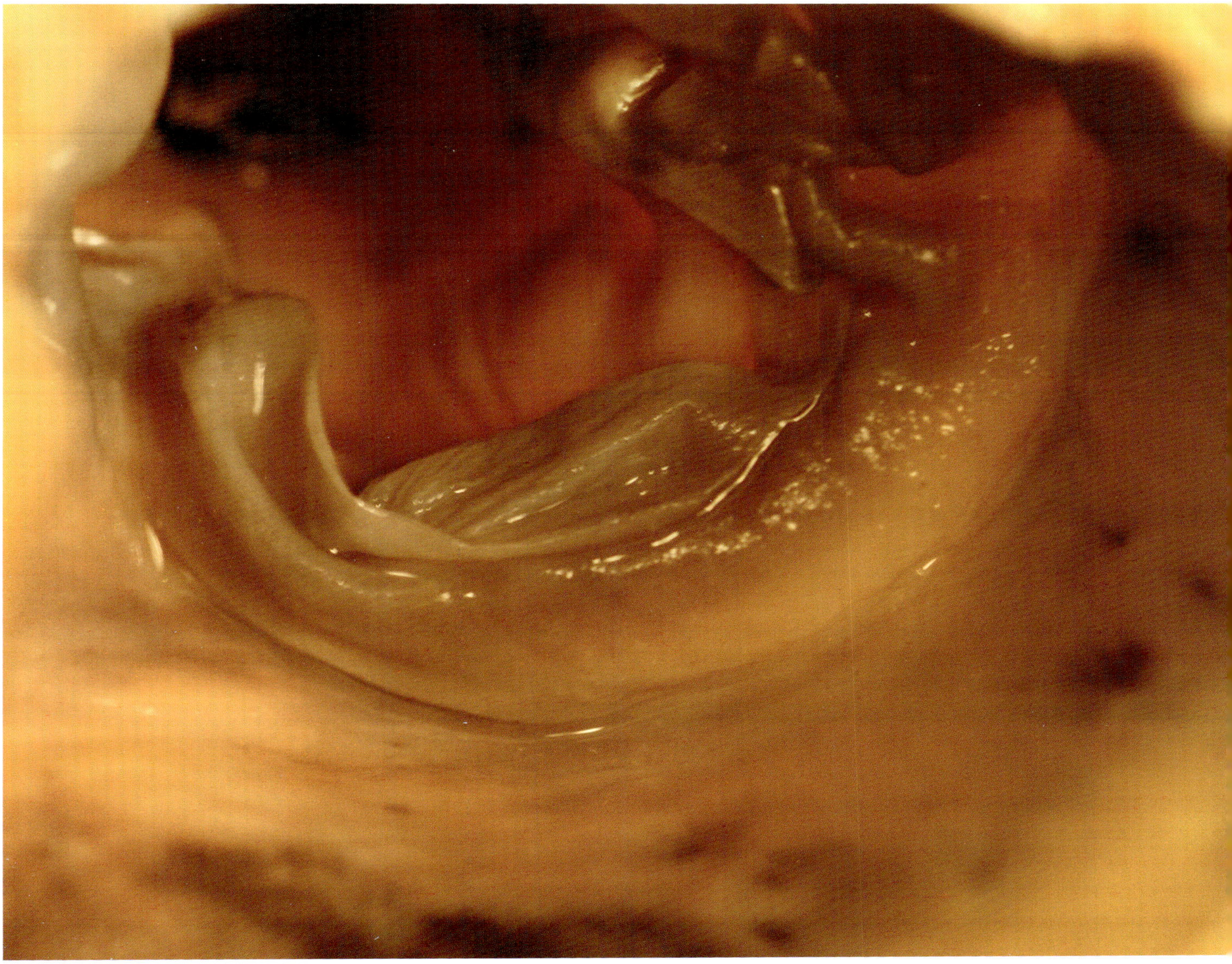

Figure 10. Valve annulus. The semilunar cusps insert into it. The muscle fibres of the infundibulum blend with it.

ANNULUS

The fibrous ring of the pulmonary valve is part of the fibrous skeleton of the heart and is attached to this latter by means of a short structure of collagen tissue named the "conus ligament", which connects it with the aortic annulus.

The muscle fibres of the infundibulum attach to its cranioventral surface, while the pulmonary trunk originates from its caudodorsal part.

The semilunar cusps are attached to it.

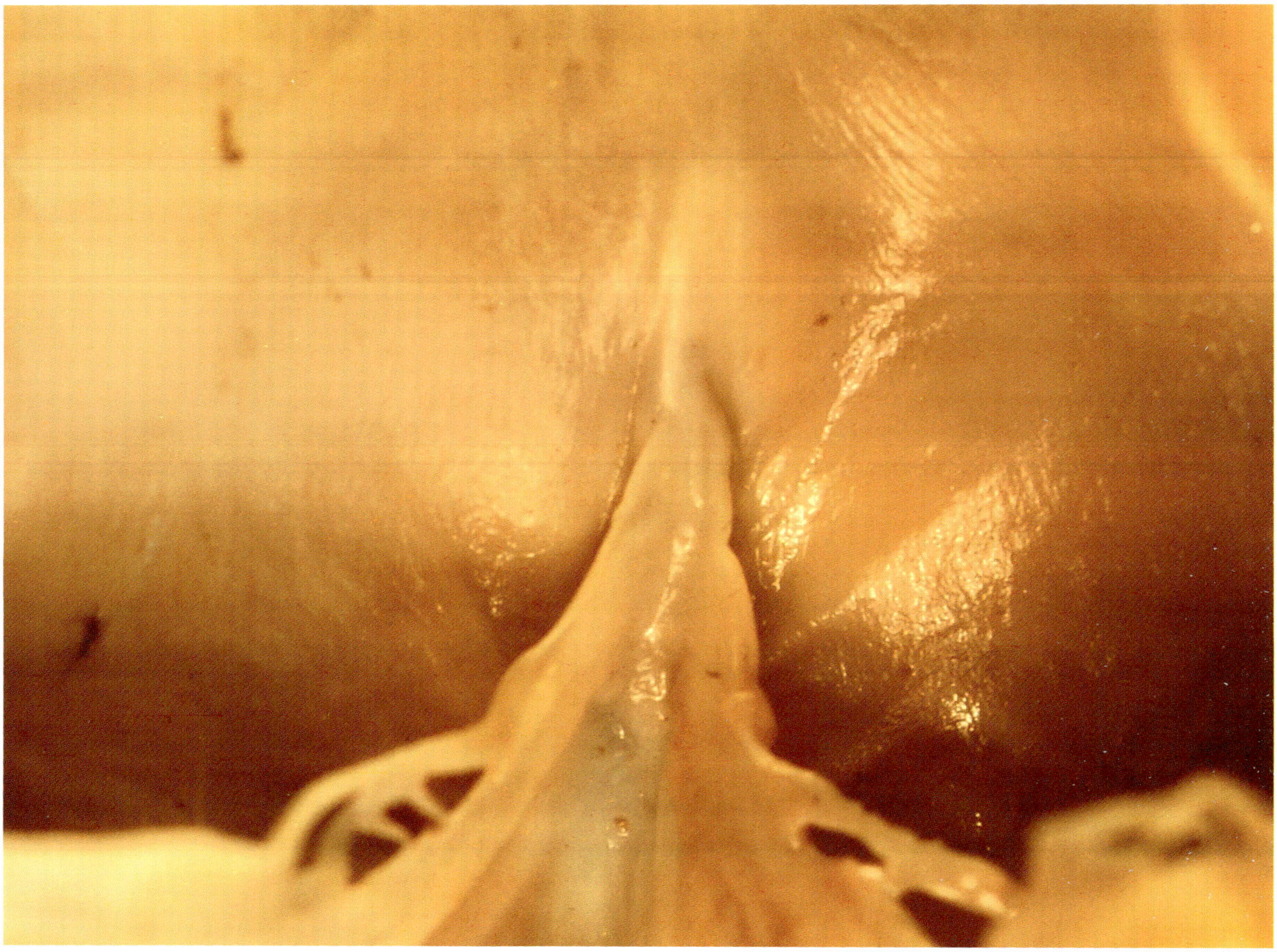

Figure 11. Commissures, the more whitish area on the left corresponds to the sinotubular junction.

CUSPS

Also named leaflets, they are three thin, semitransparent structures that attach at their base to the annulus; each of them has a fibrous nodule at the centre of their free margins, which is similar to the nodule of Arantius of the aortic valve cusps. They form three symmetric rings, which join at the centre to close the arterial orifice during diastole. They are named left, right and intermediate or cranial cusps. The right and left cusps are partly adjacent to the right and left cusps of the aortic valve.

COMMISSURES

They correspond to the junction of two valve cusps at the sinotubular junction.

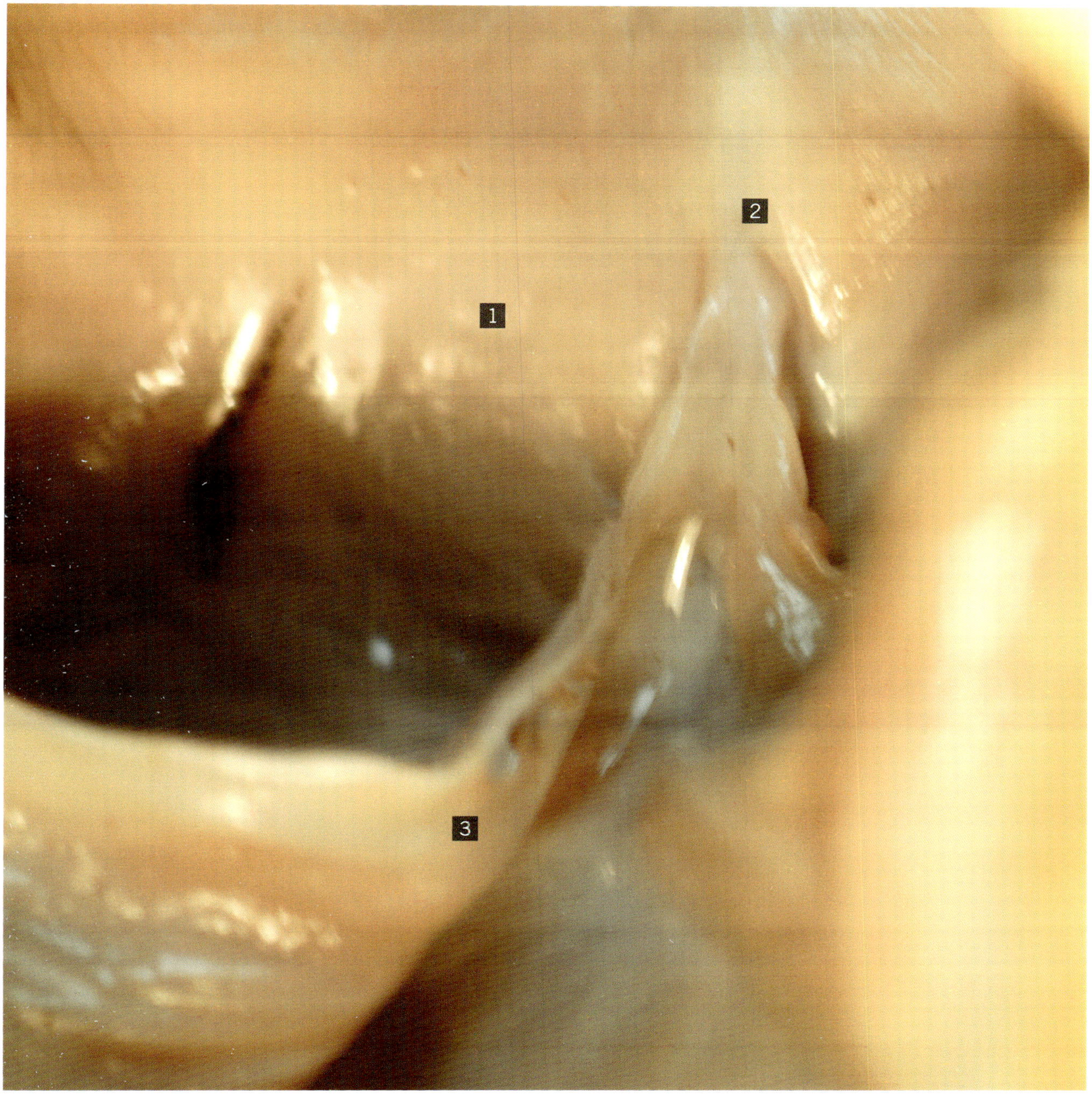

Figure 12. Area of the sinotubular junction.

[1 Sinotubular junction]

[2 Commissure]

[3 Nodule of the valve cusp]

SINOTUBULAR JUNCTION

It is the point of junction, rich in elastic fibres, between the pulmonary root and the pulmonary trunk.

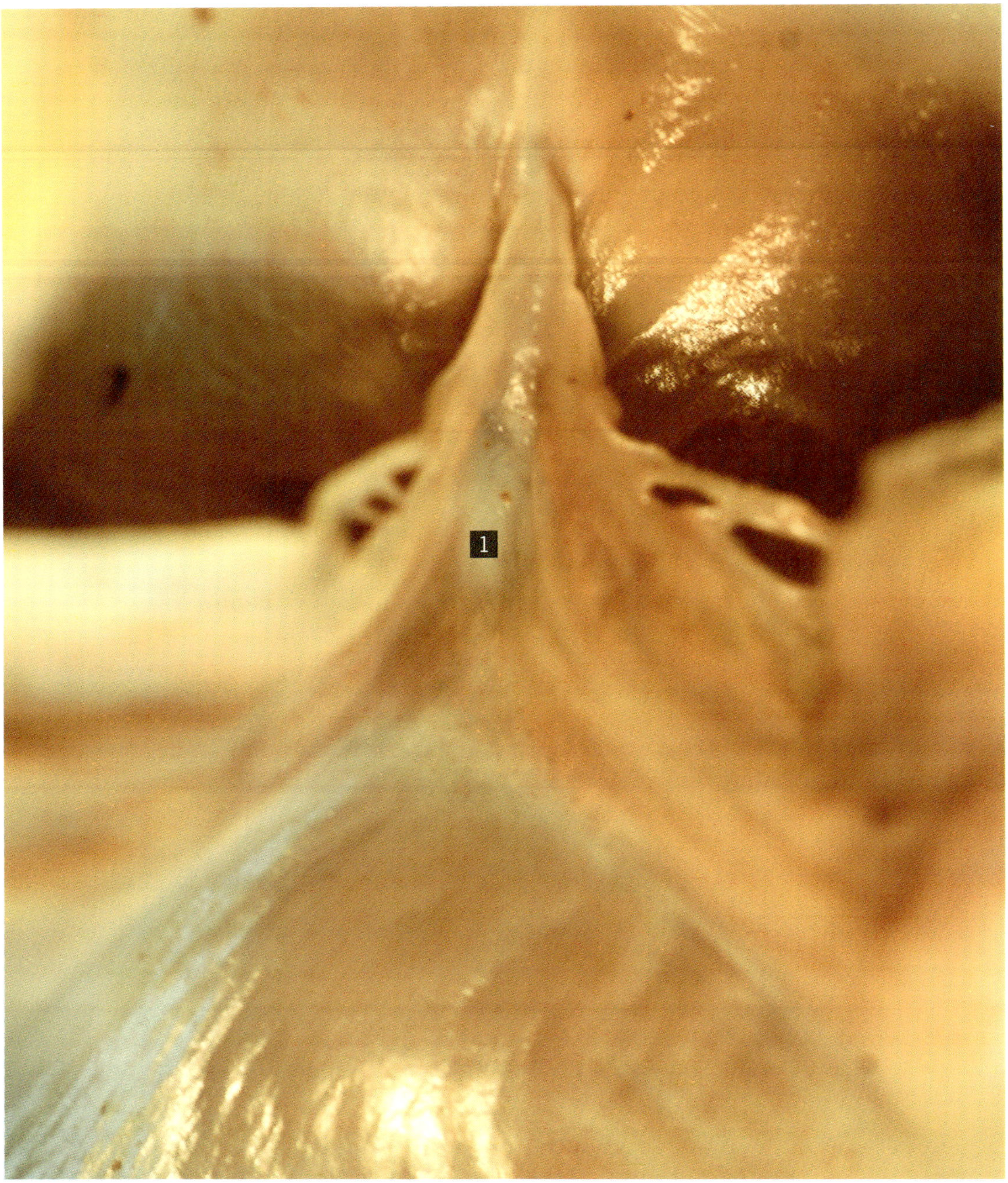

[1 Trigone]

Figure 13. Subcommissural trigone.

SUBCOMMISSURAL TRIGONES

Area of the arterial wall located below the commissures and subject to ventricular pressures.

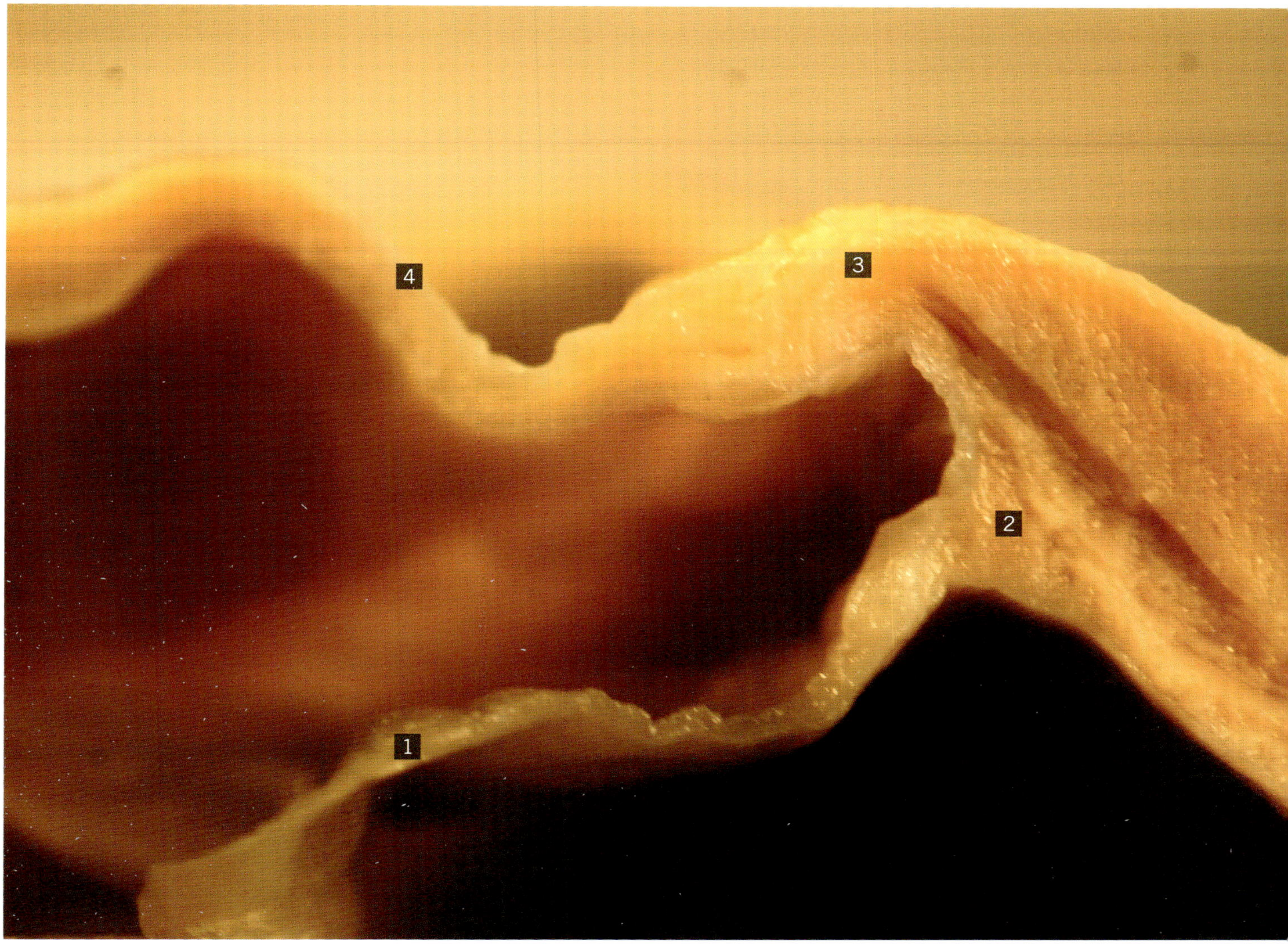

Figure 14. Sagittal section of a pulmonary valve cusp.

[1 Cusp] [2 Annulus] [3 Ventriculopulmonary junction] [4 Sinus of Valsalva]

SINUSES OF VALSALVA

Slight dilation of the pulmonary trunk between the sinotubular junction and the ventriculopulmonary junction.

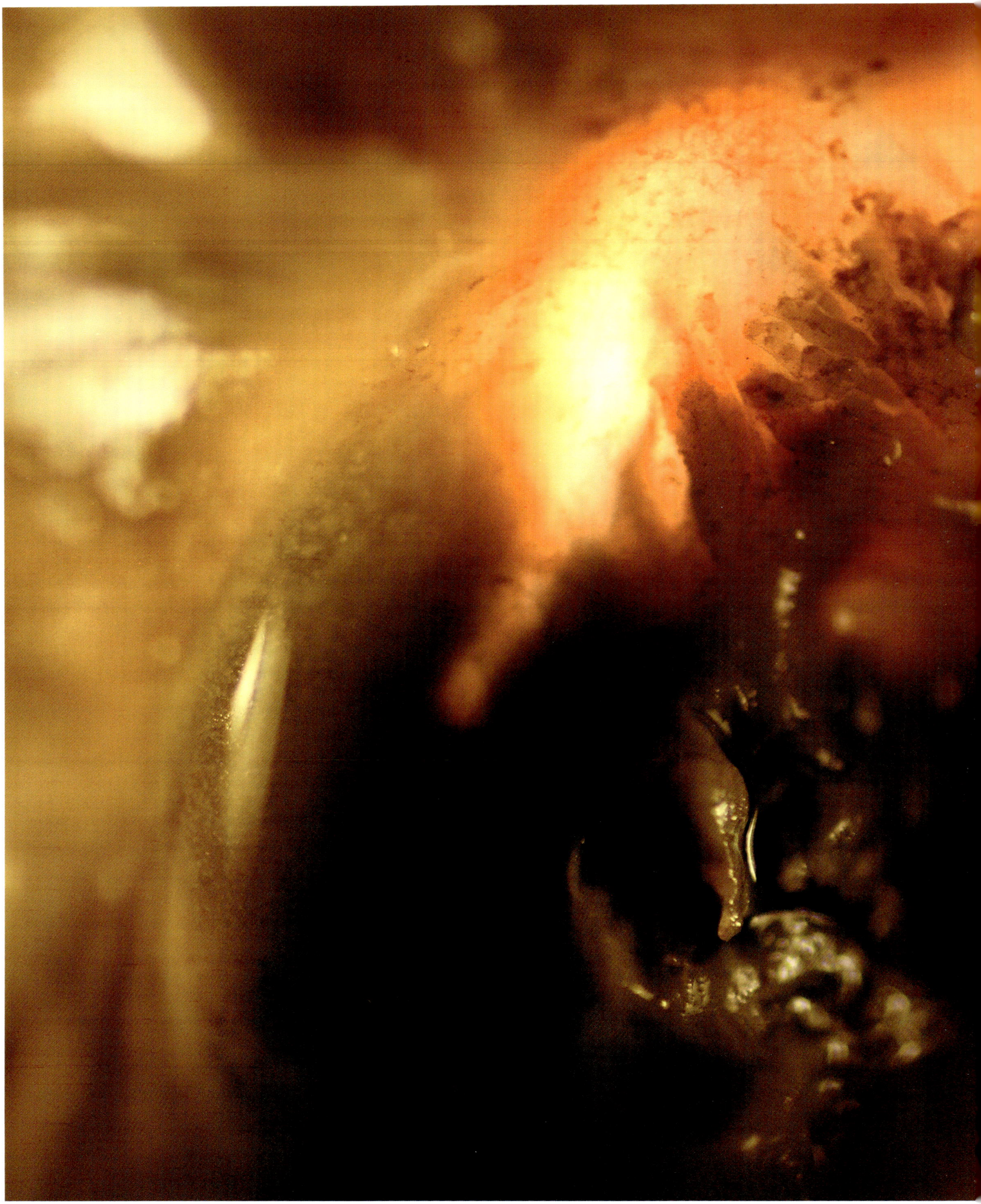

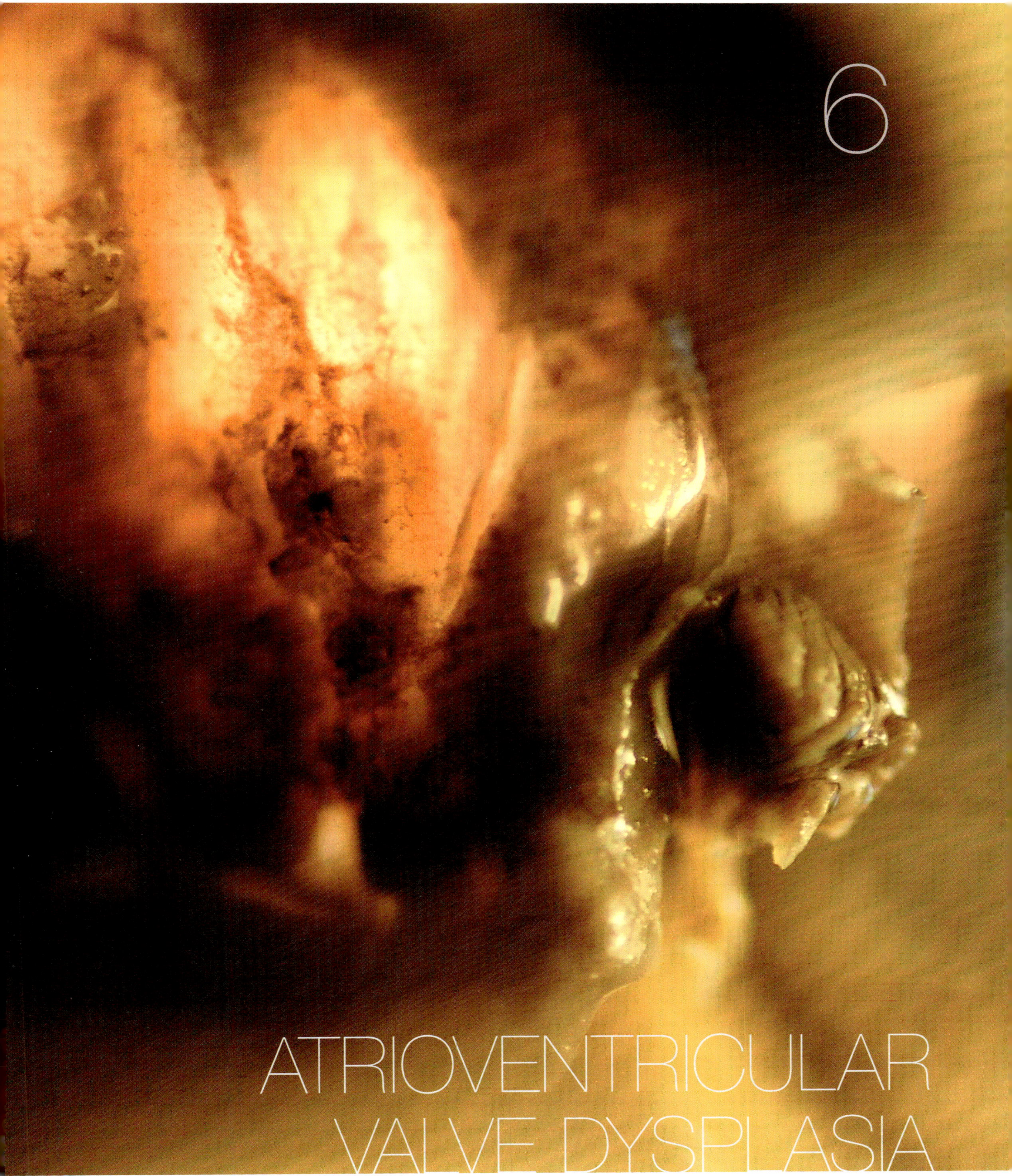

6

ATRIOVENTRICULAR VALVE DYSPLASIA

Dysplastic atrioventricular valves have a general characteristic: they are deficient. In some cases, some degree of stenosis may also be found at the same time.

For this reason, in most cases we will observe valvular regurgitation and volume overload in the chambers of the affected side, with eccentric ventricular hypertrophy, atrial dilation and reduction of the cardiac output.

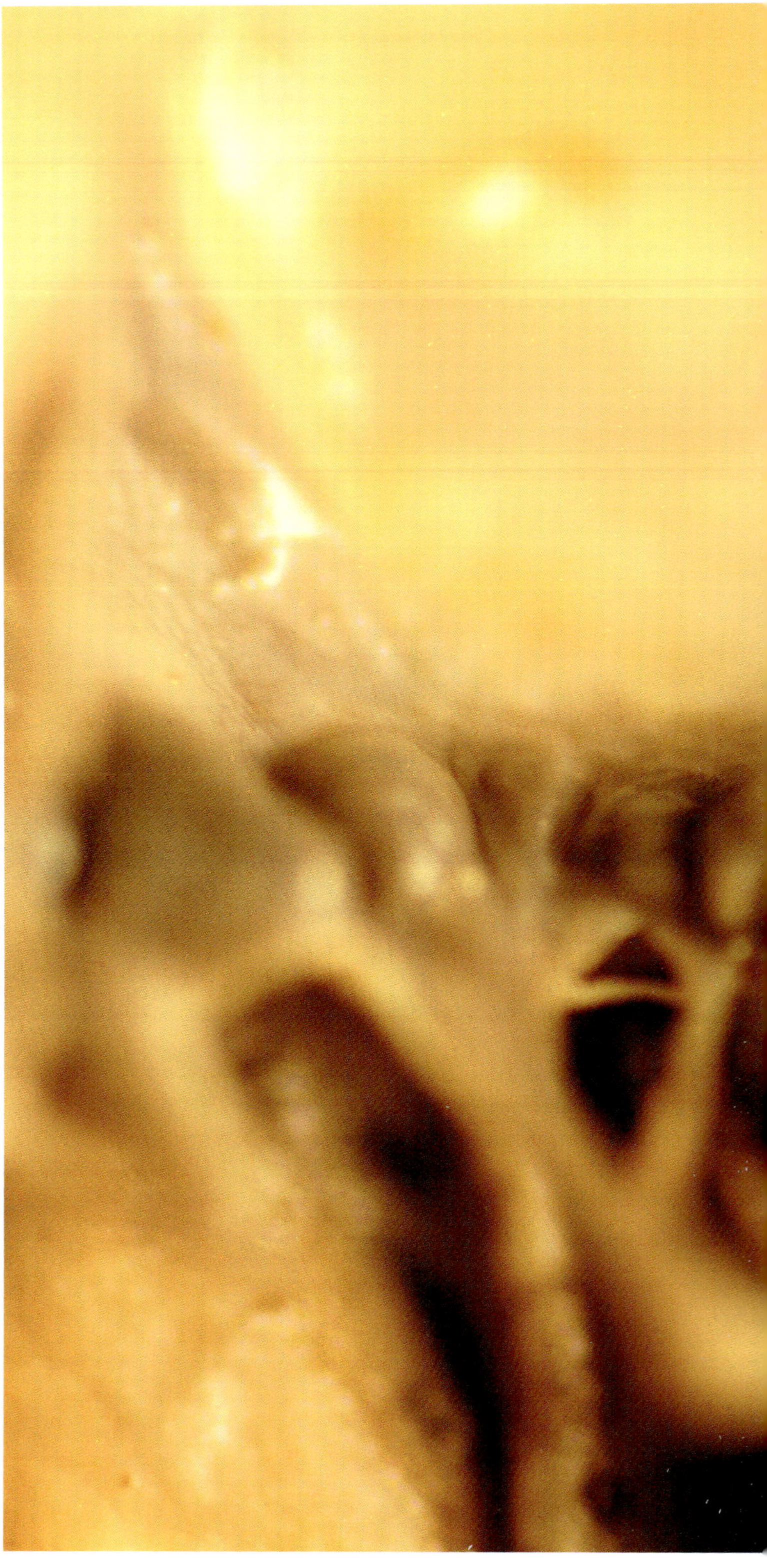

MITRAL VALVE DYSPLASIA

The malformation of the mitral valve may be seen in both dogs and cats, although in the latter it is one of the most common congenital heart diseases.

The lesions that can be found may affect one, several or all the parts of the mitral valve apparatus.

ANNULUS

In many cases, we will find that the mitral valve annulus has a larger diameter than the average diameter we should expect based on the length and weight of the animal's body and heart.

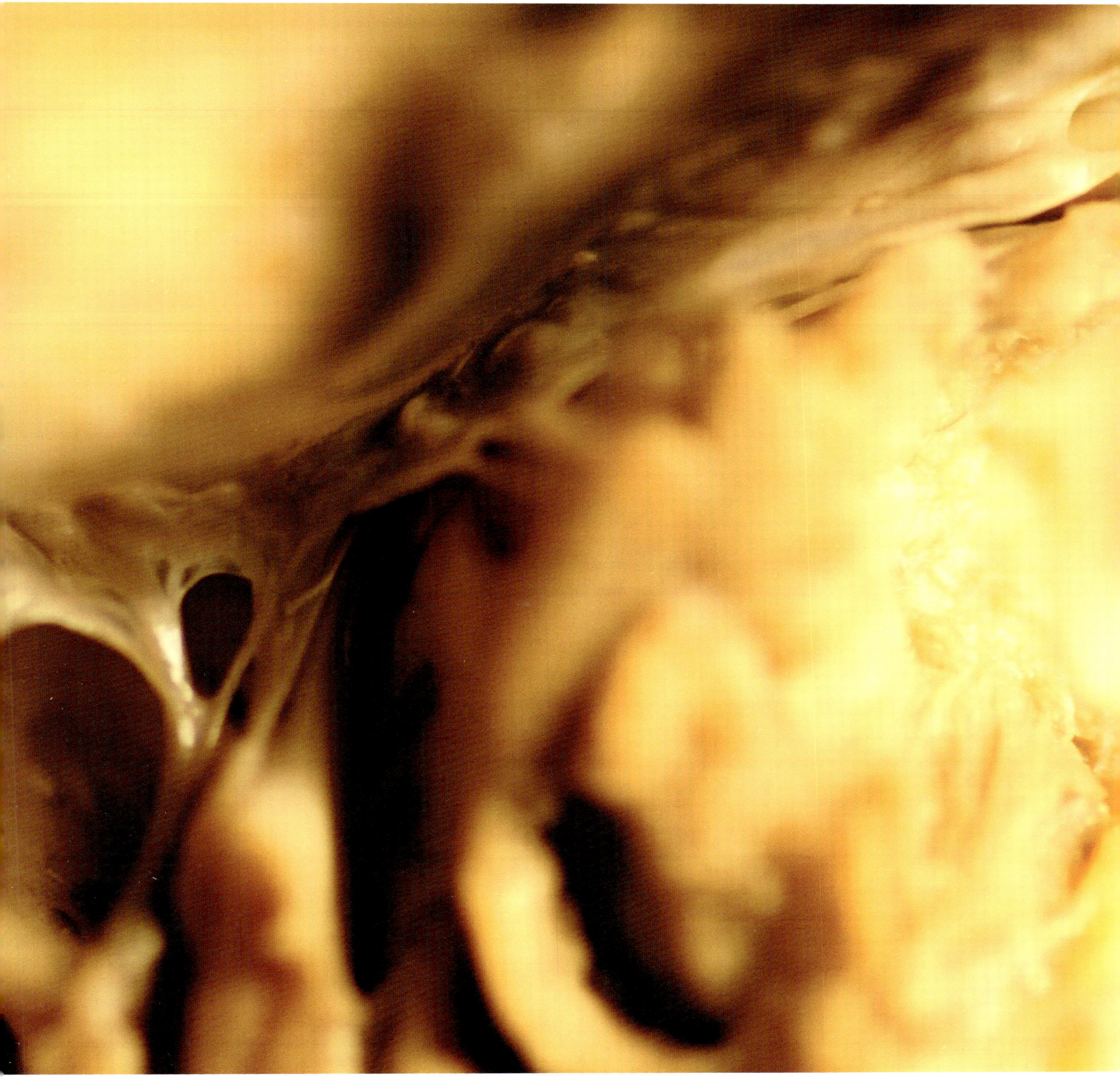

Figure 1. An increase in the diameter of the annulus may often be observed in mitral valve dysplasia. Here, it is also possible to observe a shortening of the leaflets.

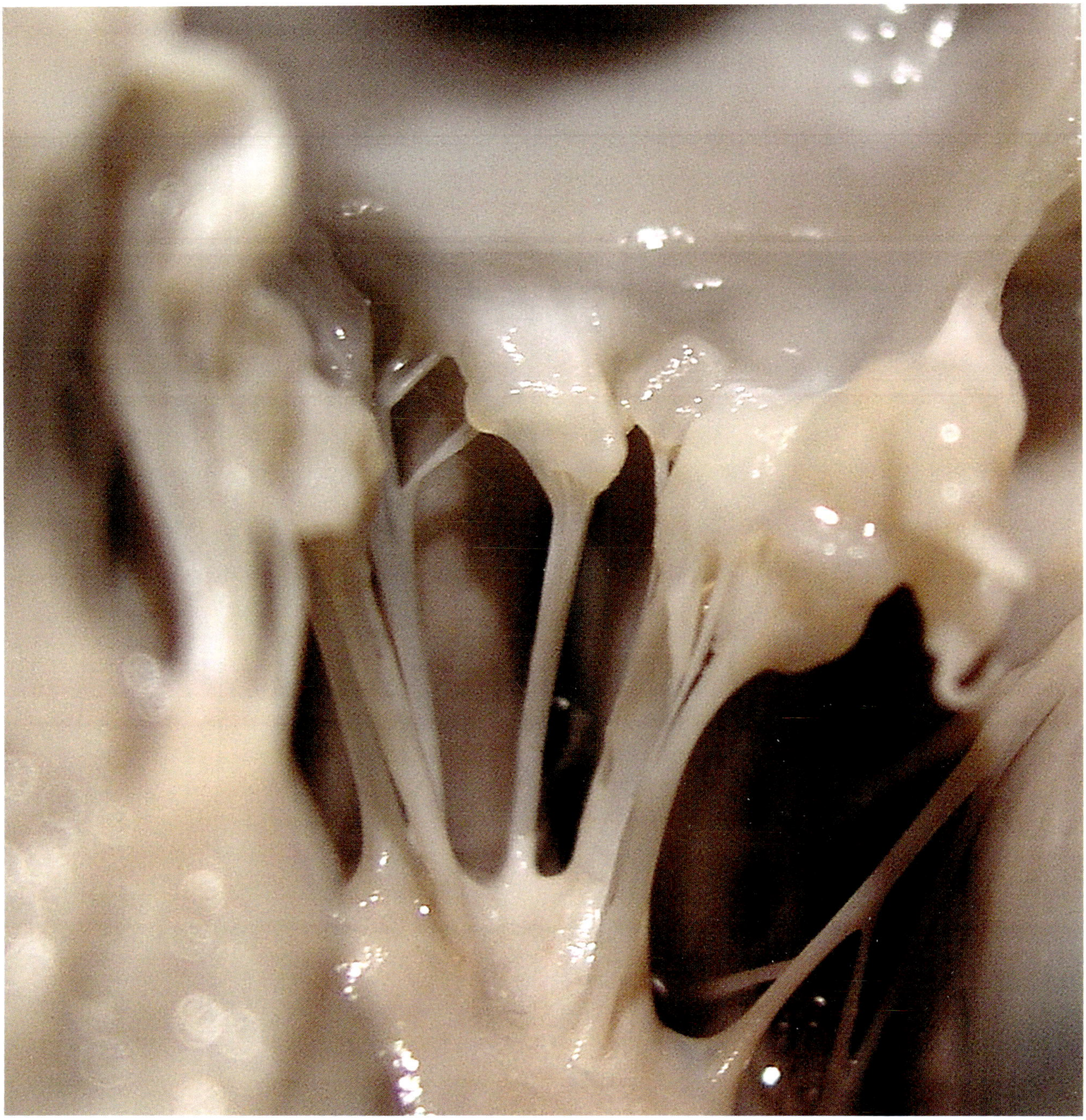

Figure 2. Mitral valve dysplasia. Nodular enlargement of the leaflets.

LEAFLETS

The shortening of the leaflets is one of the most frequent malformations; their thickening, both diffuse and localised, is also easily observed. In addition, notches or clefts may sometimes be found.

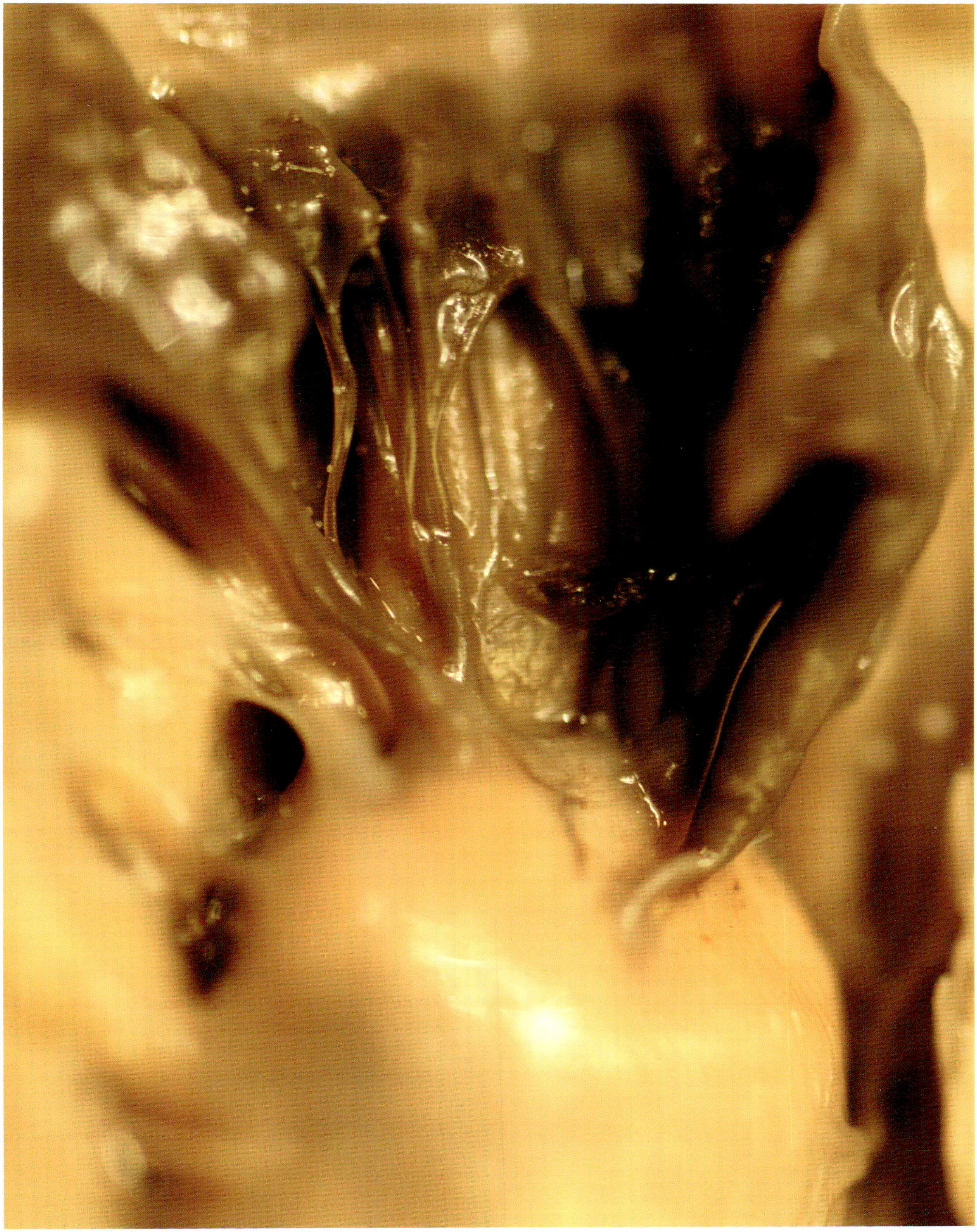

Figure 3. Mitral valve dysplasia. Shortening of the leaflets. A marked thickening of some of the chordae tendineae can also be observed.

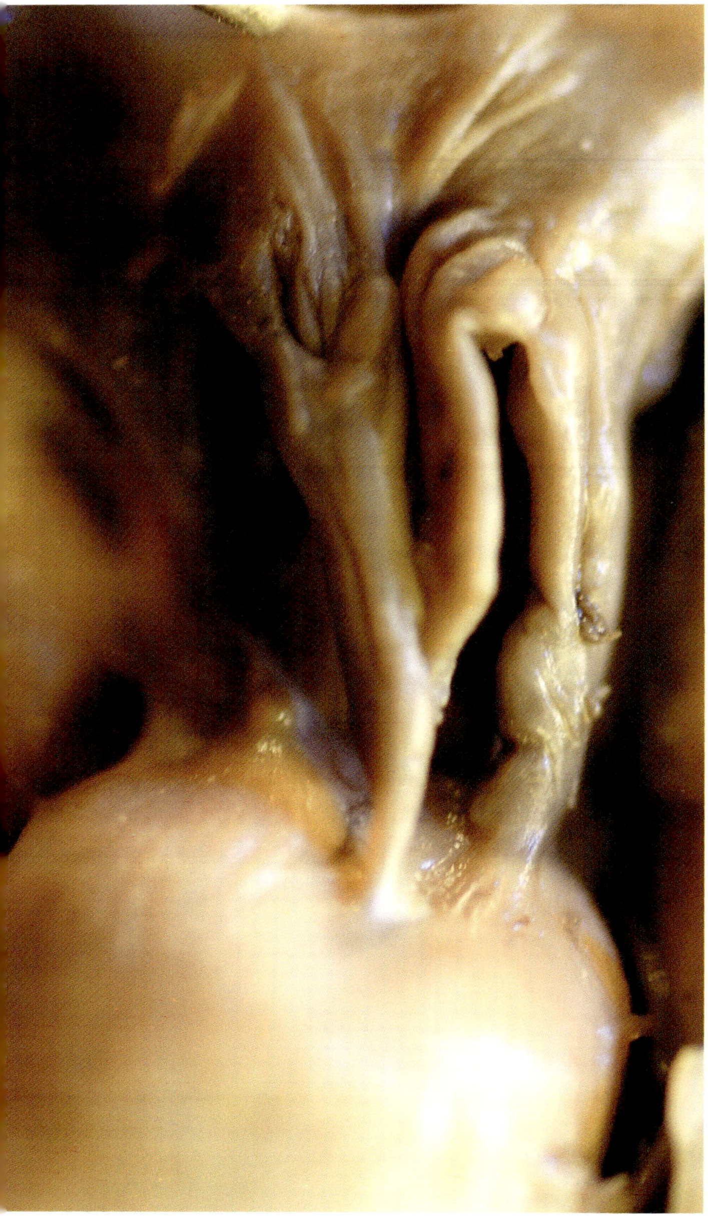

Figure 4. Mitral valve dysplasia. Thickening and shortening of the chordae tendineae.

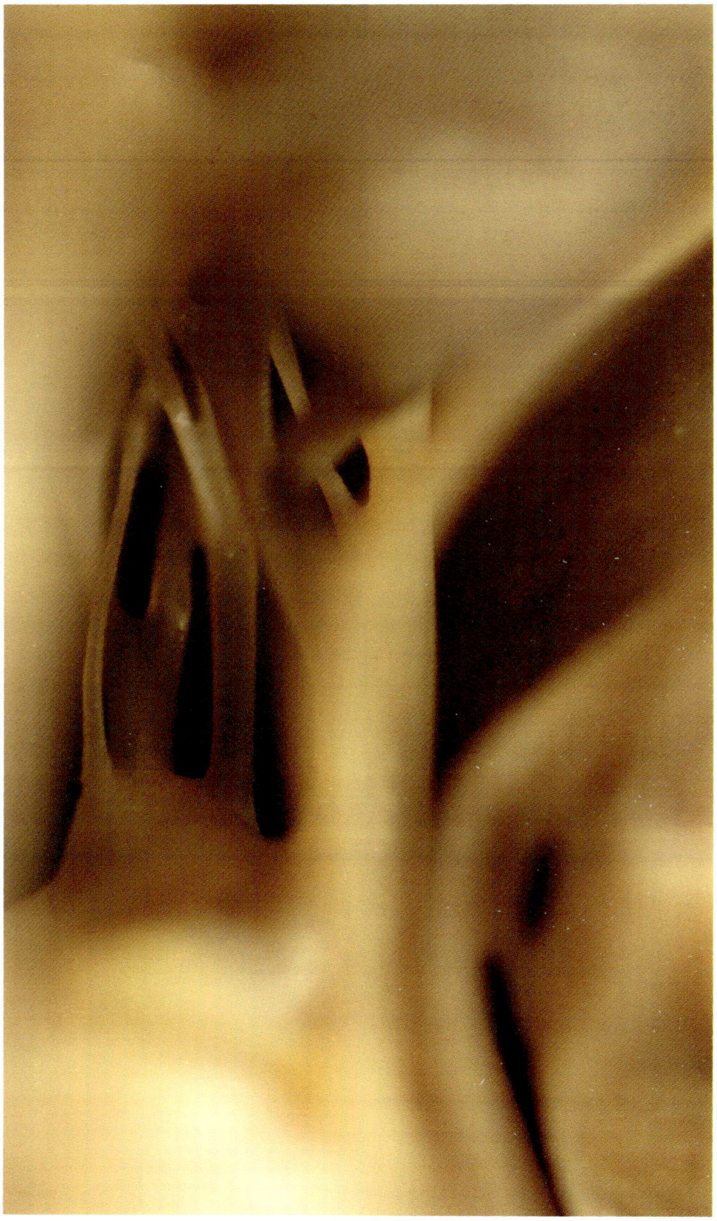

Figure 5. Mitral valve dysplasia. Thickening of the chordae tendineae.

CHORDAE TENDINEAE

The fusion of one or several chordae, their shortening or lengthening and their thickening may be observed. It is also sometimes possible to see the leaflet inserting directly into the papillary muscle.

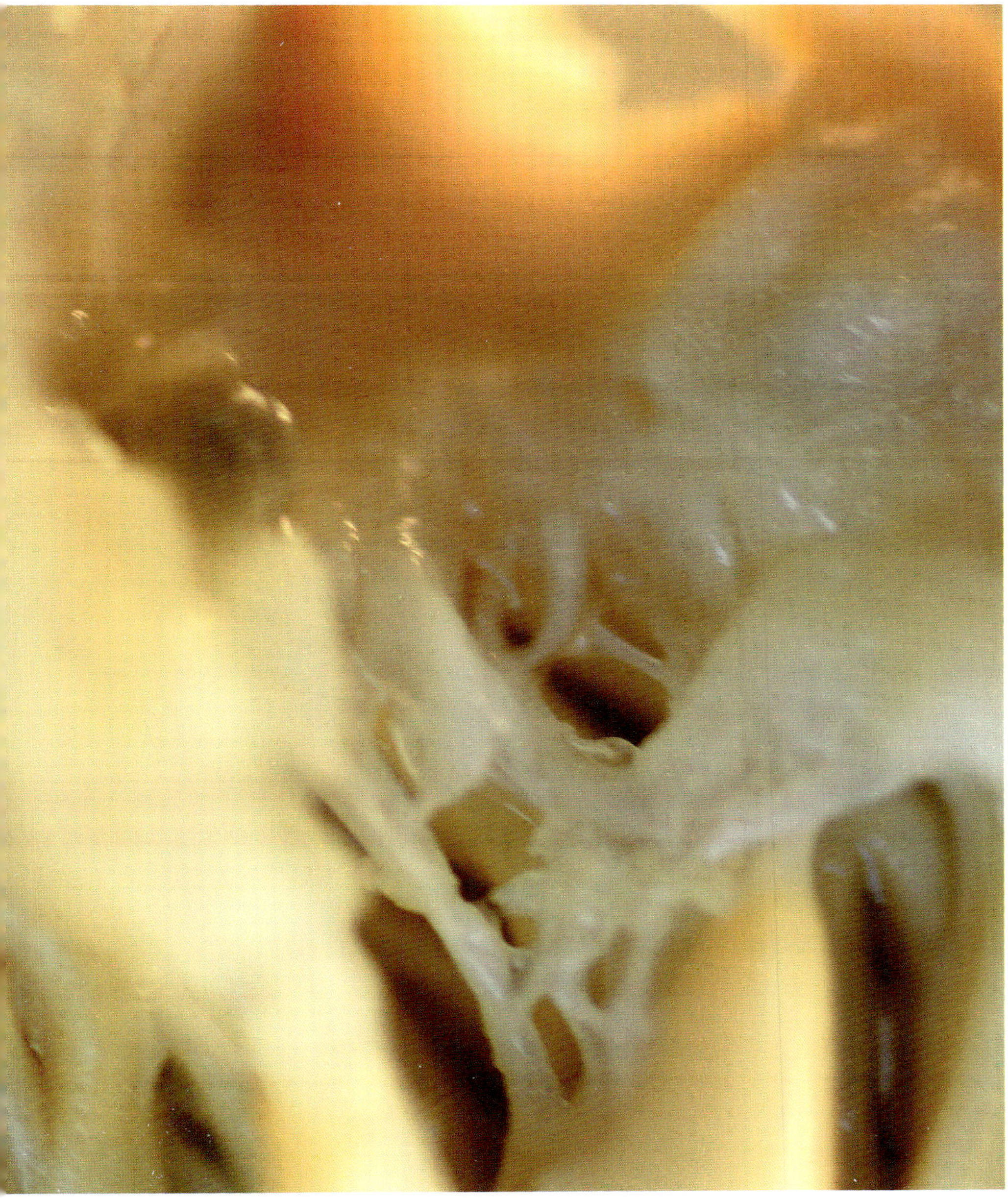

Figure 6. Mitral valve dysplasia. Shortening and fenestration of the leaflets, shortening and abnormal orientation of the chordae tendineae. Almost direct attachment of parts of the leaflet into the papillary muscles, which are displaced.

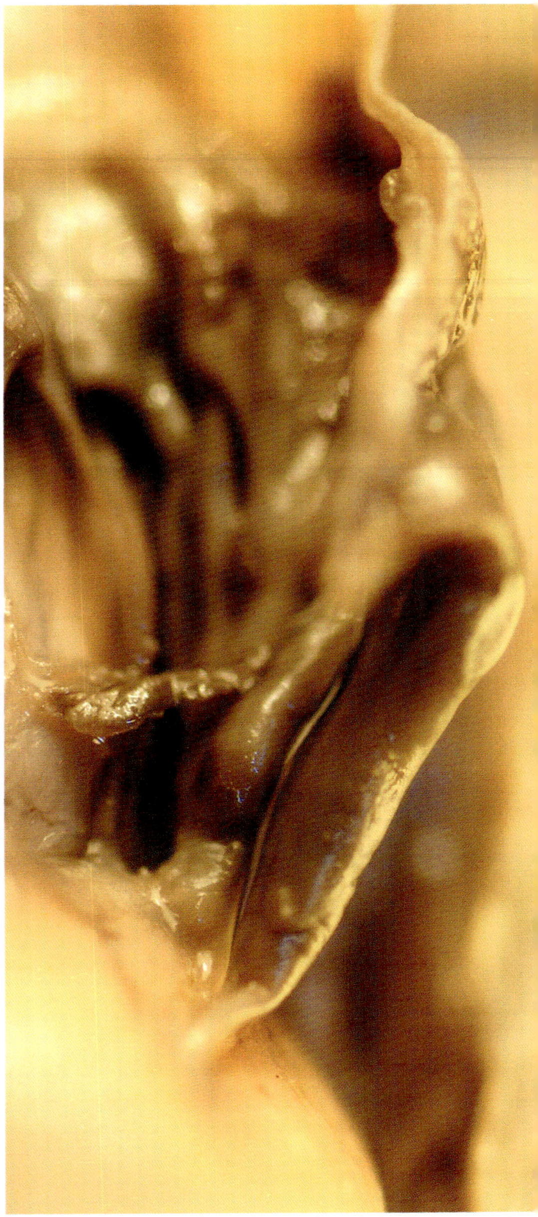

Figure 7. Mitral valve dysplasia. Thickened and fused chordae tendineae.

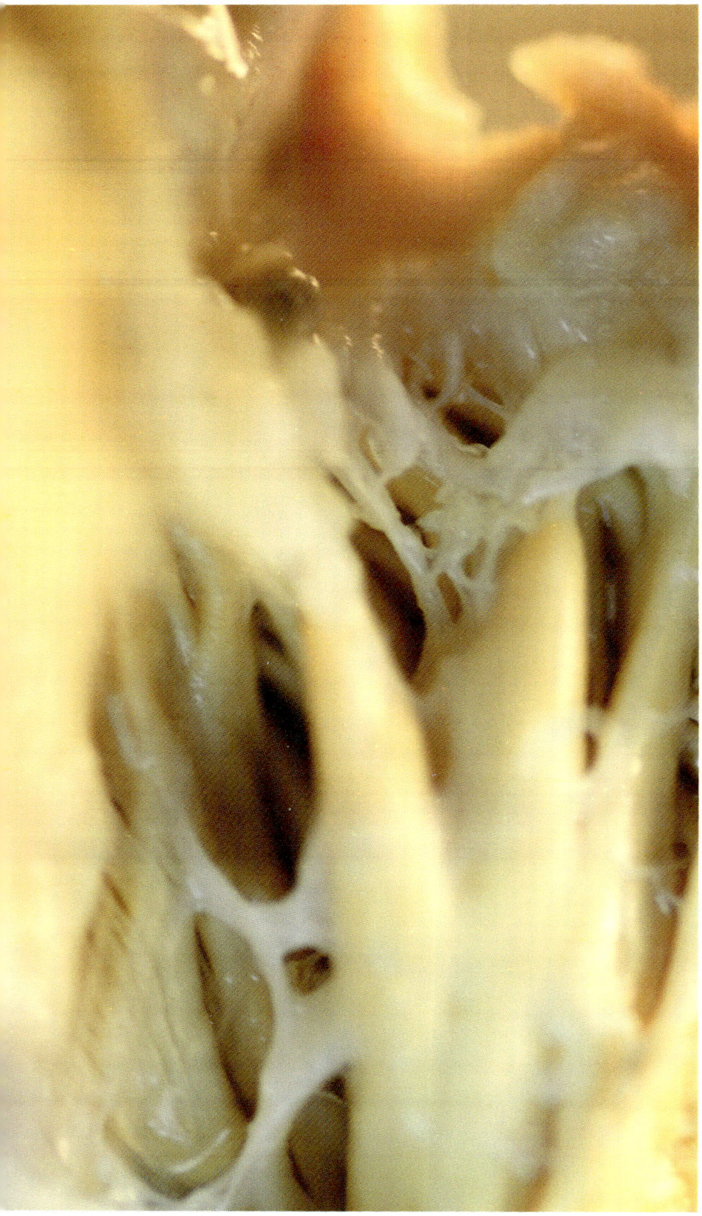

Figure 8. Abnormal papillary muscles with an abnormal position.

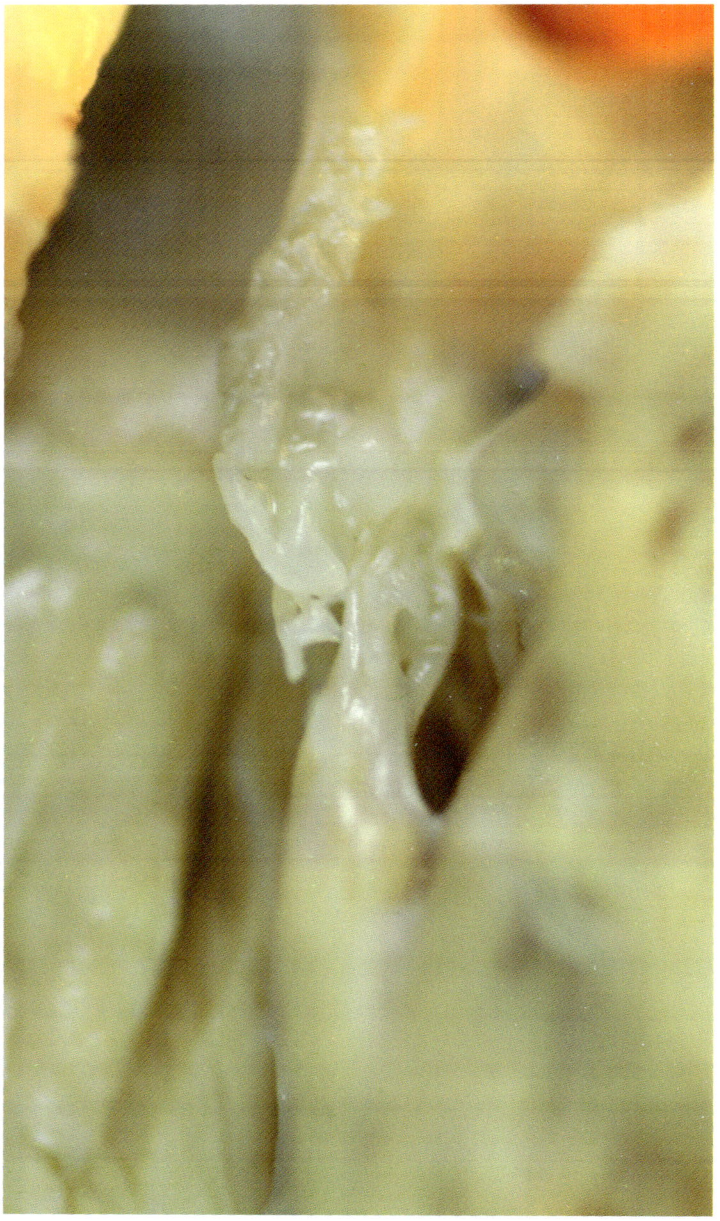

Figure 9. Atrophied papillary muscle and leaflet that inserts directly into it.

PAPILLARY MUSCLES

Malformations such as atrophy (thinner or smaller muscles), hypertrophy and an abnormal position leading to changes in the alignment of the chordae tendineae may be found.

Some breeds such as the Great Dane, Golden Retriever and German Shepherd seem to be more prone to suffer from this dysplasia.

[1 Annulus where only a small opening can be observed]

[2 Thickened leaflets]

[3 Since there are no papillary muscles, the leaflets insert, in some cases, either directly or through short and thick chordae tendineae, into the ventricular wall]

[4 In other cases the chordae tendineae, which are more or less normal, connect the leaflet with small papillae on the free wall of the ventricle]

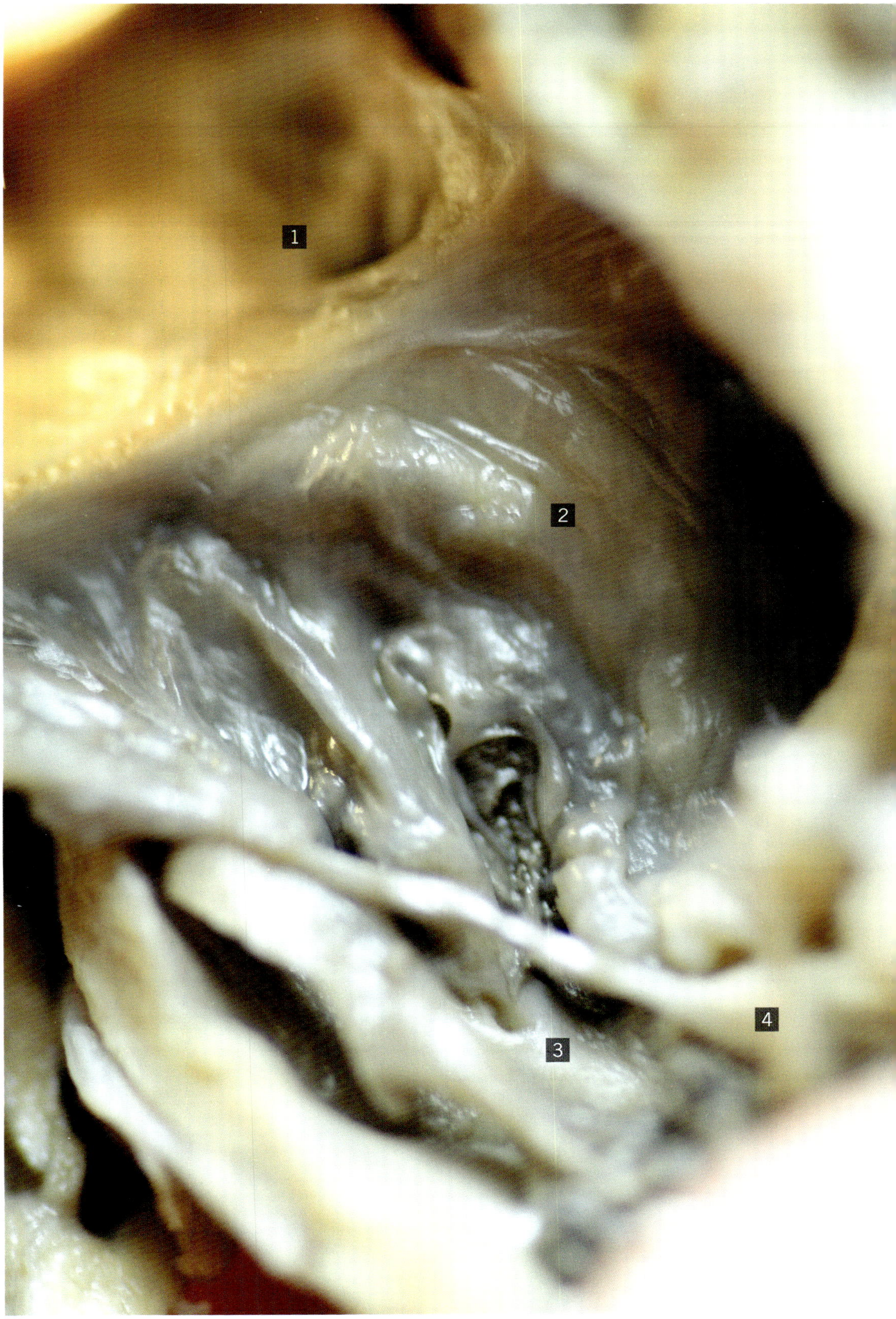

Figure 10. Mitral valve hypoplasia.

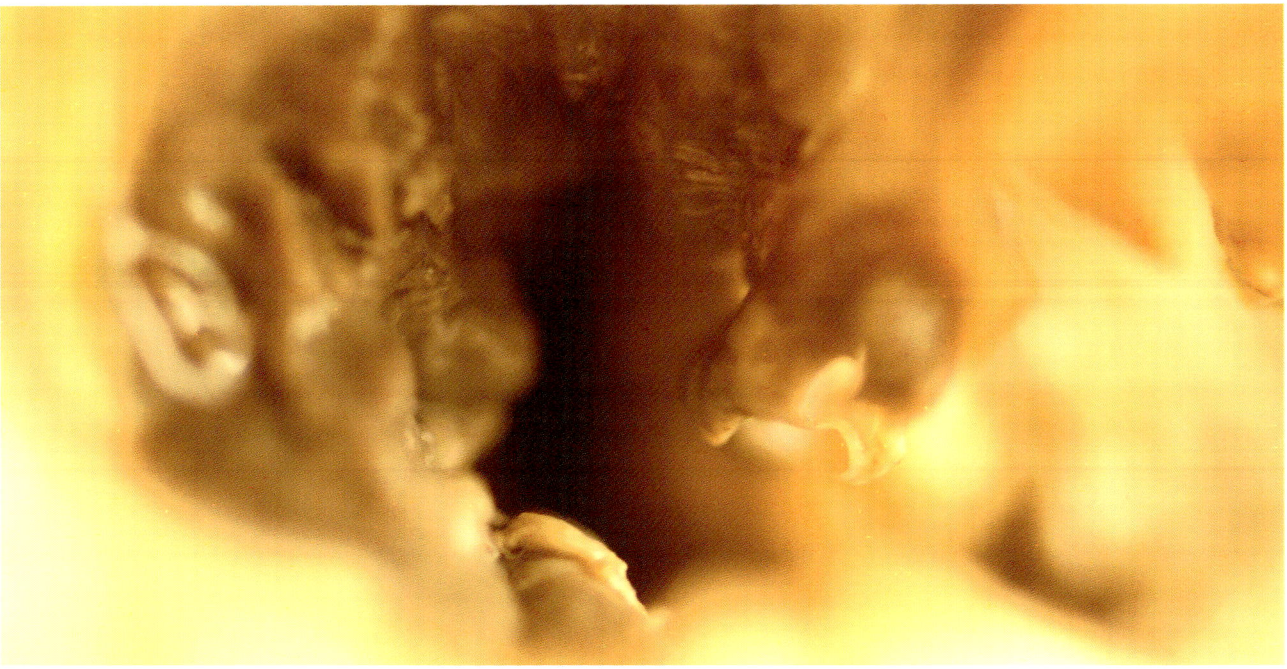

Figure 11. Tricuspid dysplasia. Reduced annulus.

TRICUSPID VALVE DYSPLASIA

The malformation of the tricuspid valve may be observed in both dogs and cats and, as occurs with mitral valve dysplasia, it may affect part of or the whole tricuspid valve apparatus.

ANNULUS

Although it is rare, in dogs it is sometimes possible to observe Ebstein's anomaly, in which the origin of the leaflets is displaced to the inside of the ventricle. The annulus may also be reduced in size. A dilation of the coronary sinus may be found as part of the dilation of the right atrium that will almost always be observed in this disease.

LEAFLETS

A great variety of alterations of the leaflets may be seen: focal or diffuse thickening, focal agenesis, muscular infiltration and fenestrations. The septal leaflet may be adhered to the ventricular septum. Fusion of the leaflets has also been described.

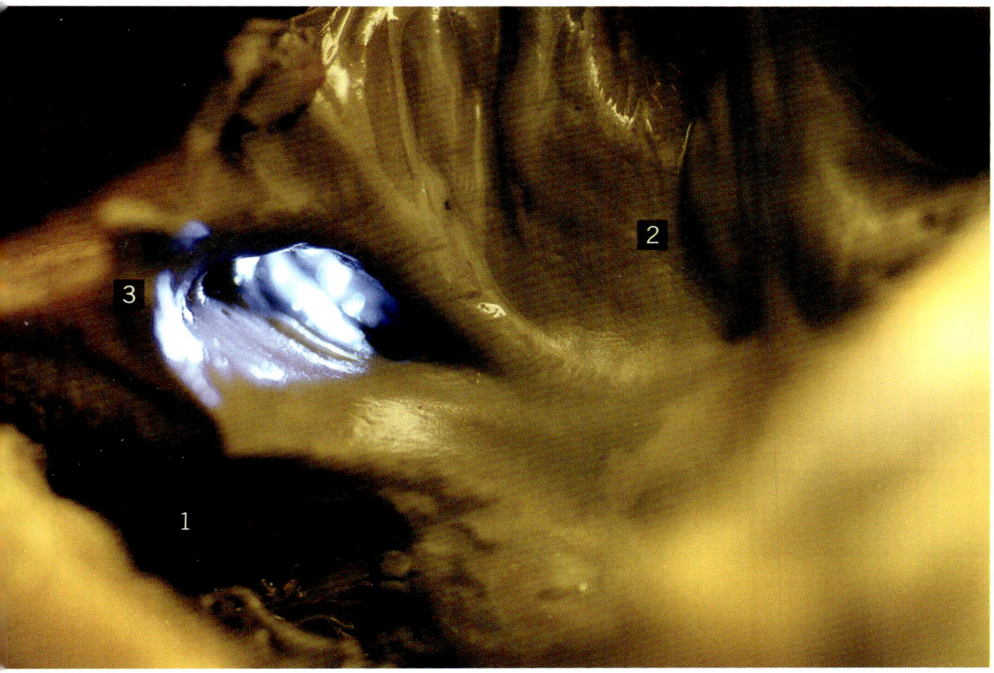

Figure 12. Tricuspid valve dysplasia.

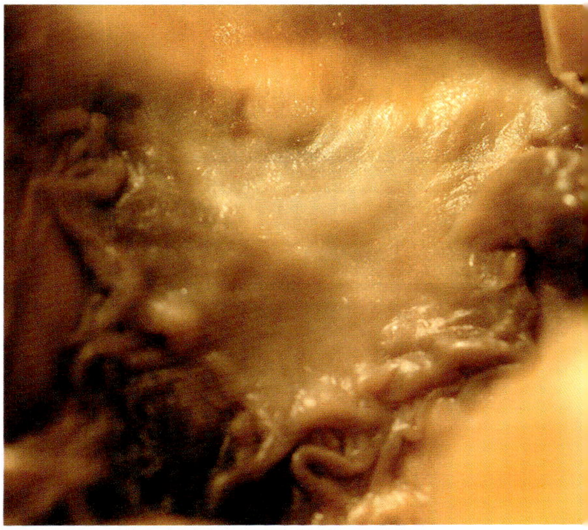

Figure 13. Tricuspid valve dysplasia. Thickened septal leaflet, which is adhered to the interventricular septum.

[1 Reduced tricuspid valve annulus] [2 Dilation of the right atrium] [3 Dilated coronary sinus]

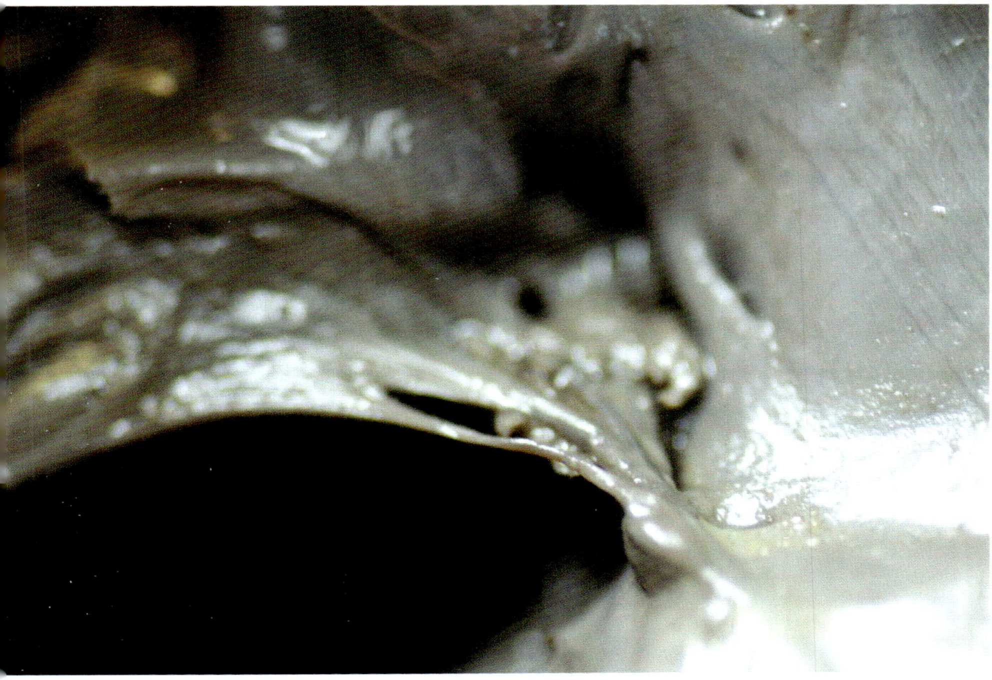

Figure 14. Tricuspid valve dysplasia. Papillary muscle of the conus. Thickening and fenestration of the mural leaflet.

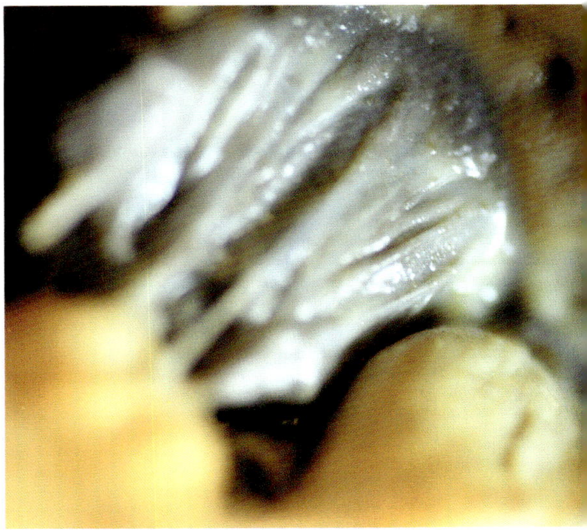

Figure 15. Tricuspid valve dysplasia. Thickened mural leaflet that is almost directly attached to the papillary muscles, which are hypertrophied.

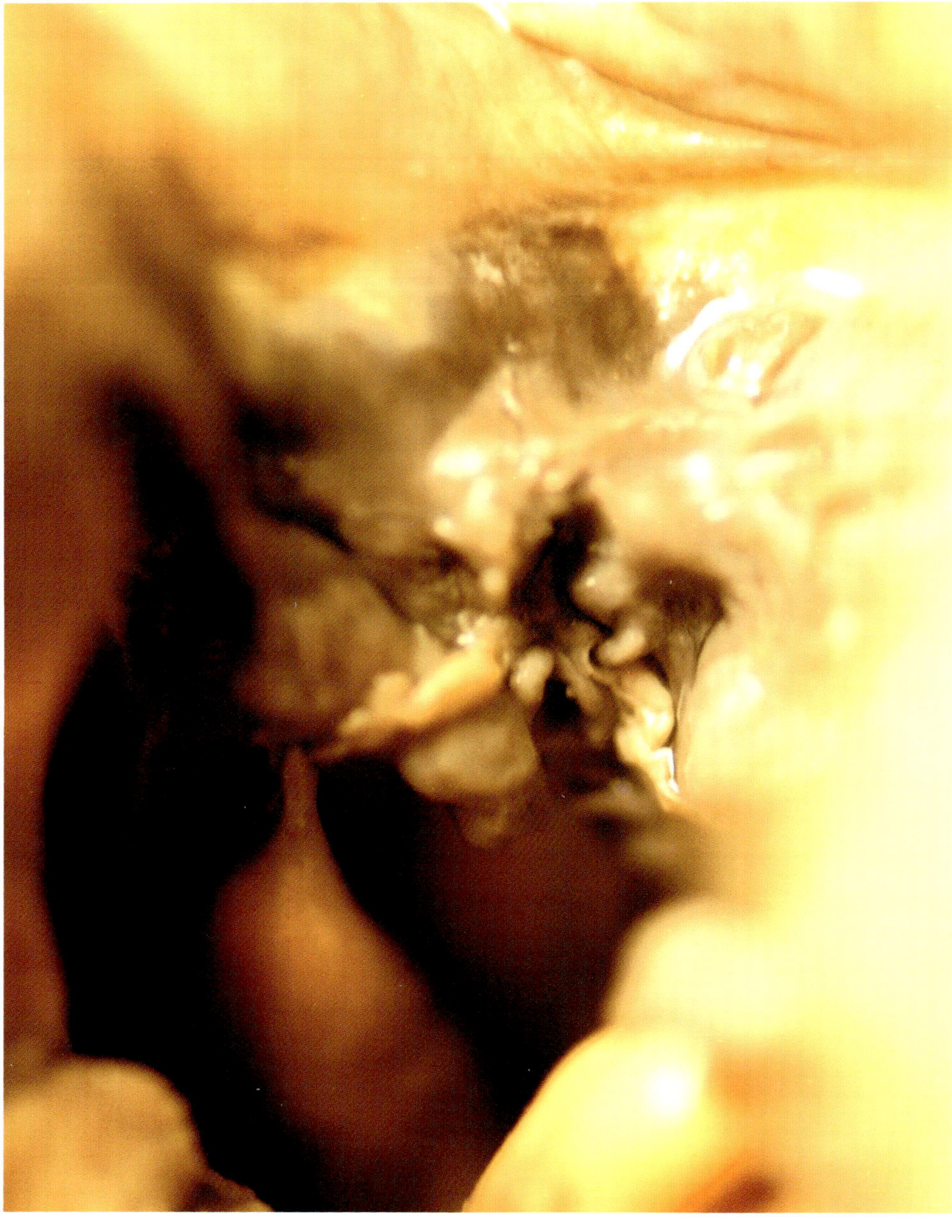

Figure 16. Tricuspid valve dysplasia. Thickening and focal agenesis of the leaflets. Absence of chordae tendineae.

CHORDAE TENDINEAE

They may be almost completely absent, thus leading to the leaflets inserting directly into the papillary muscles, or extremely short.

PAPILLARY MUSCLES

They may be hypertrophied, absent or fused.

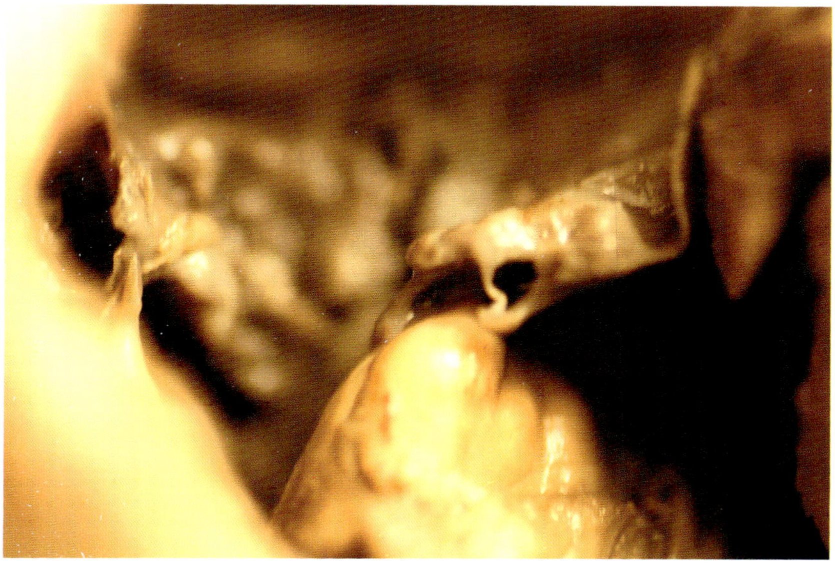

Figure 17. Tricuspid valve dysplasia. Hypertrophy of the papillary muscle.

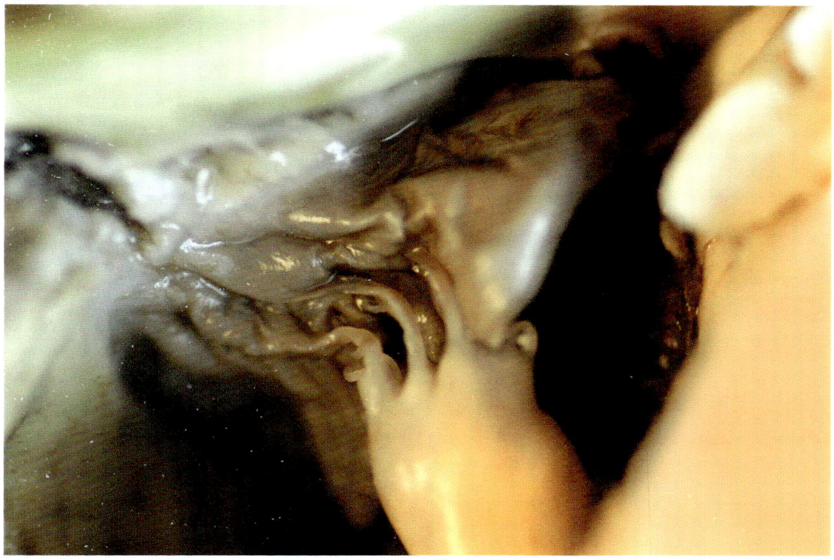

Figure 18. Tricuspid valve dysplasia. Hypertrophied papillary muscle, thickened and shortened chordae tendineae and thickened mural leaflet.

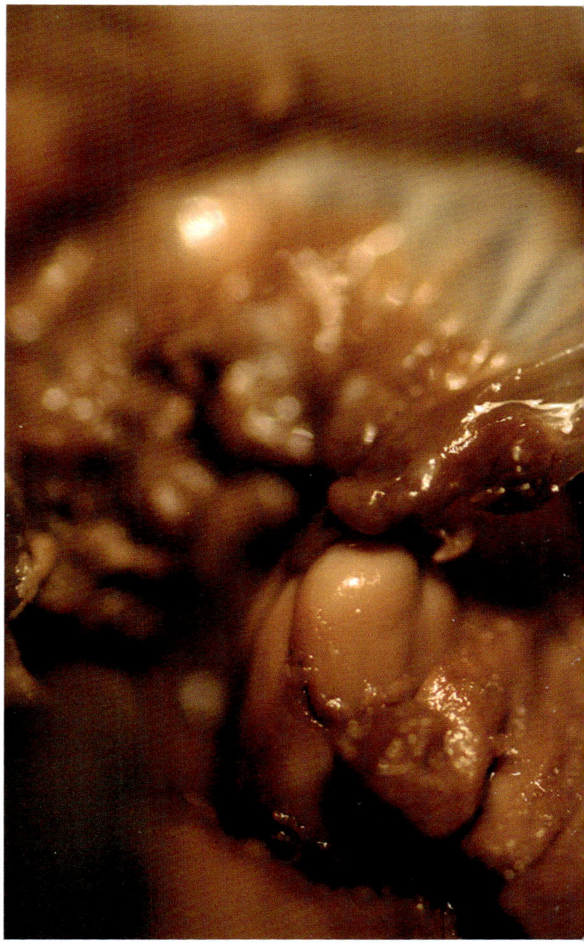

Figure 19. Tricuspid valve dysplasia. Hypertrophy and fusion of the papillary muscle. The leaflet is directly attached to the muscle.

German Shepherds, Great Danes, Bobtails and Weimaraners are among the most commonly affected breeds. In cats, as with mitral valve dysplasia, there is no breed predisposition and the disease frequently appears in crossbred cats.

Both mitral valve dysplasia and tricuspid valve dysplasia are not usually isolated defects and other congenital diseases such as dysplasia of the two atrioventricular valves, septal defects, subaortic stenosis and pulmonary stenosis are often observed.

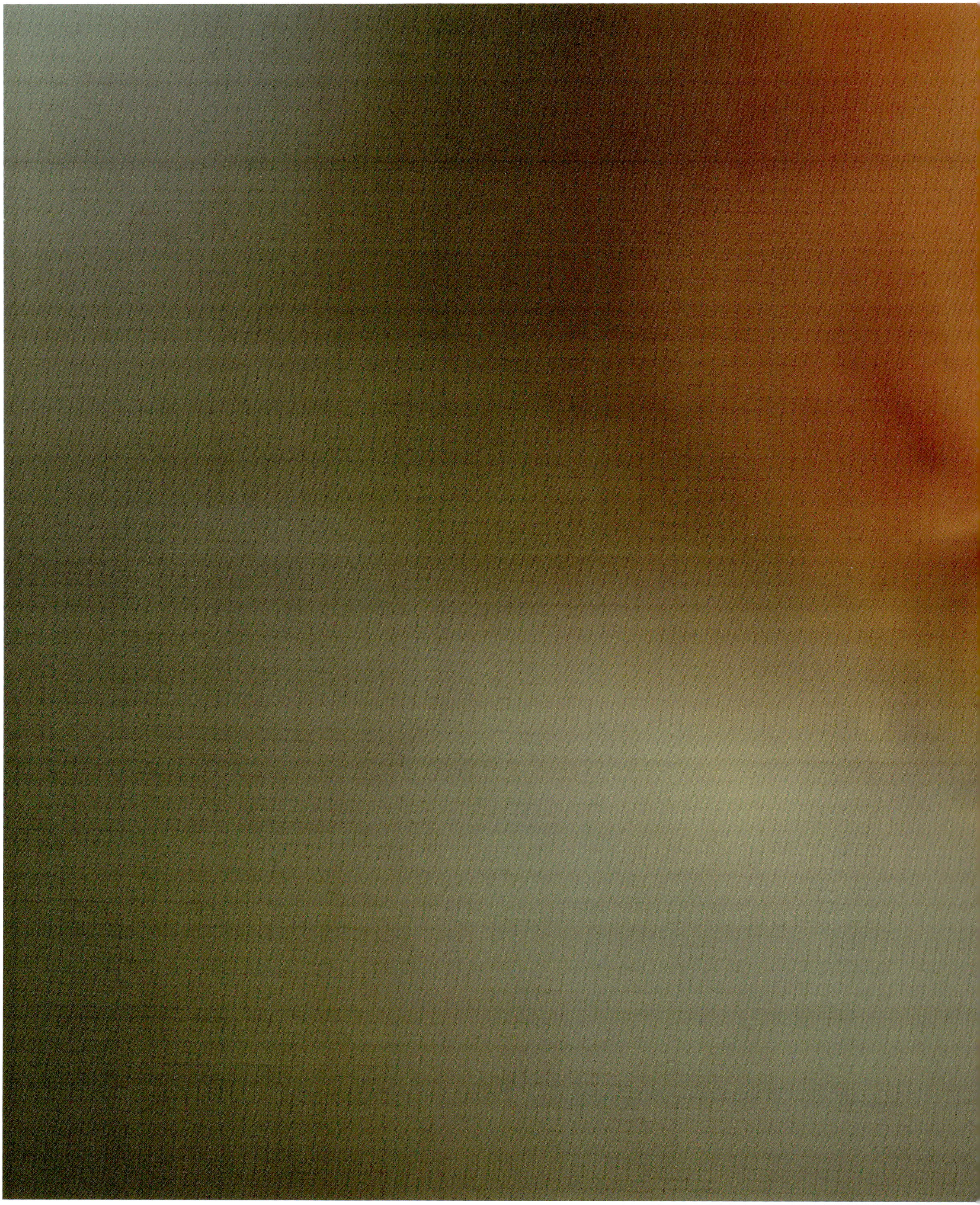

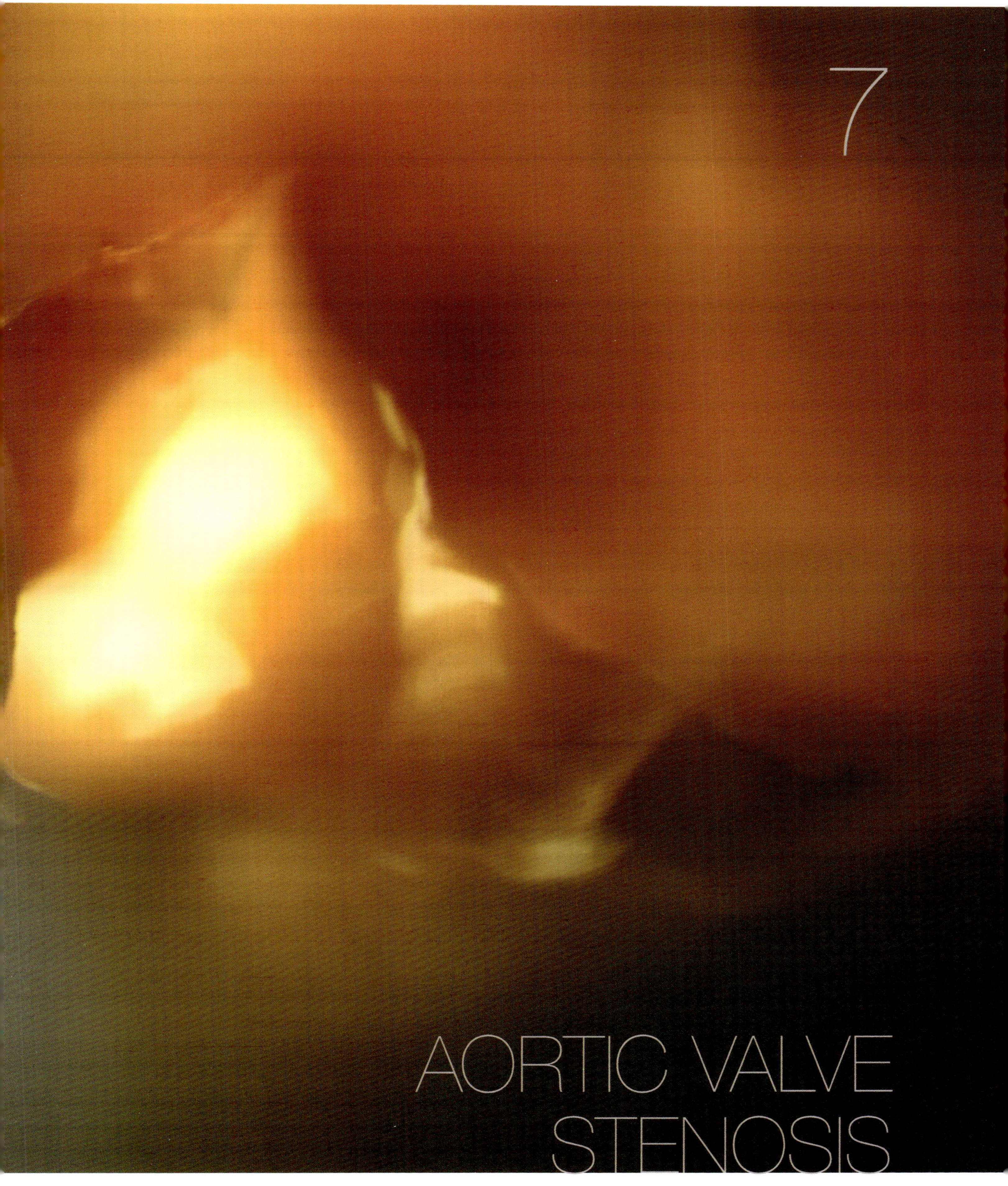

7

AORTIC VALVE STENOSIS

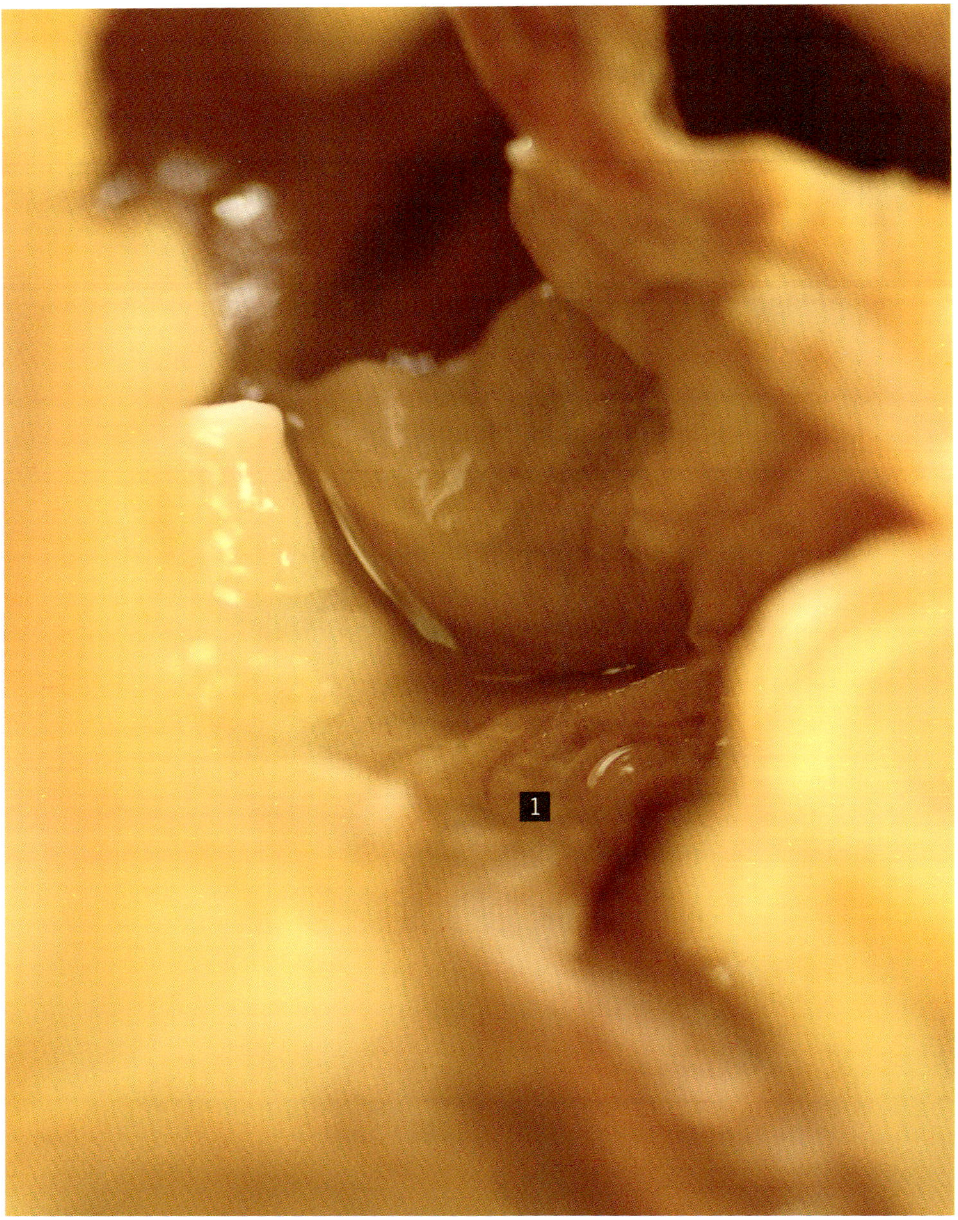

Figure 1. Small lesions located just below the valve cusp (1).

Aortic valve stenosis is one of the most common congenital heart diseases in dogs, with an incidence between 22 % and 34 % of the total of these diseases.

The predisposition of certain breeds (Terranova, Boxer) and families to suffer from this disease reveals a genetic component with dominant transmission and variable expression.

Of the three types of fixed lesions, the subvalvular type is the one that has most commonly been described, while the supravalvular type is extremely rare and the valvular type, with a thickening of the cusps and/or their fusion, is also very uncommon.

[1 Valve cusps]

[2 Small nodular lesions just below the cusps]

[3 Small endocardial ridges]

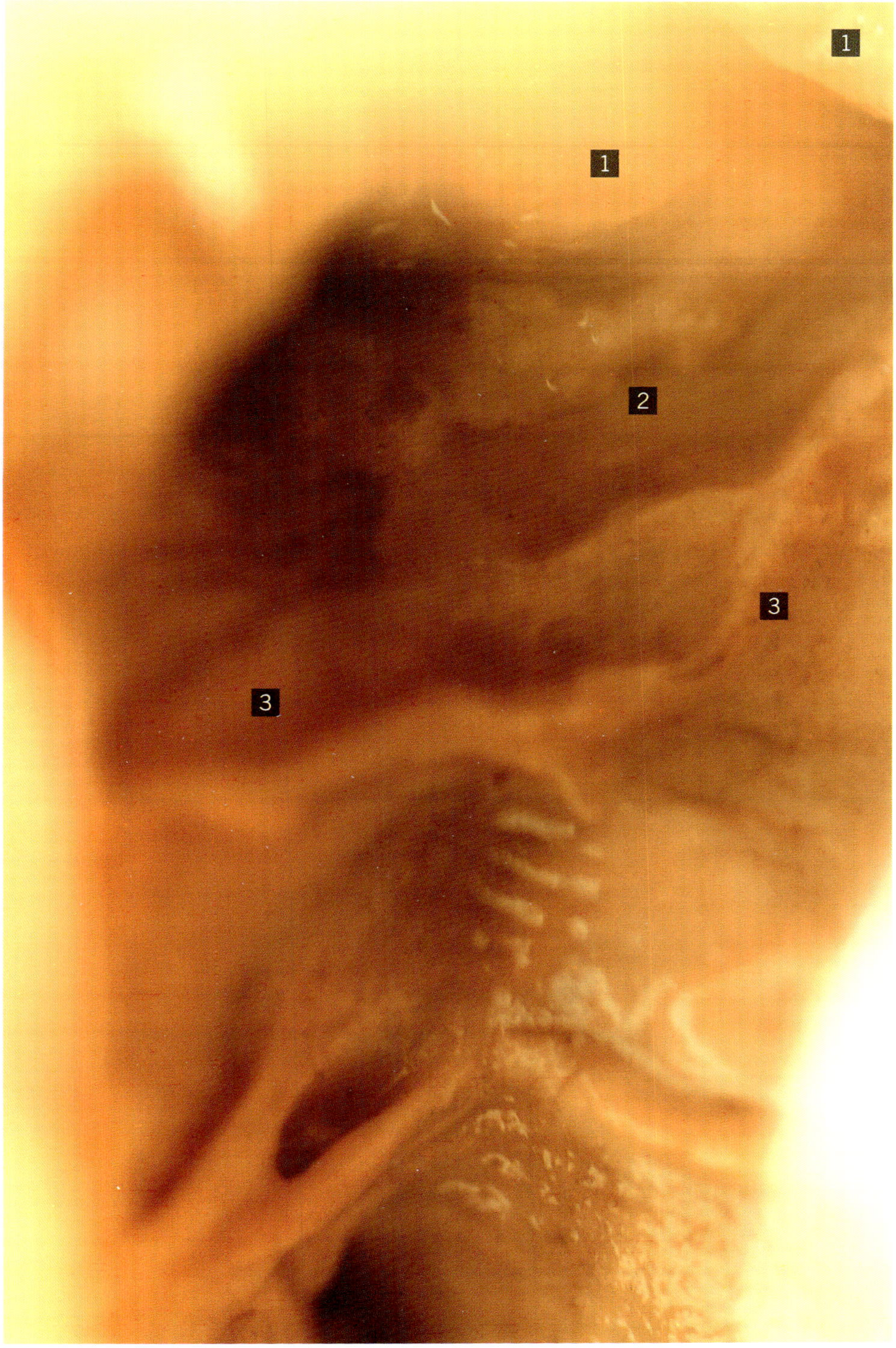

Figure 2. Lesions along the outflow tract.

Subvalvular lesions (subaortic stenosis) may be present at birth or develop during the postnatal period, in the first 3-8 weeks of life. In some cases, they may evolve and worsen until adulthood.

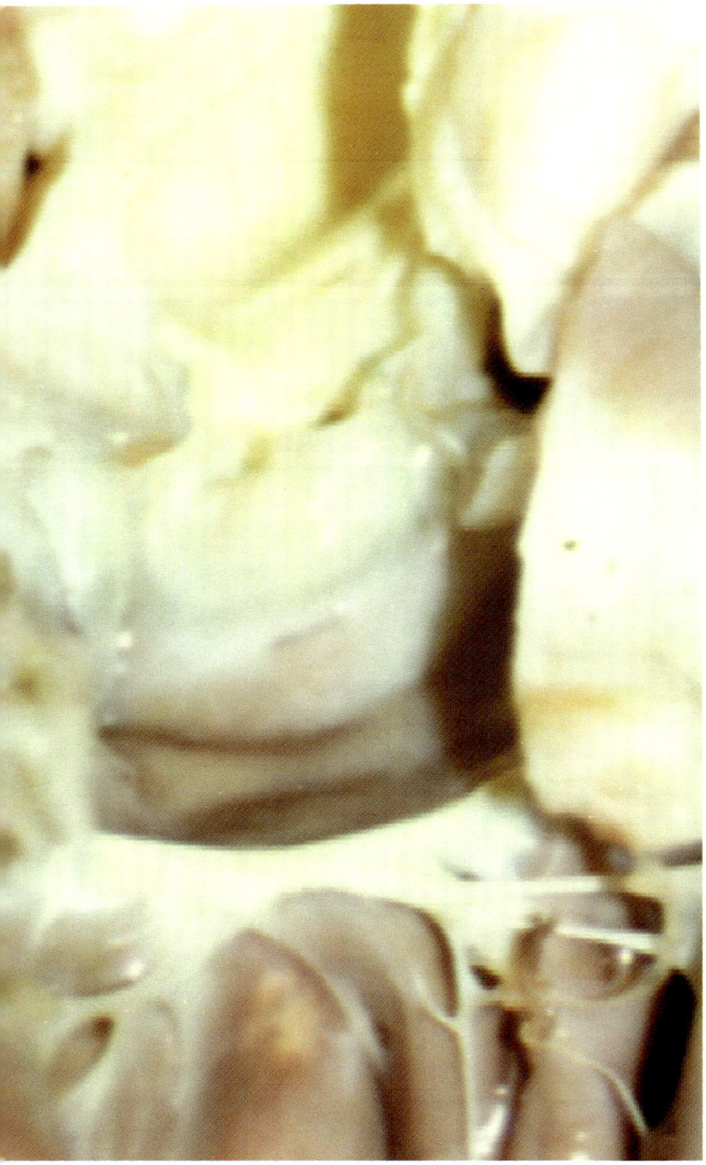

Figure 3. Fibrous ring located at the beginning of the outflow tract of the left ventricle. It goes from the left coronary cusp to the cranial leaflet of the mitral valve.

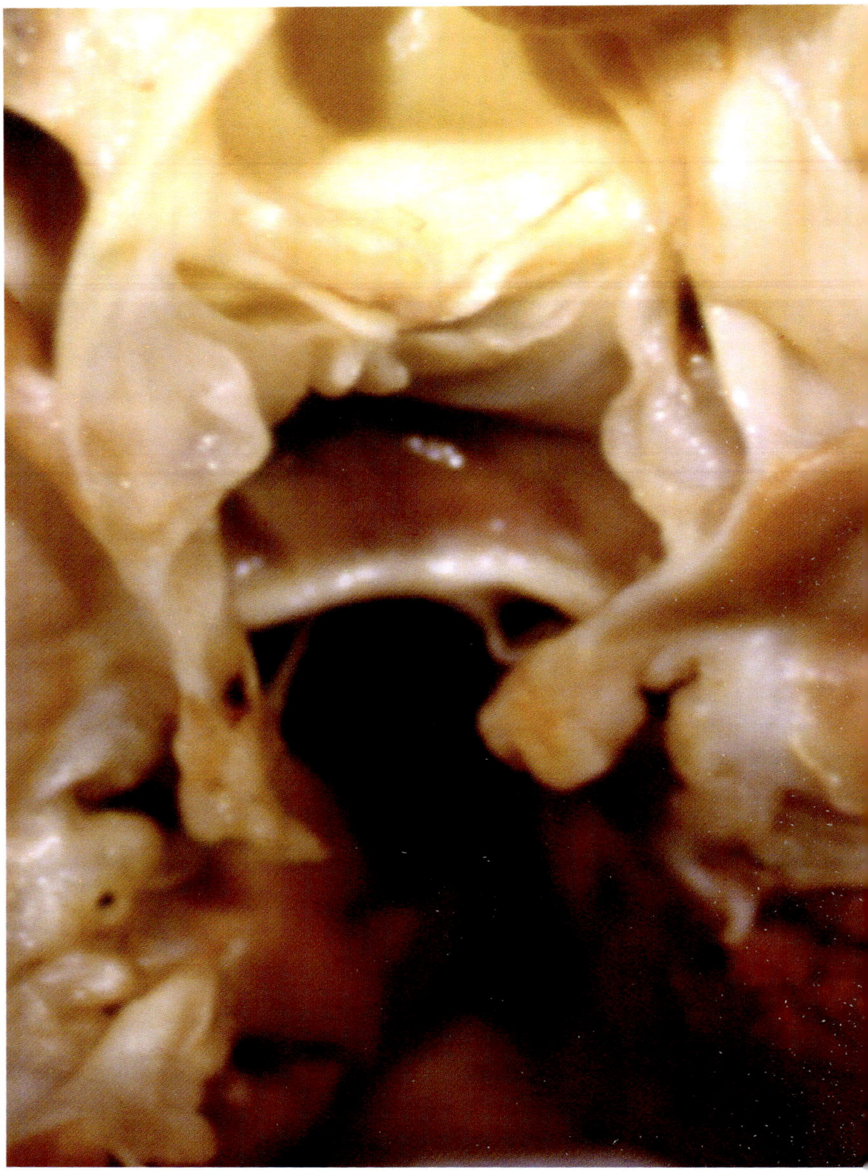

Figure 4. Important fibromuscular ring that nearly occupies the whole outflow tract of the left ventricle.

The outflow tract of the left ventricle originates from the embryonic development of the conotruncal septum, ventricular septum and cranial leaflet of the mitral valve; any alteration in the development of these structures may lead to subaortic stenosis. The most common type is probably due to a failure in the development of the region from the conus to the aortic trunk; the fibrous ring may be derived from persistent embryonic endocardial tissue that maintains its proliferative capacity and chondrogenic potential after birth.

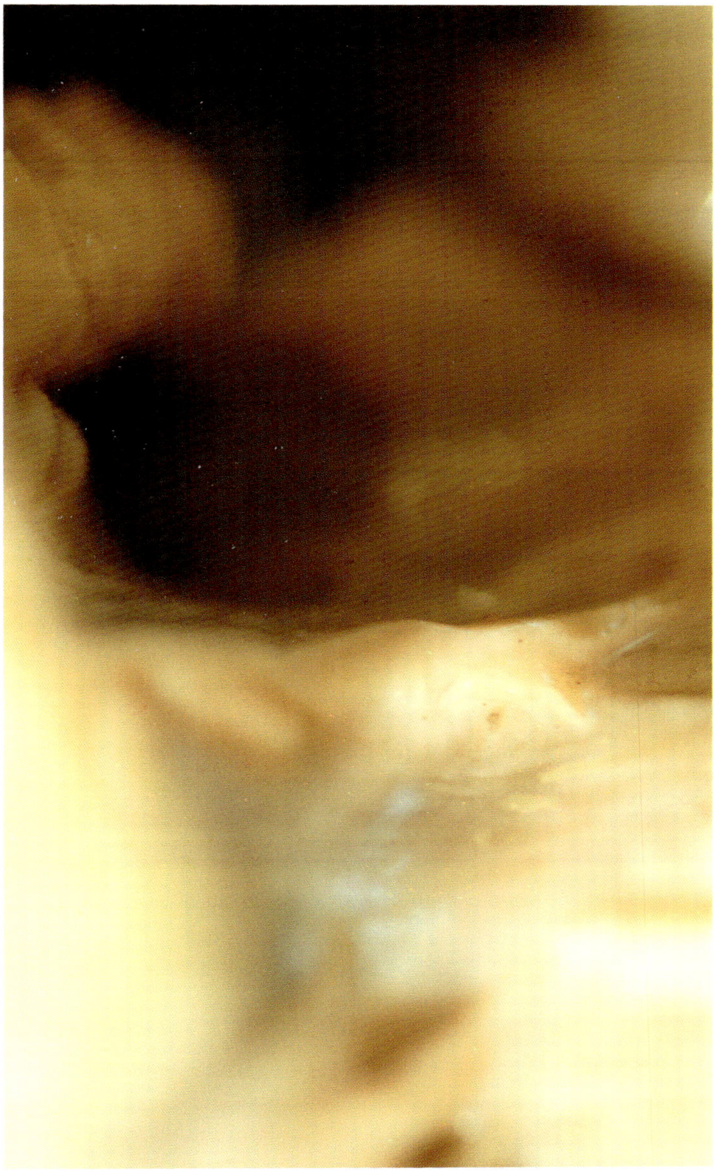

Figure 5. Small endocardial ridge located in the septum. The valve cusps can be seen at the back.

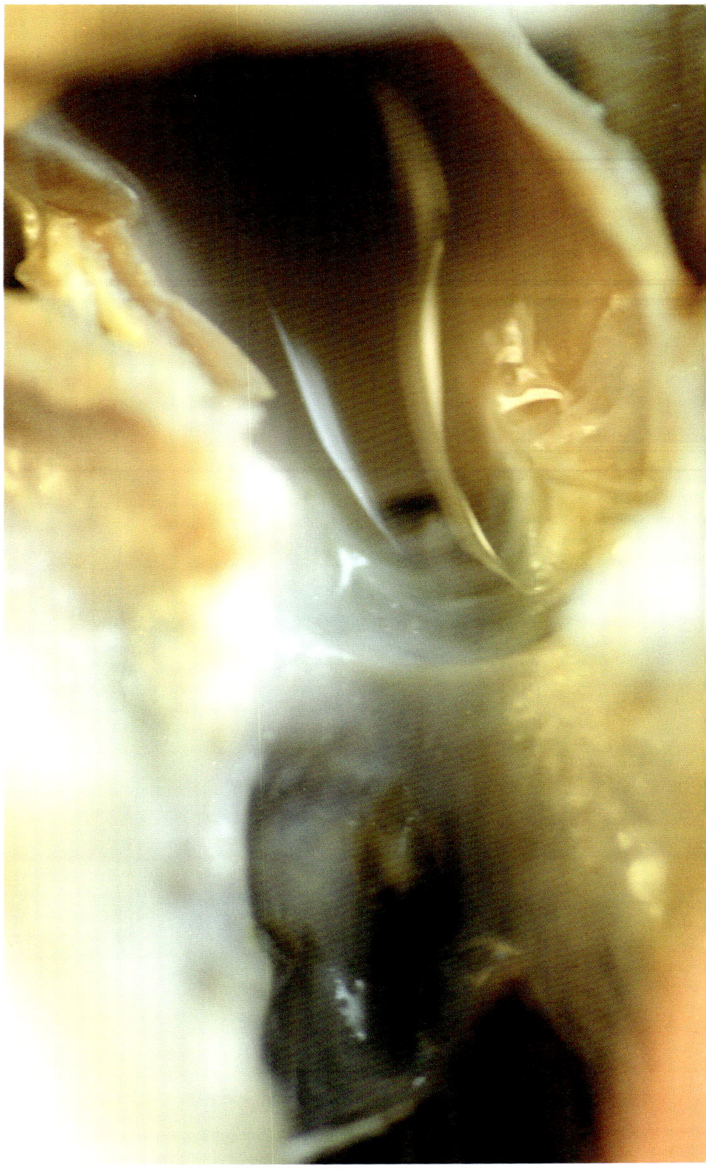

Figure 6. Complete and wide fibrous ring, which encircles almost the whole outflow tract of the left ventricle.

Subvalvular lesions have been classified into three types:

- Type I consists in small nodular lesions on the endocardial surface of the interventricular septum, just below the valve.
- Type II consists in a narrow and whitish band on the endocardium, which extends to the outflow tract of the left ventricle. Its location is variable, although it usually affects the area from the cranial leaflet of the mitral valve to the left coronary cusp of the aorta.
- Type III is the most severe type of subvalvular stenosis. It consists in a complete fibromuscular ring, which completely surrounds the outflow tract of the left ventricle.

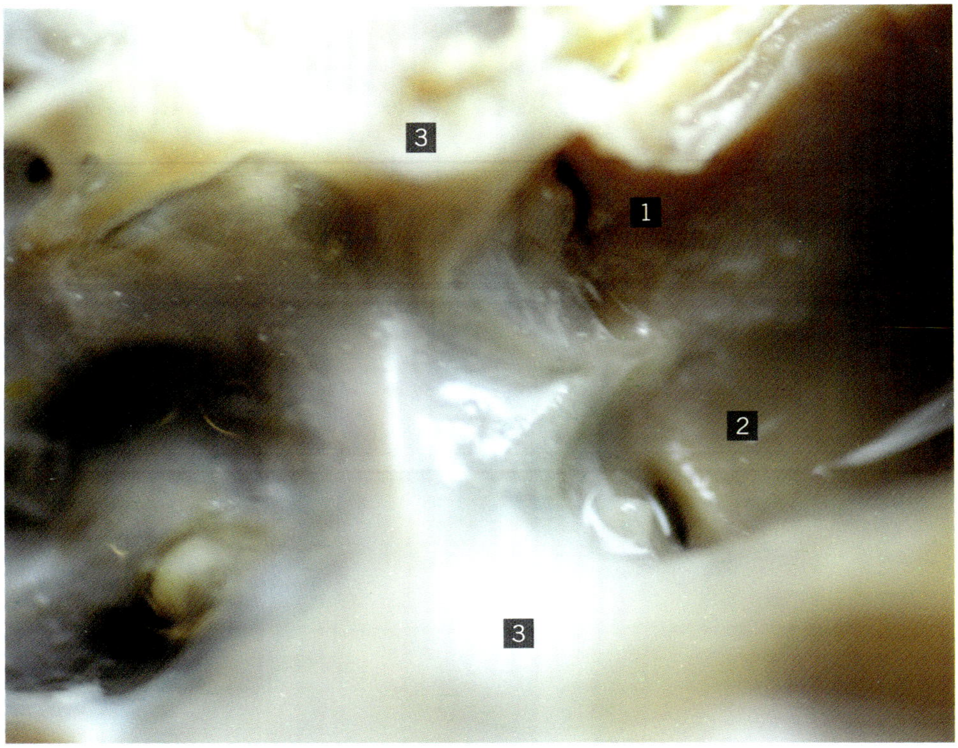

[1 Left coronary cusp]

[2 Right coronary cusp]

[3 Ring that extends to the cranial leaflet of the mitral valve]

Figure 7.

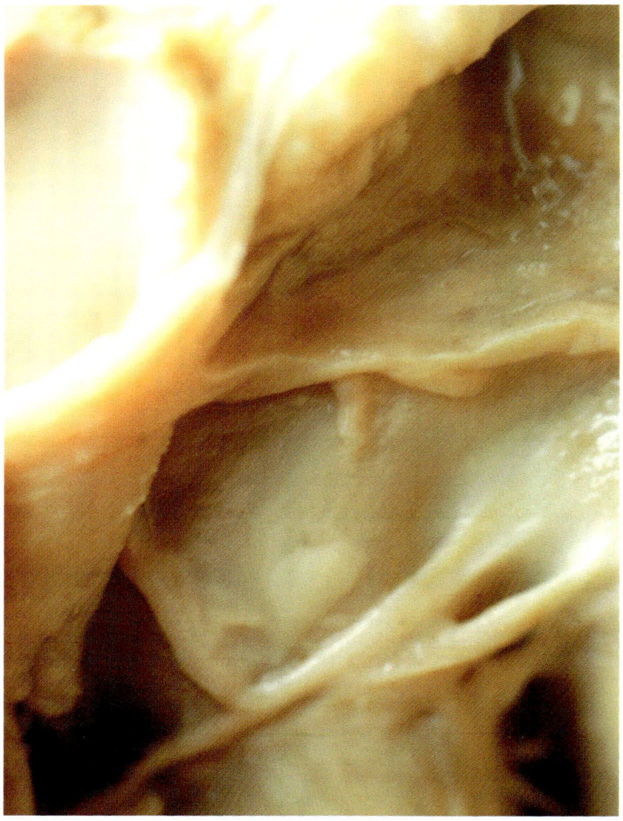

Figure 8. Ring extending to the cranial leaflet of the mitral valve.

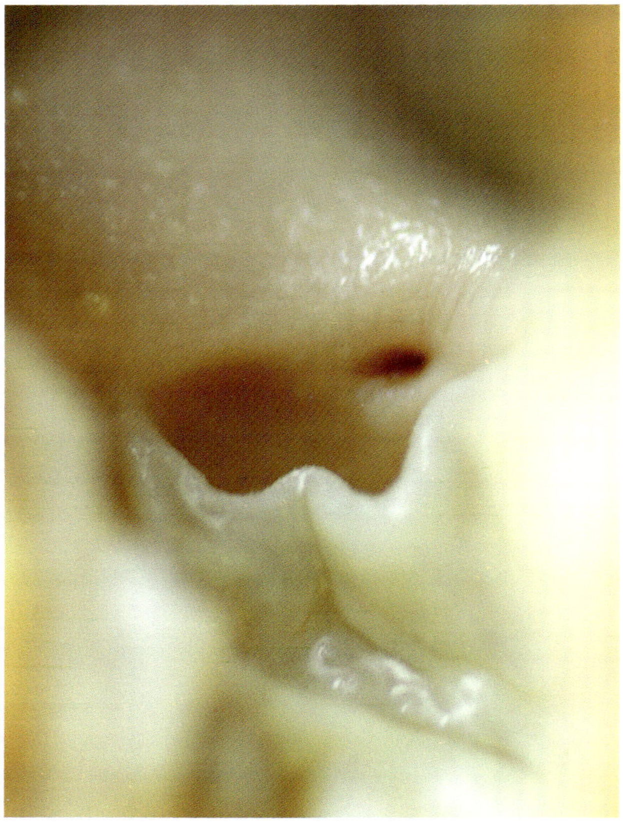

Figure 9. Thickening of the left coronary cusp; the fibrous ring may be observed below.

Figure 10. Large nodular lesions, which obstruct almost the whole outflow tract.

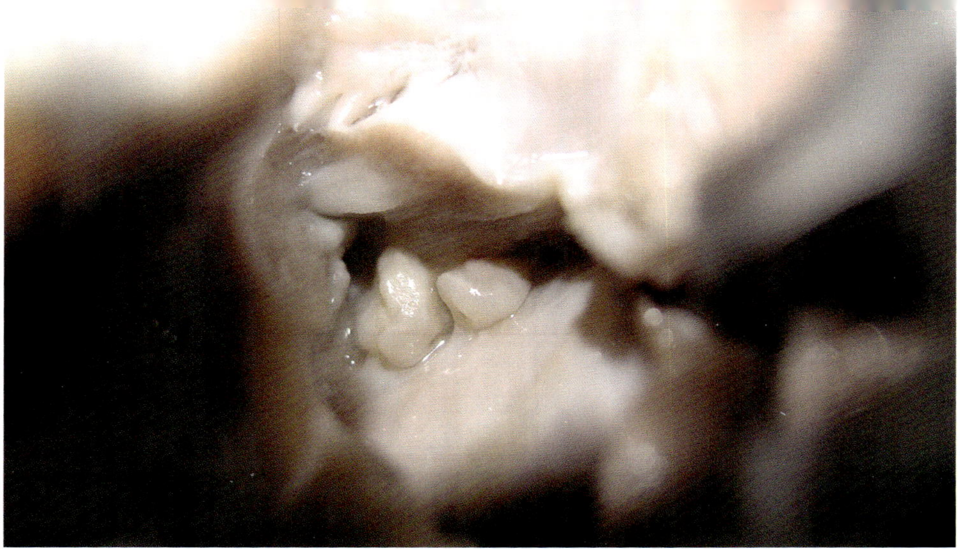

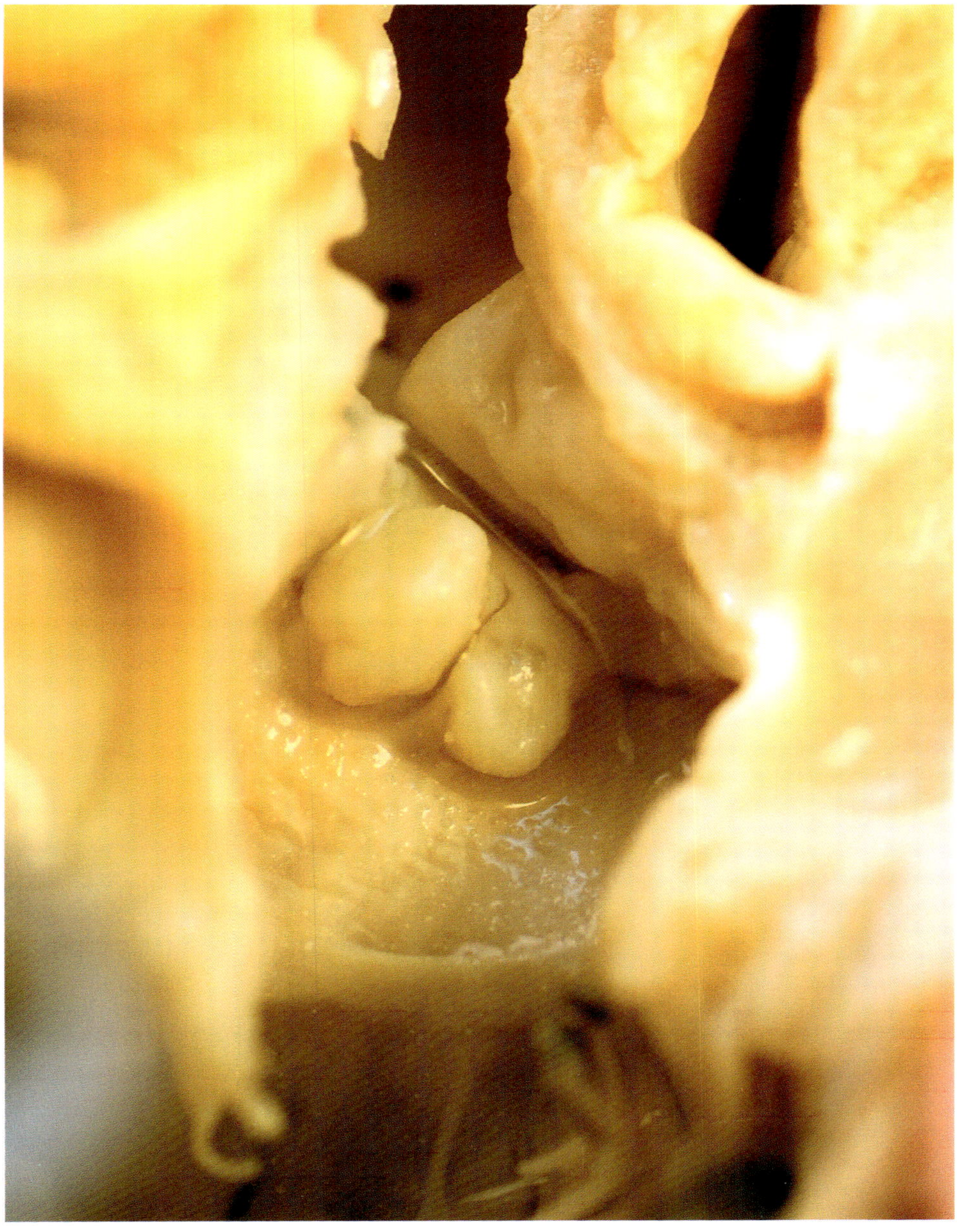

Figure 11. Sagittal section of the outflow tract and aorta of the same case as in the previous image. In addition to the nodular lesions, the presence of a fibrous ring in a more distal position may be observed.

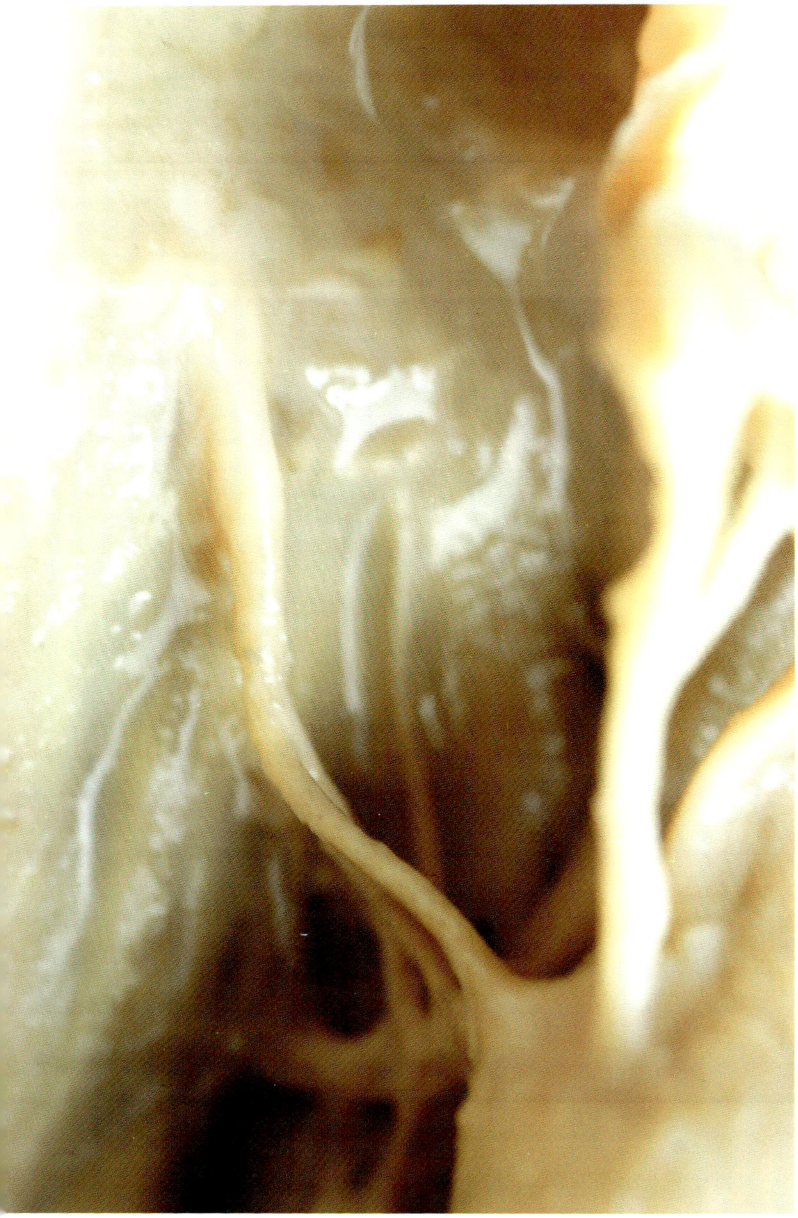

Figure 12. It is often possible to observe the presence of chordae tendineae running from the papillary muscles to the subvalvular lesions.

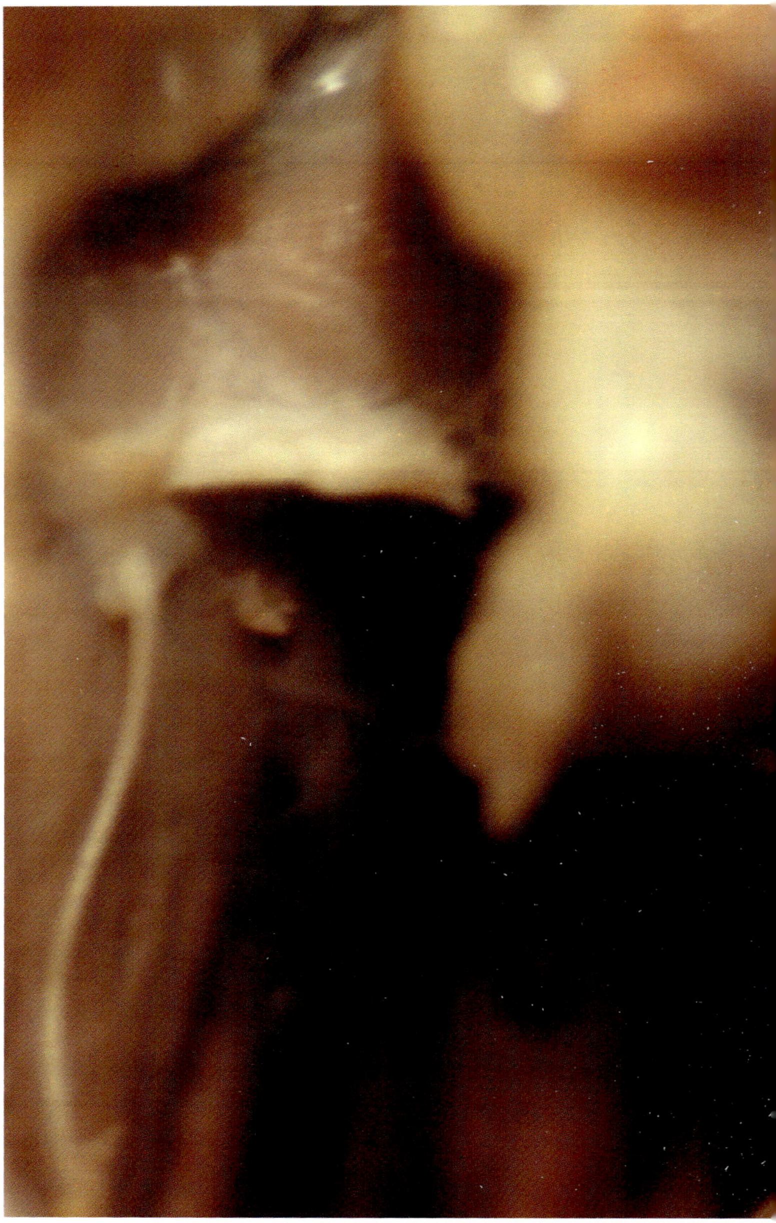

Figure 13. Chorda tendinea.

It is often possible to observe the presence of chordae tendineae running from the papillary muscles to the area of the subvalvular ring.

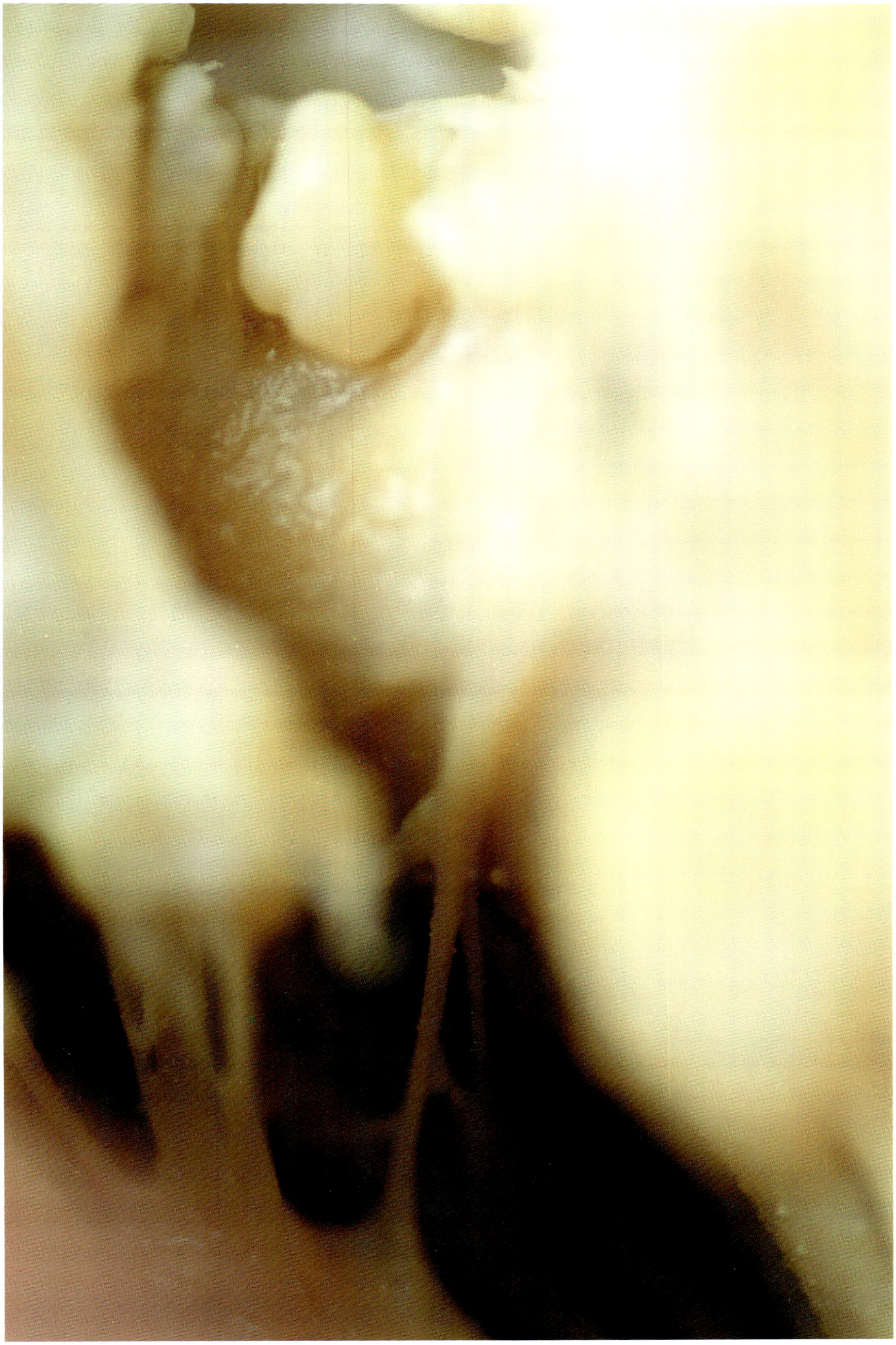

Figure 14. Chorda tendinea.

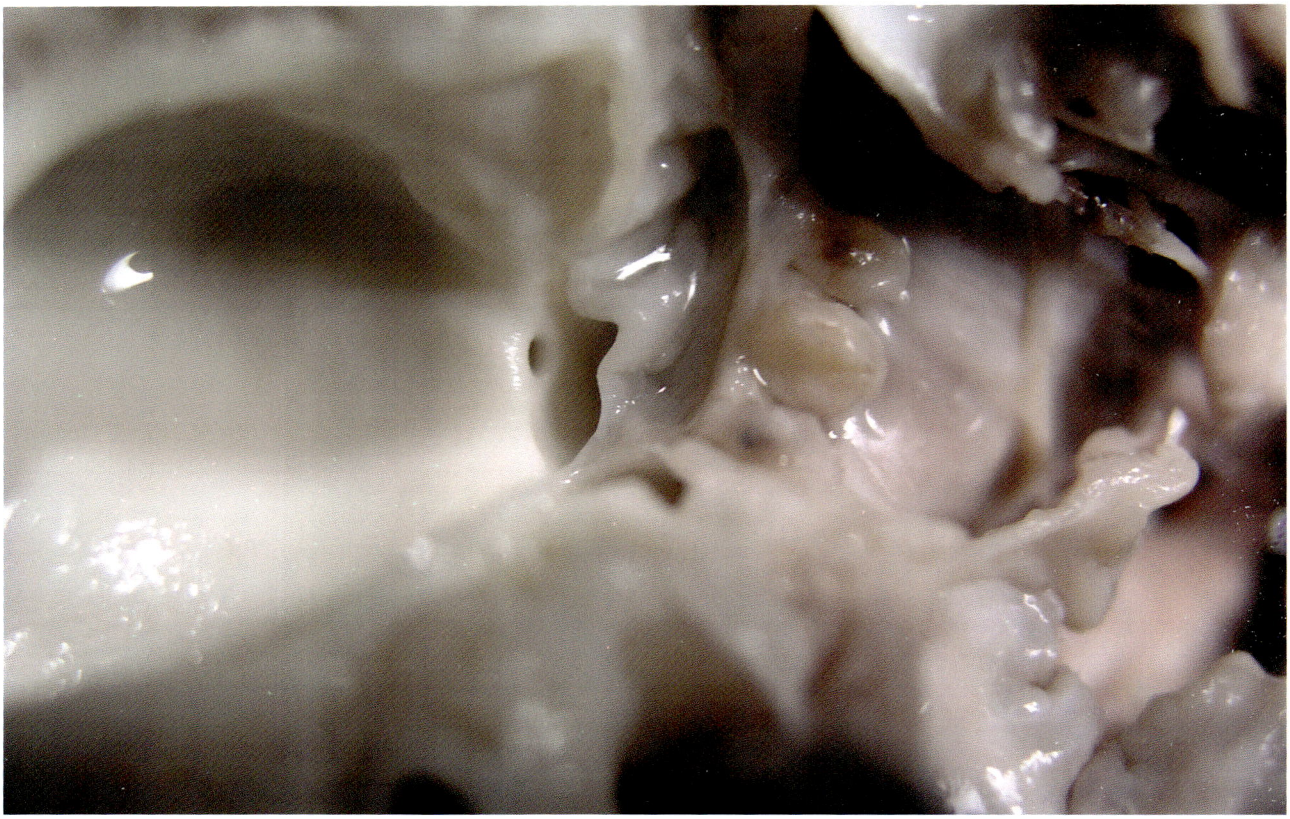

Figure 15. Dilation of the aortic arch, as a consequence of the turbulent flows subsequent to stenosis.

These lesions cause the chronic obstruction of the left ventricular outflow tract, thus generating pressure overload and systolic parietal stress, which will lead to concentric hypertrophy of the ventricle to maintain the ventricular function and cardiac output, and to a decrease in the size of the ventricular cavity.

Contrary to what may be thought, there is usually no mitral insufficiency unless the valve is affected by another disease, so it is not common to find dilation of the left atrial appendage, except in some advanced cases of the disease.

The increase in the speed of ejection and turbulence originated by the stenosis may lead to dilation of the aortic arch.

The coronary arteries and arterioles are narrowed due to an increase of the intramural pressure, which causes a proliferation of the muscle tissue of the intima.

The increase in the ventricular muscle mass and the alterations of the coronary flow favour the appearance of myocardial ischaemia and fibrosis with the presence of ventricular arrhythmias.

The obstruction also causes incapacity to increase the volume of ejection, which leads to intolerance to exercise and the presentation of syncope. There may also be sudden death caused by severe ventricular arrhythmias.

Figure 16. Left ventricular hypertrophy and outflow tract in a Golden Retriever with dynamic subaortic stenosis.

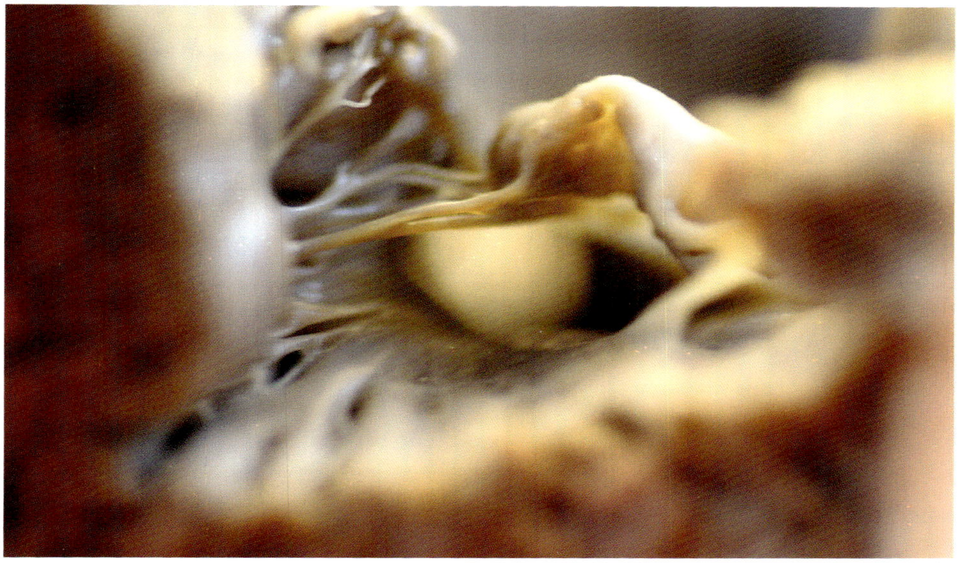

A "dynamic" obstruction has been described in Golden Retrievers, in which the size of the outflow tract varies during systole from one heartbeat to another. There is usually a marked hypertrophy of the ventricular septum with fibrosis of the endocardium just in front of the cranial leaflet of the mitral valve, which is often thickened. The most common characteristic of this type of obstruction, which contributes to a worsening of the problem, is the "systolic anterior movement of the mitral valve".

The breeds most commonly affected by subaortic stenosis are: the Terranova, Boxer, German Shepherd, Golden Retriever, Rottweiler and Bull Terrier.

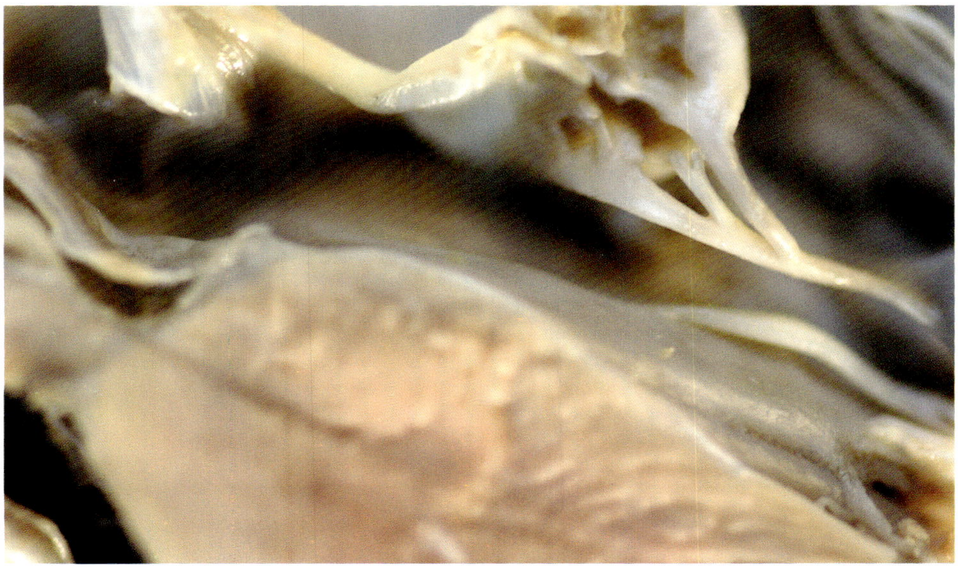

Figure 17. Dynamic subaortic stenosis. Note the marked thickening of the septum just at the subvalvular level. The Venturi effect caused by the increase of the velocity in this area is going to lead to the cranial leaflet of the mitral valve being displaced towards the outflow tract, causing the "systolic anterior movement of the mitral valve", which contributes to the aggravation of the obstruction.

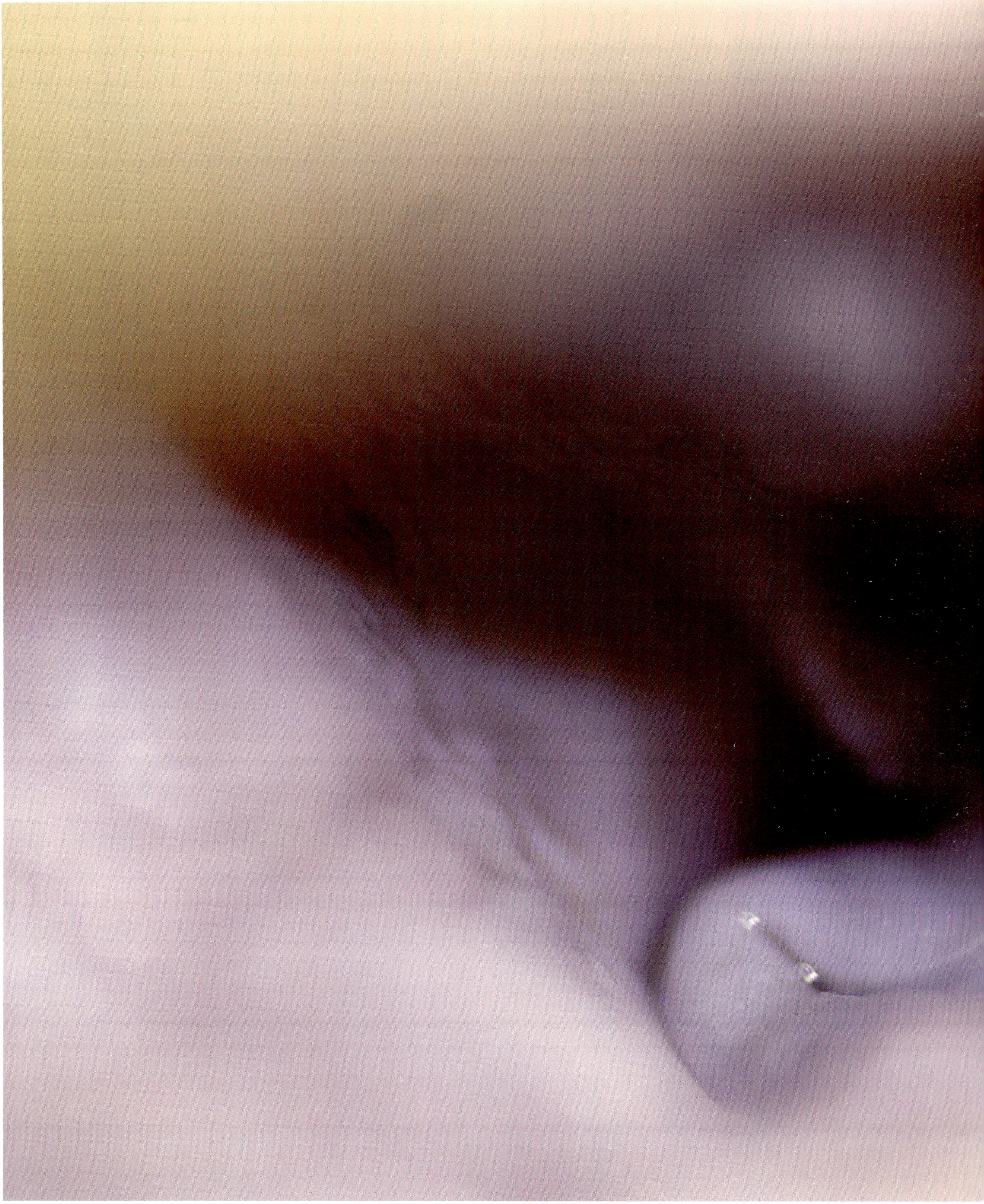

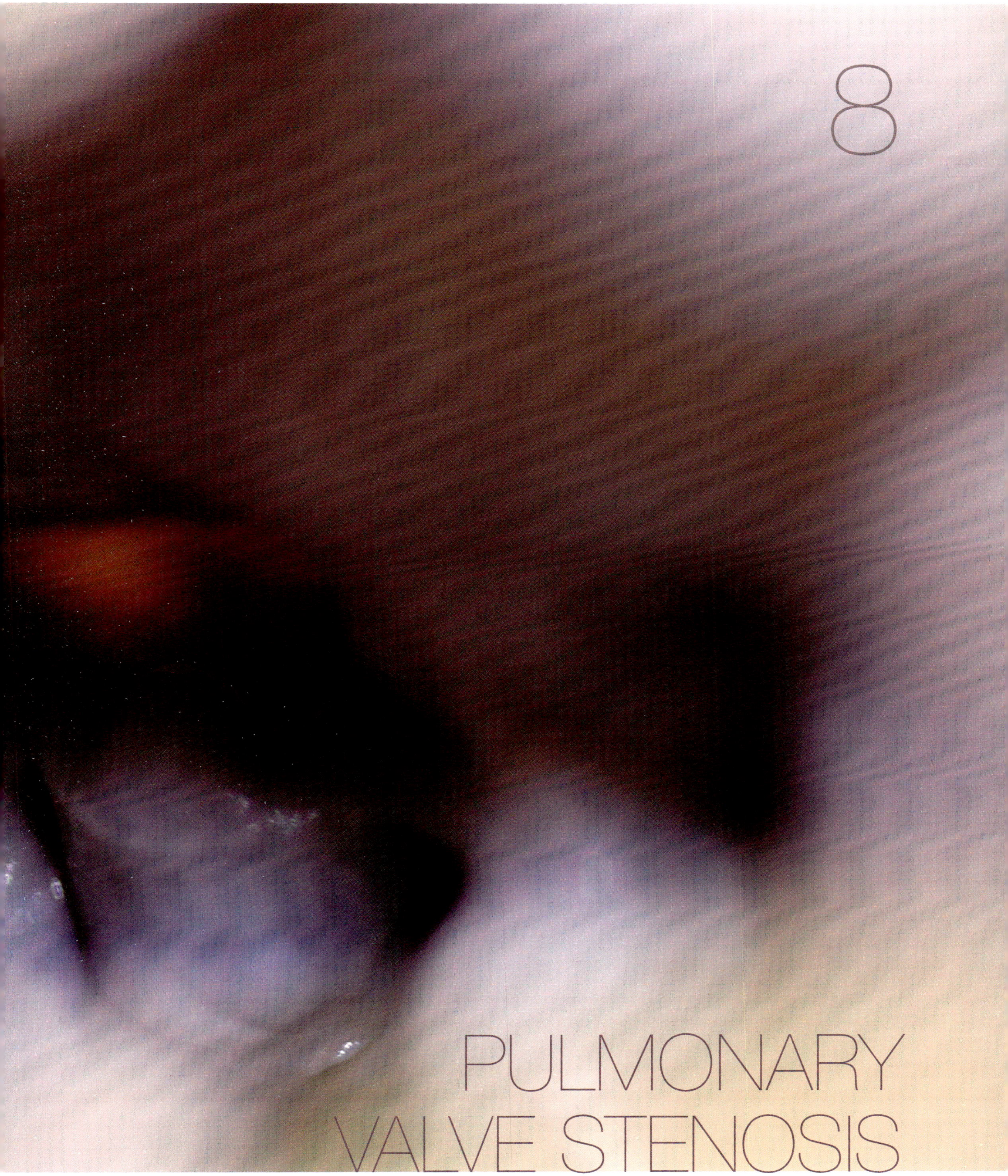
8
PULMONARY
VALVE STENOSIS

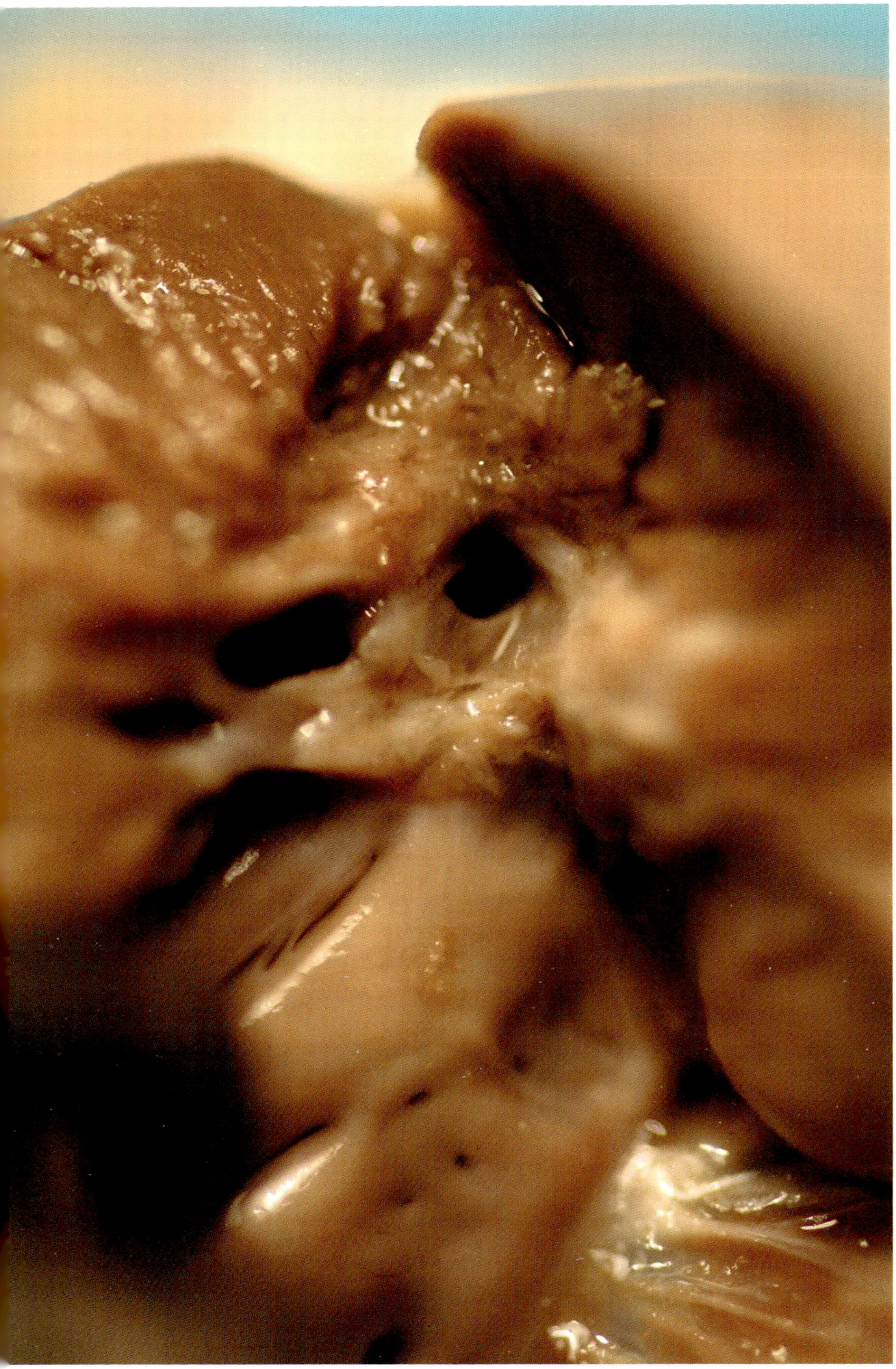

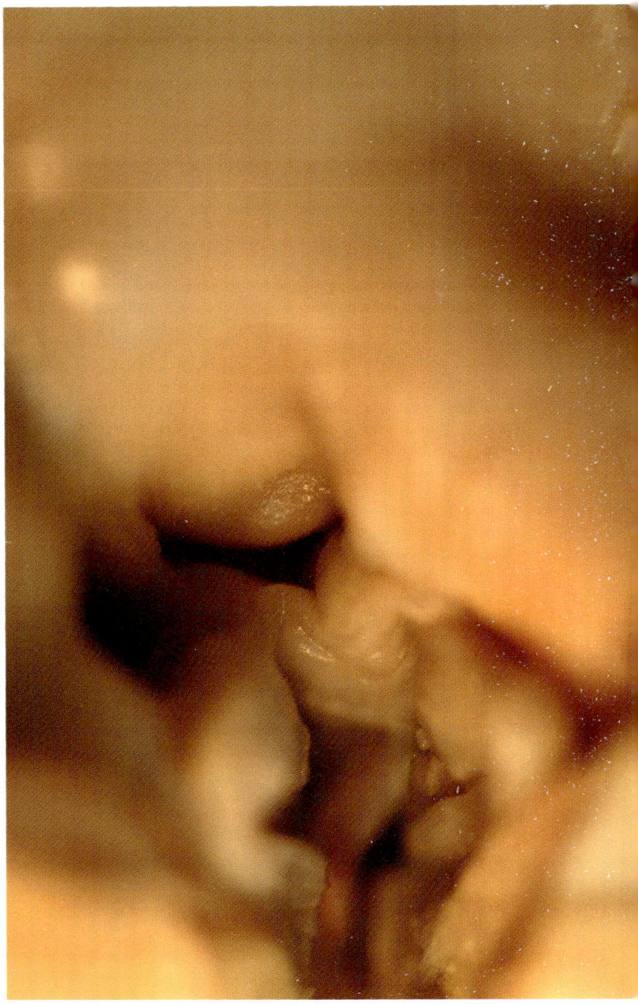

Figure 2. Valvular stenosis with thickening of the valve cusps and fusion of the commissures.

Figure 1. Fibromuscular band, which creates a division of the outflow tract of the right ventricle, causing subvalvular stenosis.

Pulmonary valve stenosis is a congenital defect that is commonly observed in dogs and uncommon in cats. This disease is often associated with other defects such as tricuspid valve dysplasia, tetralogy of Fallot or division of the outflow tract of the right ventricle by fibromuscular bands.

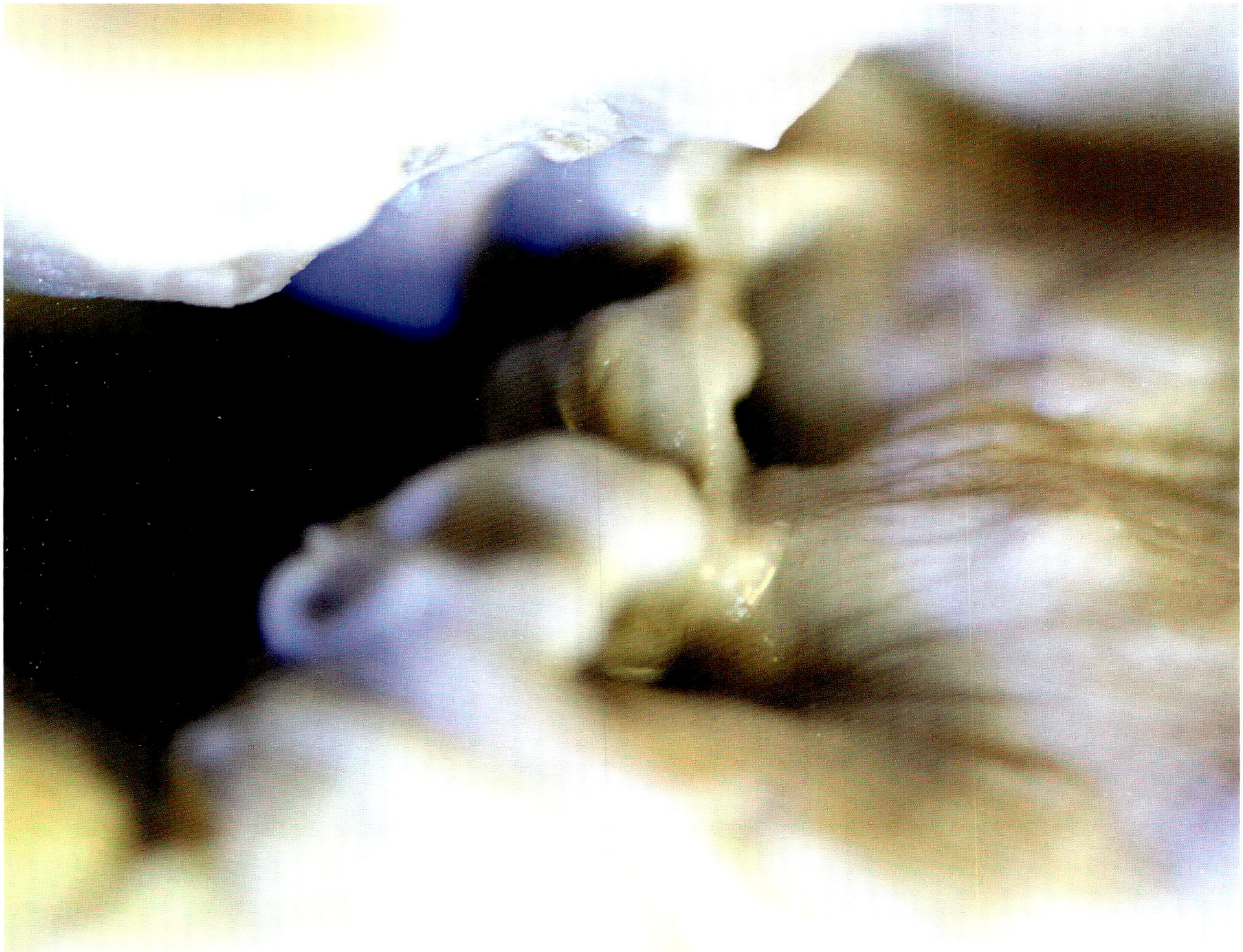

Figure 3. Valvular stenosis, sagittal section. Thickening of the valve cusps.

We can find three types of lesions:

- The most frequent type consists in a **valvular lesion** with a thickening of the leaflets and fusion of their commissures, which can be accompanied by different degrees of valvular and annular hypoplasia.
- The **subvalvular type** is usually characterised by the presence of a fibrous ring located at the base of the valve, which is often accompanied by valvular deformity. A fibromuscular narrowing sometimes occurs in the infundibular region. A particular form of subvalvular obstruction occurs in English Bulldogs and Boxers due to an abnormal origin of the left coronary artery in the right coronary artery (R2A coronary artery anomaly). This artery surrounds and compresses the outflow tract of the right ventricle before dividing into the left descending and circumflex arteries.
- **Supravalvular estenosis** is very rare and is usually the consequence of hypoplasia of the pulmonary trunk.

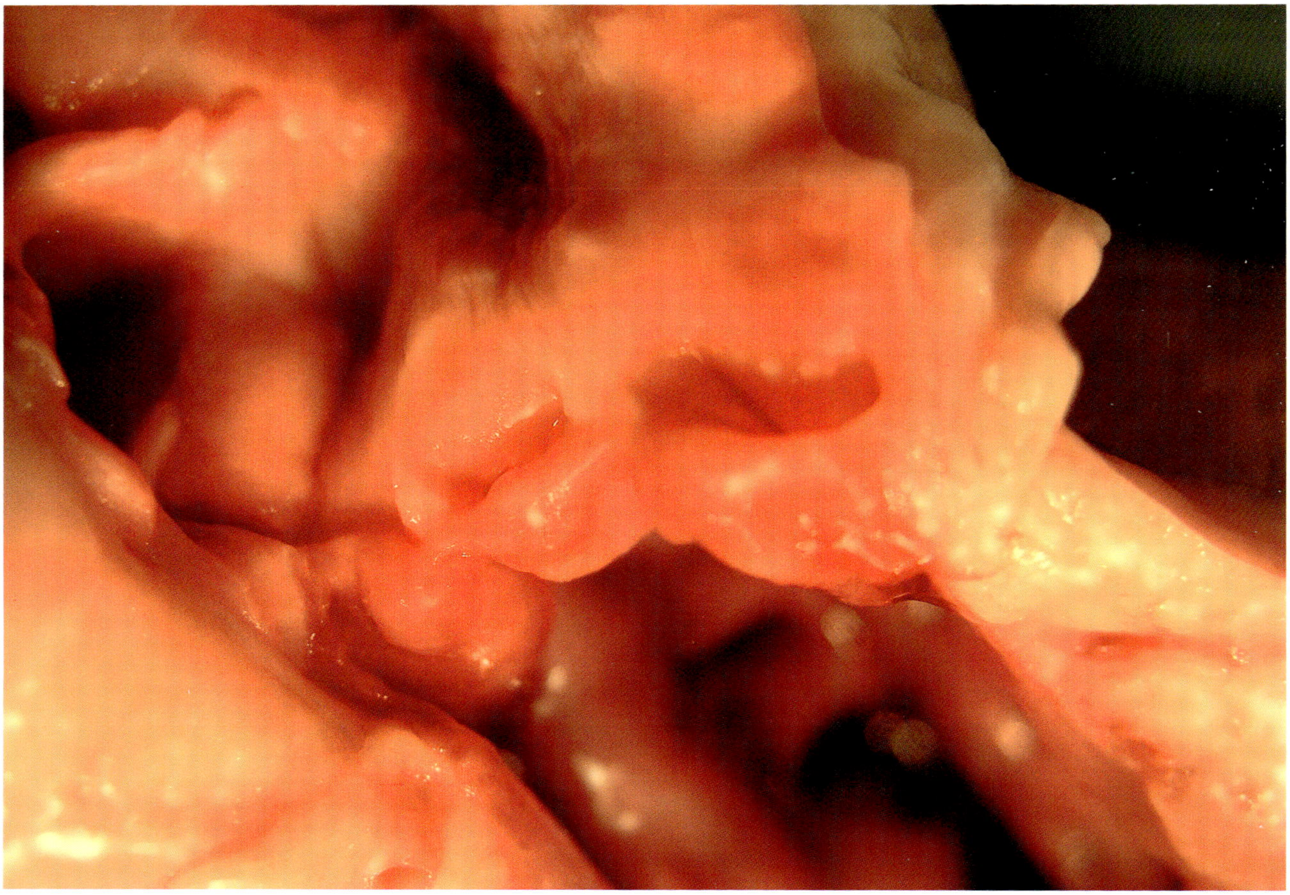

Figure 4. Thickening of the cusps and fusion of the commissures.

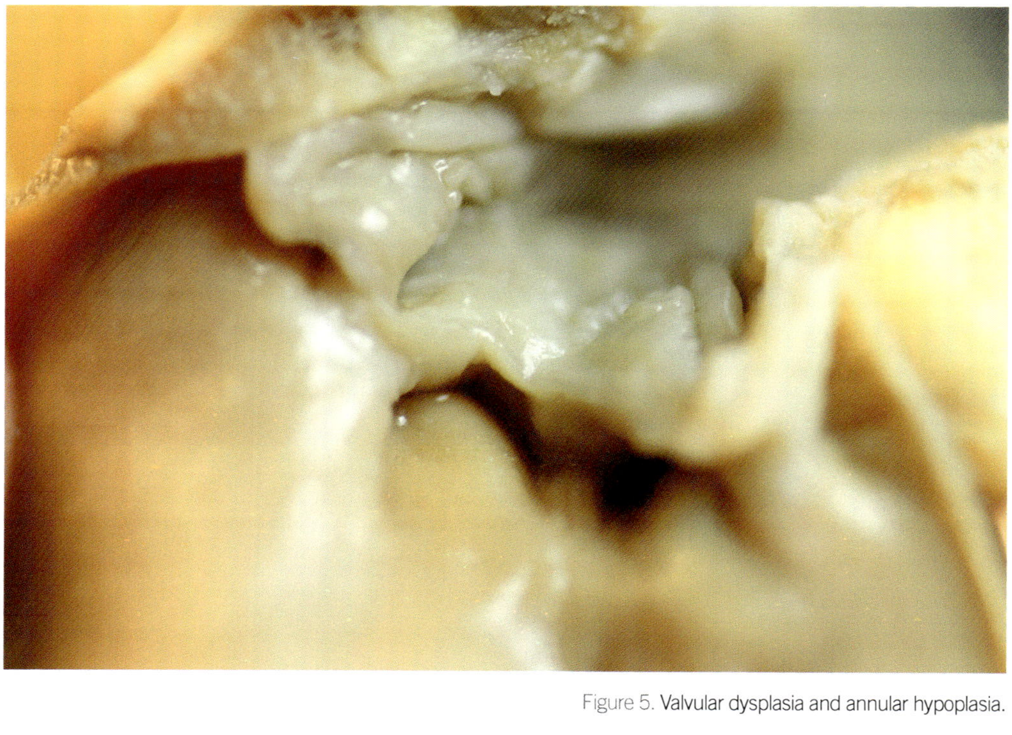

Figure 5. Valvular dysplasia and annular hypoplasia.

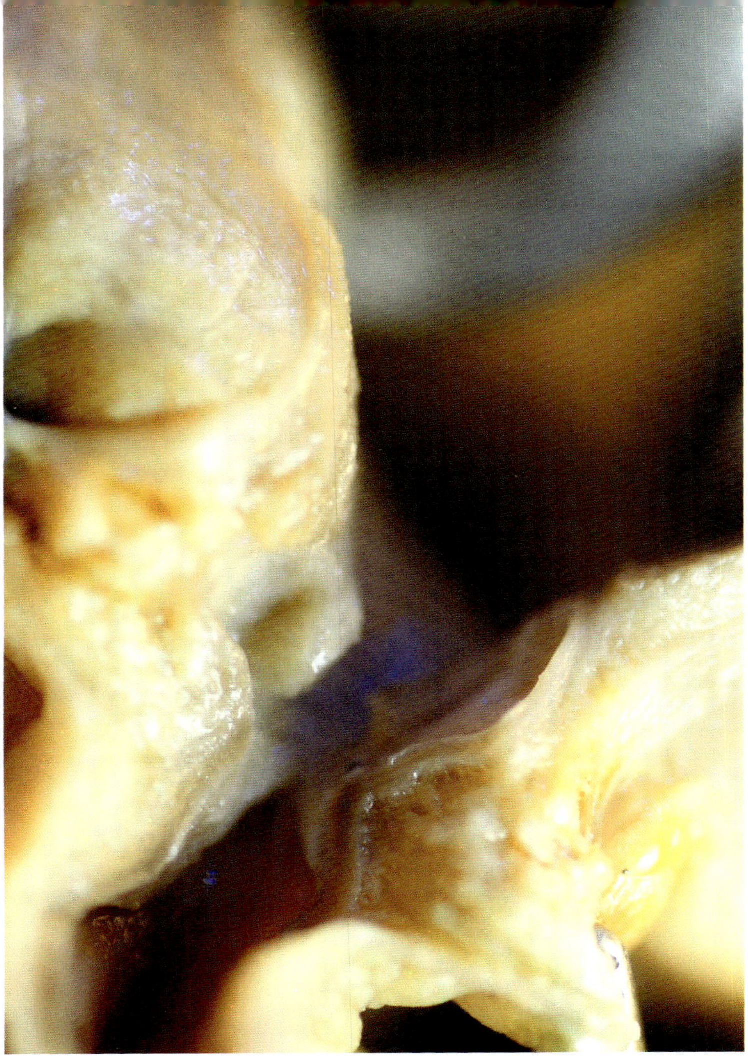

Figure 6. Marked valvular and annular hypoplasia, up to the point that there is virtually no pulmonary valve apparatus.

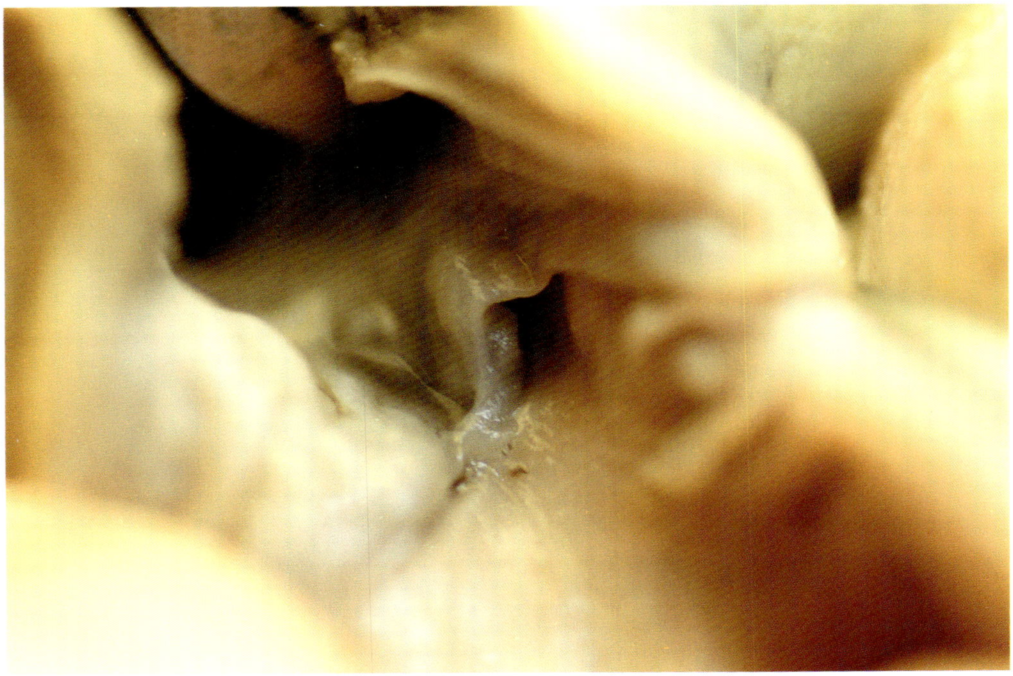

Figure 7. Valvular dysplasia with incomplete development of two of the three valve cusps.

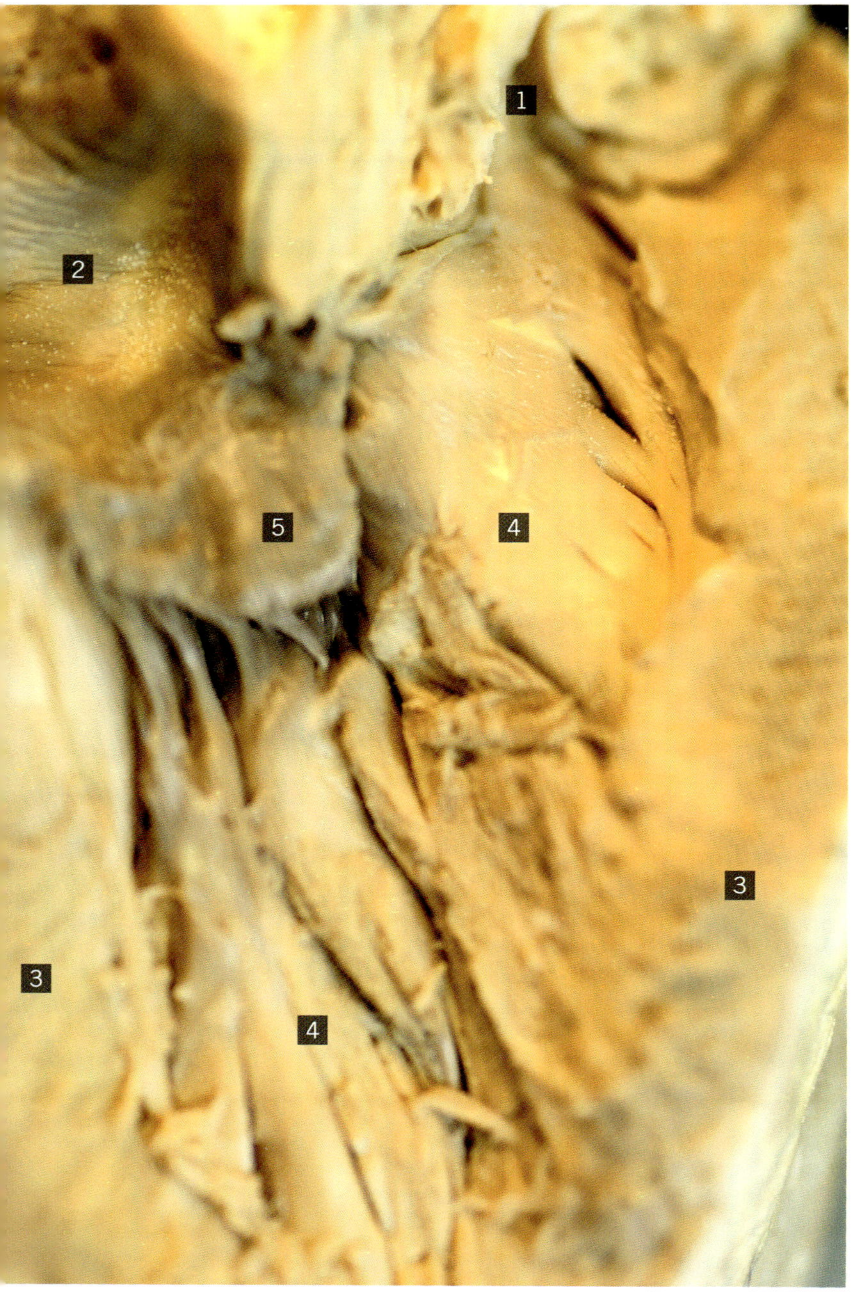

Figure 8. Infundibular subvalvular stenosis in which it is possible to observe, in addition, hypertrophy of the right ventricle.

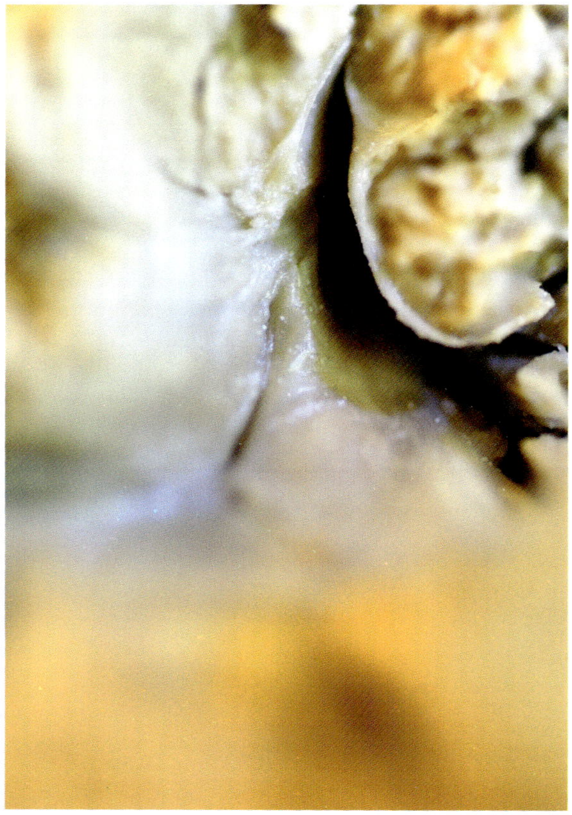

Figure 9. Close view of the infundibular stenosis of the previous image.

[1 Infundibulum]

[2 Right atrium]

[3 Free wall of the right ventricle]

[4 Interventricular septum]

[5 Septal leaflet of the tricuspid valve]

It seems that malformations in the distal part of the bulbus cordis are directly related to pulmonary valve stenosis, while subvalvular and infundibular stenoses may be the consequence of an abnormal division of the bulbus cordis during the formation of the ventricular septum, and supravalvular stenosis may be due to alterations in more distal parts, in the truncus arteriosus.

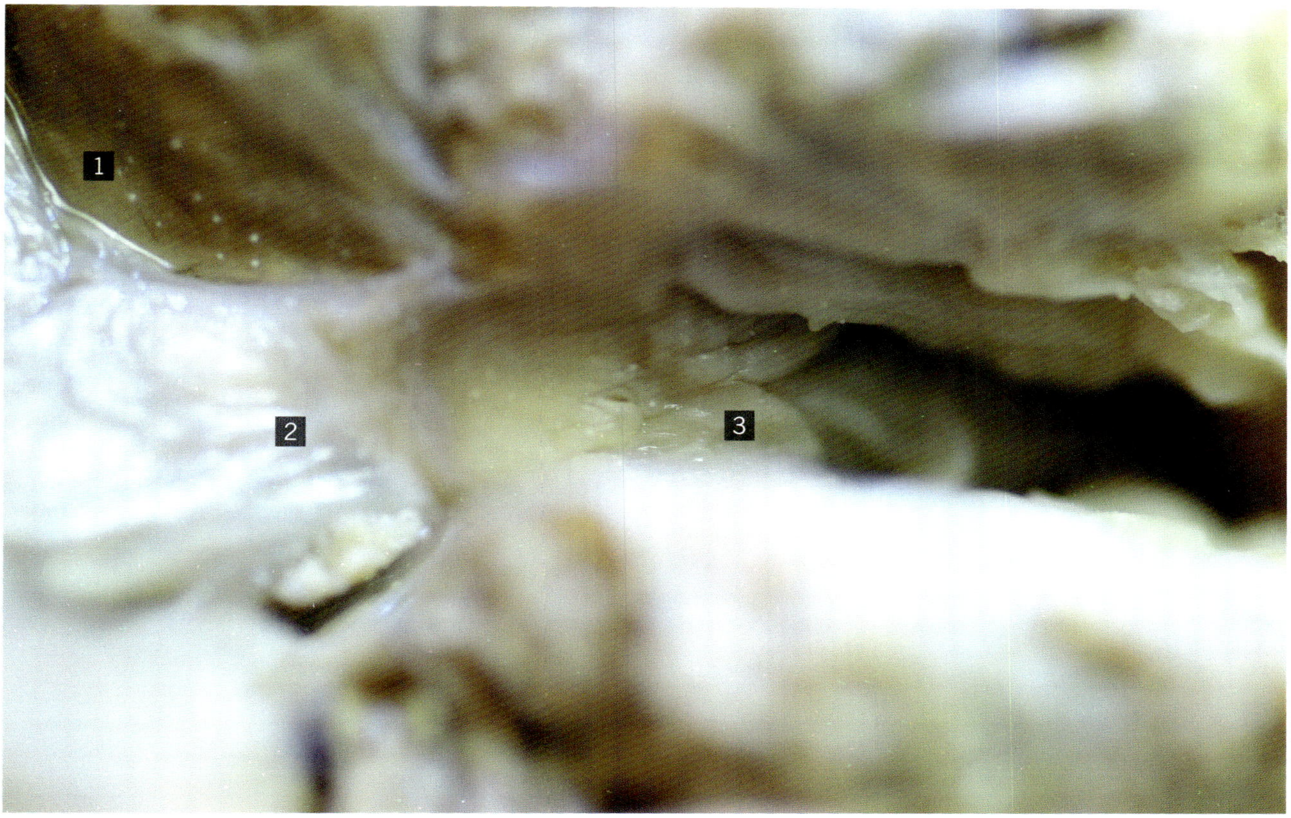

Figure 10. Subvalvular stenosis.

[1 Infundibulum]

[2 Fibrous ring at infundibular level]

[3 Marked valvular hypoplasia]

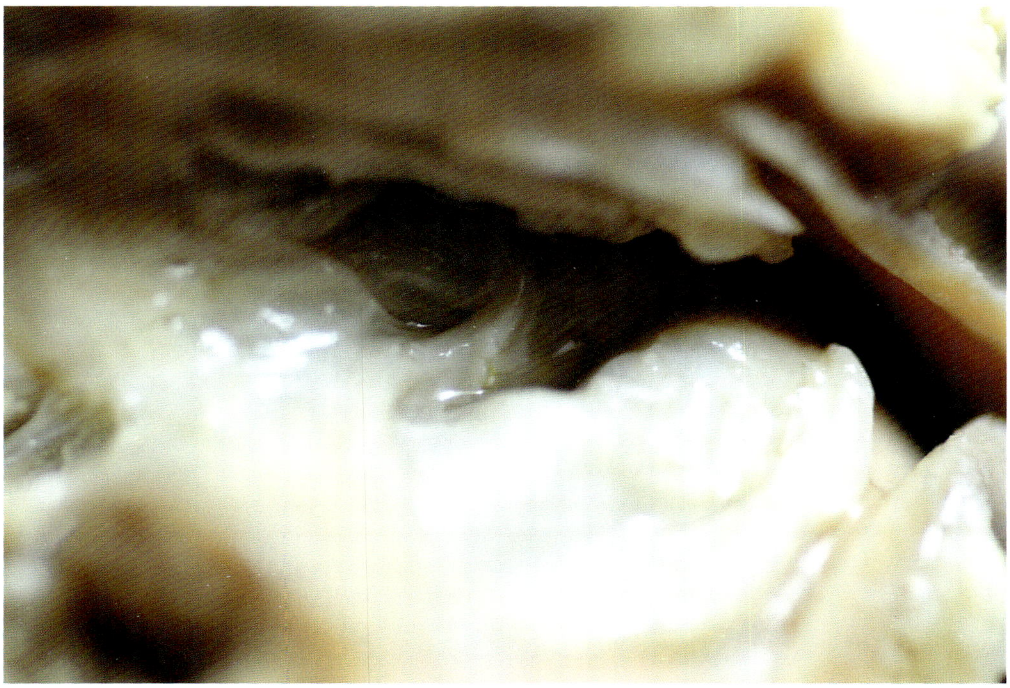

Figure 11. Hypoplastic pulmonary valve apparatus of the same case as in the previous image.

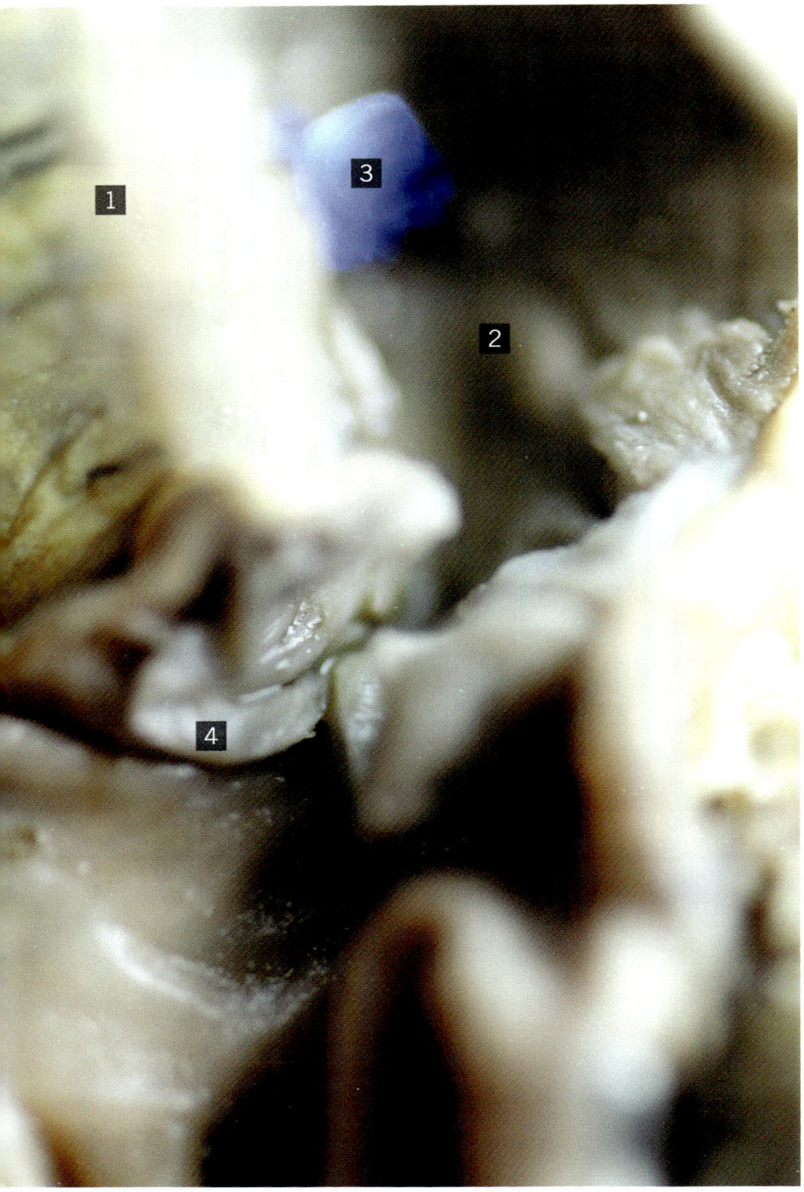

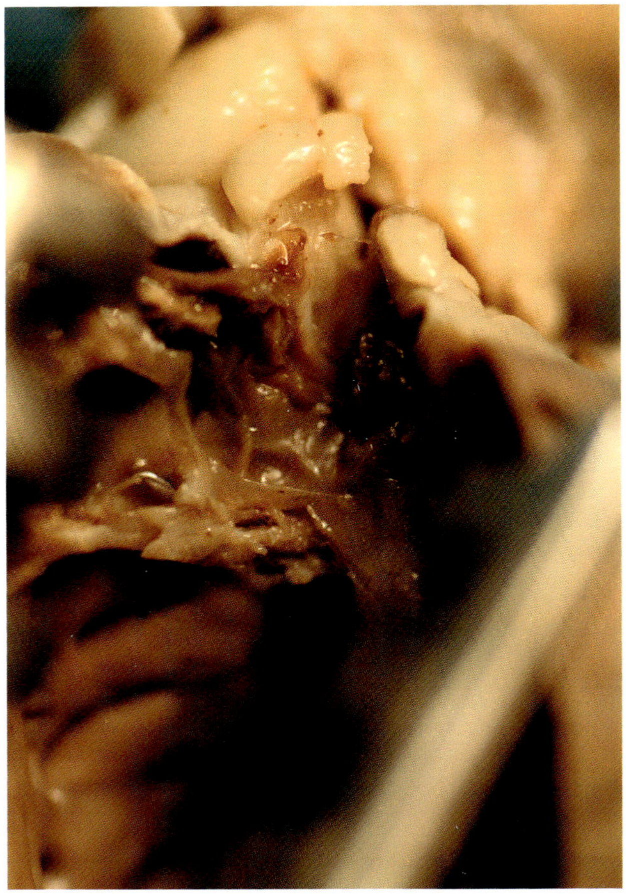

Figure 13. Marked subvalvular fibrosis with valvular hypoplasia.

Figure 12. Sagittal section of a pulmonary valve stenosis in which part of the infundibular area has been removed, which reveals how right ventricular hypertrophy contributes to worsening the narrowing.

Regardless of what its origin is, pulmonary valve stenosis causes an increase in the resistance to the outflow from the right ventricle and thus in ventricular systolic pressure, while pressure values in the pulmonary artery are normal or even decrease if the flow is significantly reduced. The pressure gradient between these two points –right ventricle and pulmonary trunk– will provide information about the severity of the lesion.

The right ventricle will respond to pressure overload with concentric hypertrophy in order to maintain systolic function but, in severe cases, it will decrease the final diastolic volume and limit the volume of ejection.

[1 Free wall of the right ventricle]

[2 Infundibulum]

[3 Ventricular cavity]

[4 Valve apparatus]

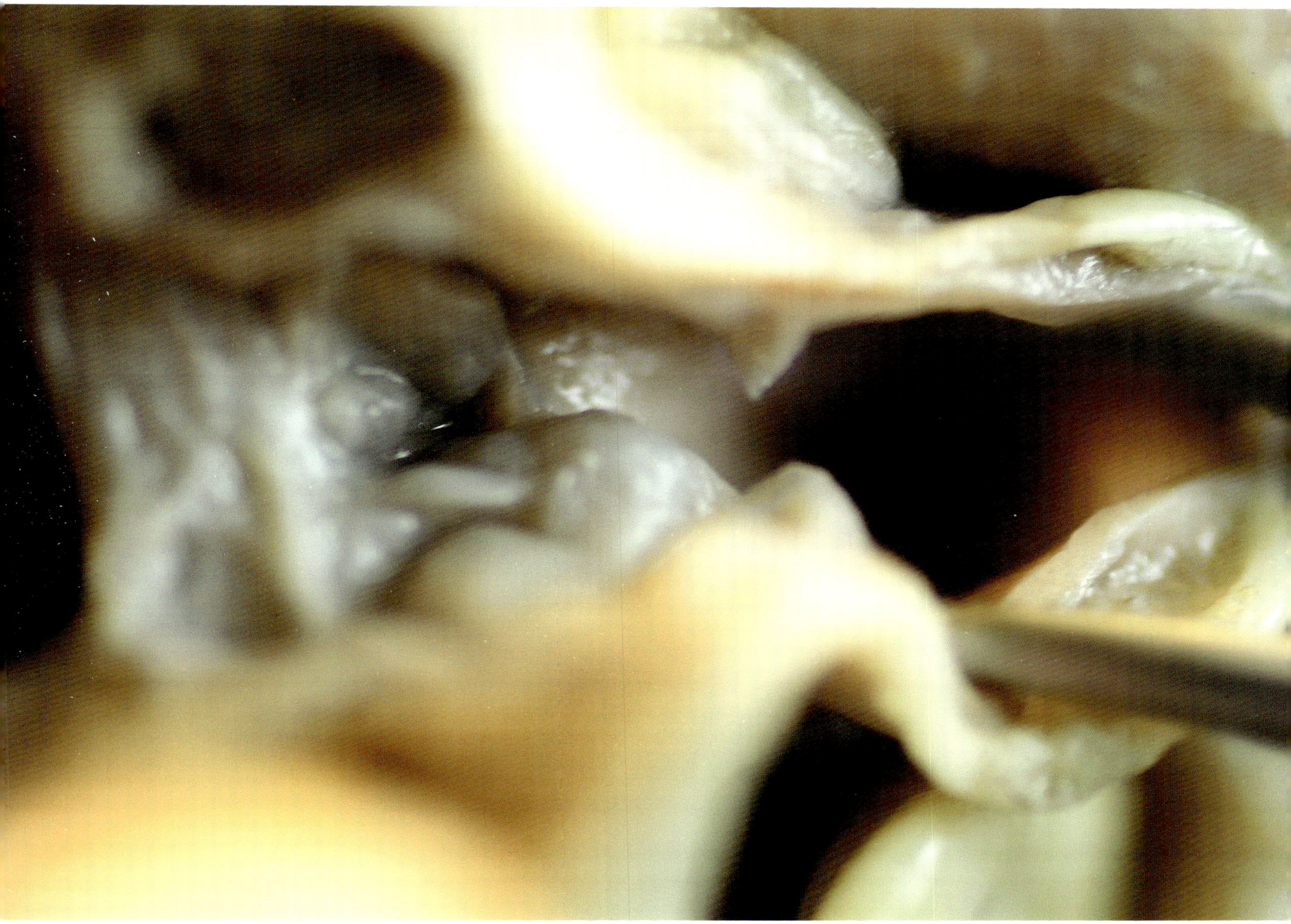

Figure 14. Subvalvular fibrous ring in a case of pulmonary valve stenosis in a tetralogy of Fallot.

The hypertrophy, which causes an increase in the rigidity of the ventricular wall, will lead to strong contractions of the right atrium, which may even be noticed in the jugular vein. It may also sometimes lead to dilation of this structure as a result of a high ventricular diastolic pressure and of tricuspid regurgitation caused by these pressure changes as well as by morphological changes in the ventricle.

If the pressure in the right atrium significantly increases, right congestive heart failure will occur.

Hypertrophy may also cause changes in the coronary flow of the right ventricle.

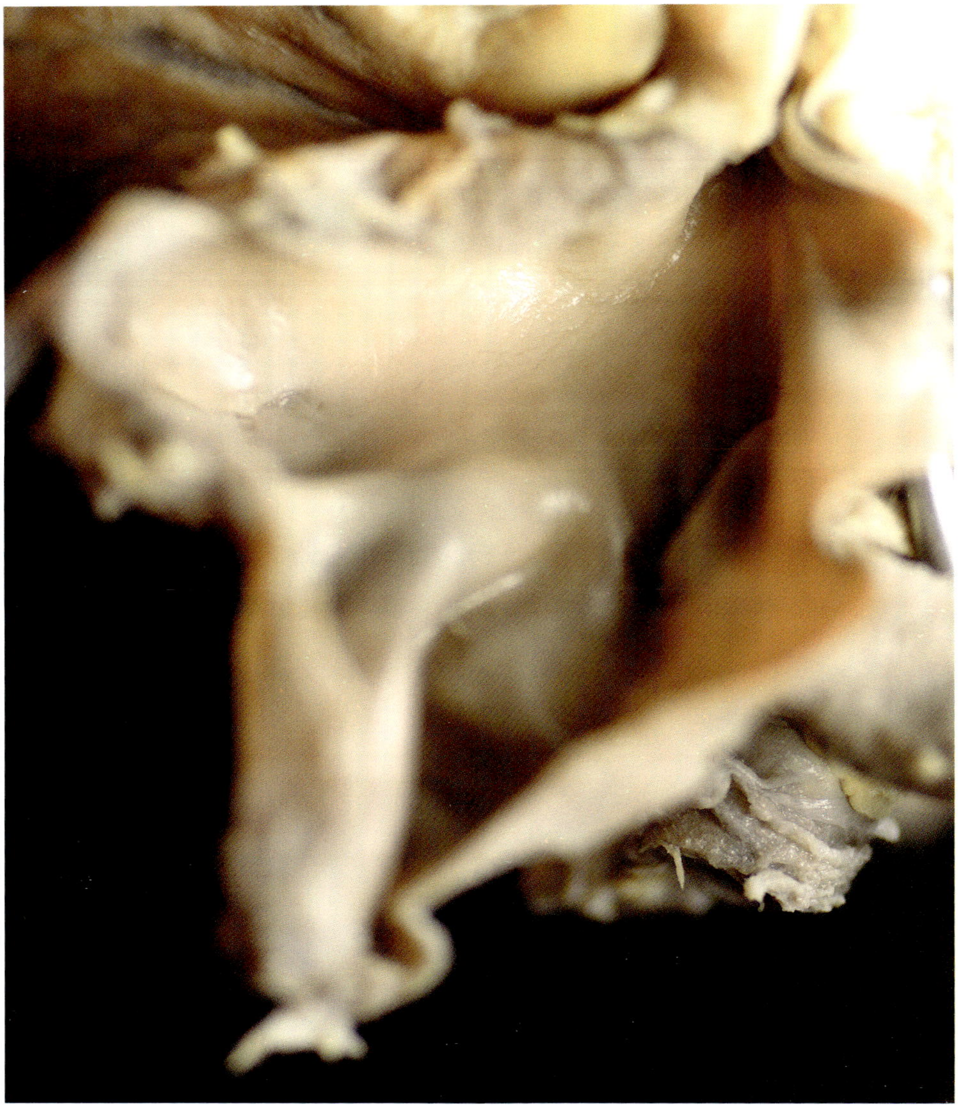

Figure 15. Pulmonary trunk, post-stenotic dilation.

The turbulent flow due to the narrowing of the valve may lead to post-stenotic dilation of the pulmonary trunk.

The presence of a patent foramen ovale with a right-left shunt is not uncommon in cases of pulmonary valve stenosis.

The Beagle, English Bulldog, Samoyed, Miniature Schnauzer, Chihuahua, Mastiff, Labrador, Chow Chow as well as the Spaniel and Terrier breeds are among the most affected breeds, although this disorder may occur in almost every breed and crossbreed.

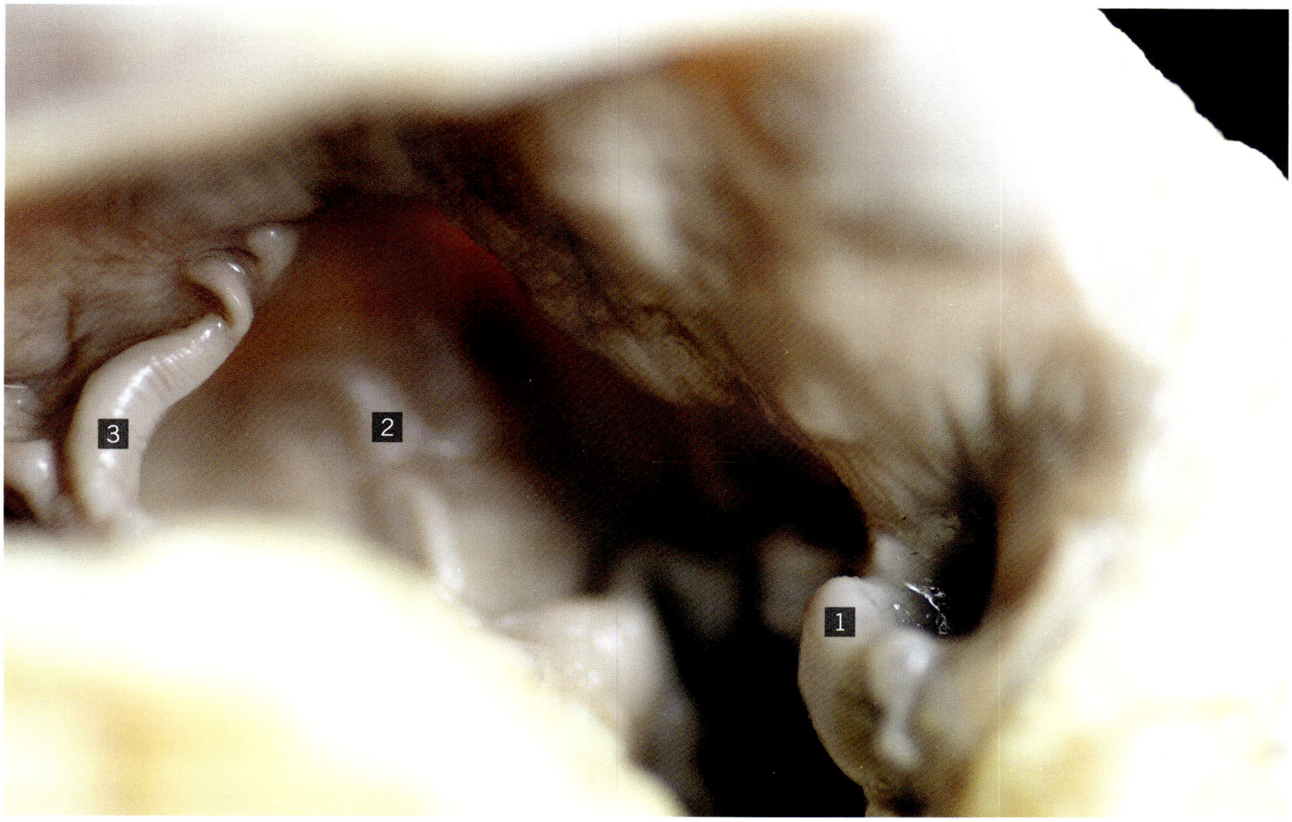

Figure 16. Dilation of the pulmonary trunk, sagittal section.

[1 Pulmonary valve] [2 Dilation] [3 Bifurcation of the pulmonary trunk]

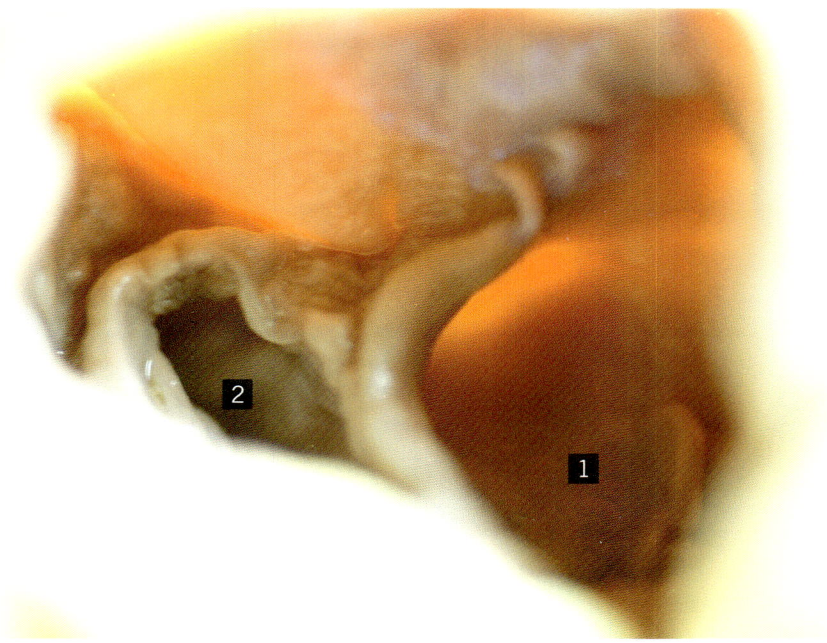

[1 Left pulmonary artery]

[2 Right pulmonary artery]

Figure 17. Bifurcation of the dilated pulmonary trunk.

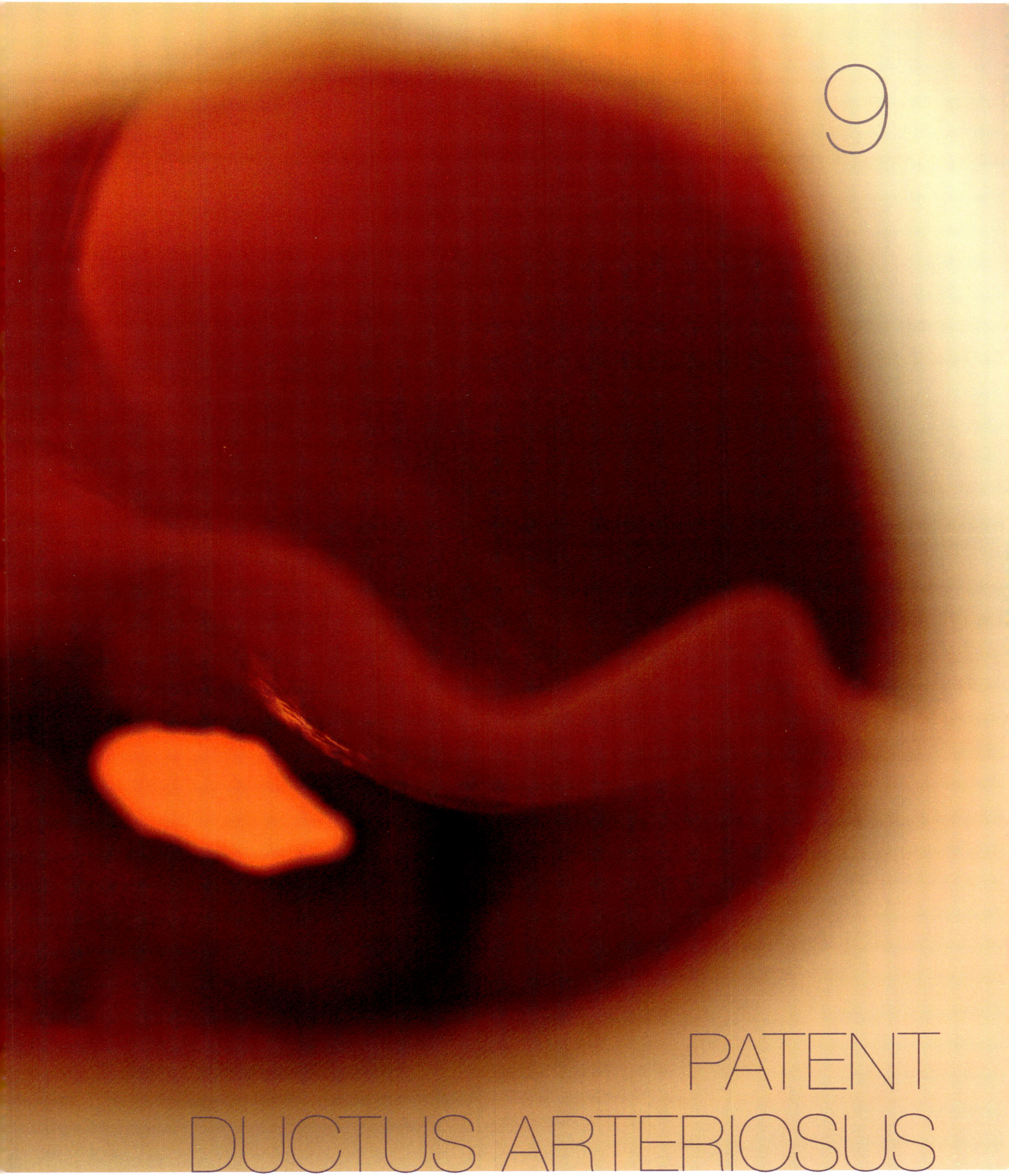

9

PATENT DUCTUS ARTERIOSUS

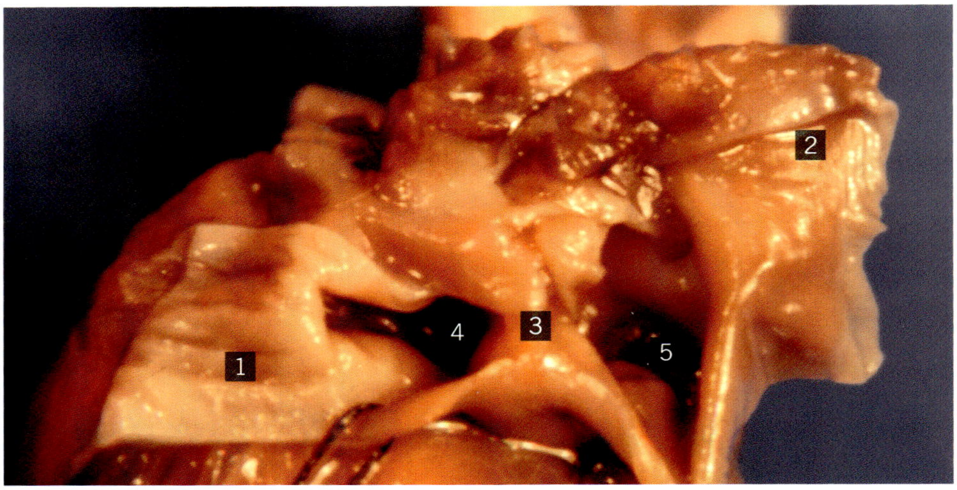

[1 Caudal vena cava]

[2 Cranial vena cava]

[3 Intervenous tubercle]

[4 Foramen ovale]

[5 Tricuspid valve]

Figure 1. Foetal heart. View of the inside of the right atrium in a craniocaudal section.

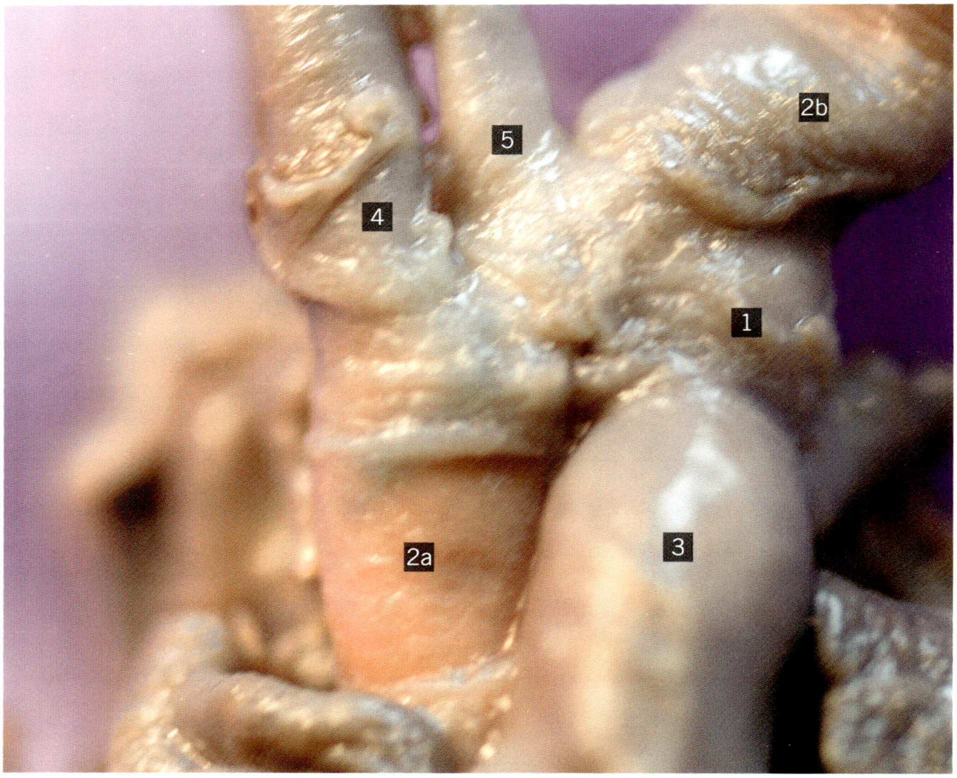

[1 Ductus arteriosus]

[2a Ascending aorta]

[2b Descending aorta]

[3 Pulmonary artery]

[4 Brachiocephalic trunk]

[5 Left subclavian artery]

Figure 2. Foetal heart. Left lateral view, exit of the great vessels.

During foetal life, the blood from the placenta reaches the right atrium from the caudal vena cava. Due to the presence of the intervenous tubercle, most of this blood goes through the foramen ovale and runs to the left atrium and ventricle, from where it will supply the head and forelimbs via the aorta, brachiocephalic trunk and left subclavian artery; this blood returns to the right atrium through the cranial vena cava and the intervenous tubercle deviates the blood again, this time to the tricuspid valve and right ventricle.

[1 Descending aorta]

[2 Left pulmonary artery]

[3 Ligamentum arteriosum]

[4 Right pulmonary artery]

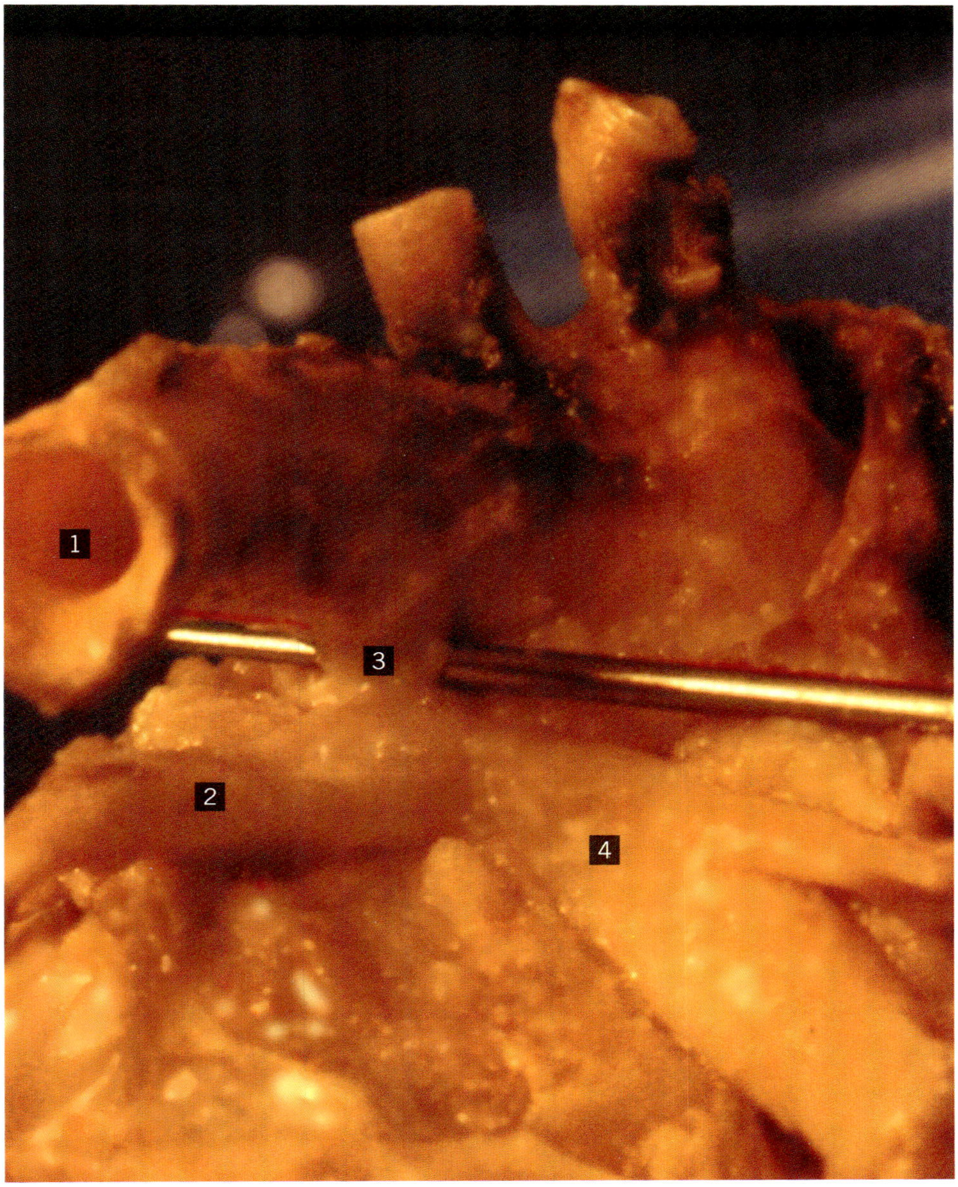

Figure 3. Ligamentum arteriosum.

The blood that reaches the right ventricle from the cranial vena cava, and to a lesser extent from the caudal vena cava, will follow two routes; a minimal part of it (approximately 12 %) will go to the high-resistance pulmonary vascular system due to the collapsed lungs and low partial oxygen pressure, which will lead to a marked vasoconstriction in this system. The rest of the blood will go, through the ductus Botalli, from the bifurcation of the pulmonary artery to the ventral aspect of the descending aorta, at a point located immediately posterior to the origin of the left subclavian artery. In this area, the size of the duct is similar to that of the aorta and pulmonary artery and offers little resistance to blood flow. Its histological structure includes a middle layer poor in elastic fibres with muscle fibres arranged in a spiral pattern; its intimal layer is thick and there is eosinophilic material known as mucoid substance in its subintimal layer.

The placental circulation disappears at birth and the systemic vascular resistances increase considerably. On the other hand, with the expansion of the lungs and the vasodilation that takes place due to the increase in the partial oxygen pressure, the resistance of the pulmonary bed significantly decreases. The blood from the pulmonary artery will go to the lungs to receive oxygen and will not be shunted to the aorta, where it will find higher pressures. The increase in the partial oxygen pressure in the duct and decrease of the vasodilator prostaglandins PgE_1, PgE_2 and PgI_2 released by the placenta will cause vasoconstriction of the ductus arteriosus (physiological closure). The anatomical closure takes place subsequently and is due to phenomena of thrombosis, proliferation of the vascular intima and fibrosis, thus transforming the duct into the ligamentum arteriosum.

A failure in the closure of the ductus arteriosus is one of the most common congenital heart diseases in dogs, although it is unusual in cats, and it has been shown to be hereditary in most cases. The main breeds predisposed to this disease are: the Dwarf Poodle, Cocker Spaniel, Collie, Shetland, Pomeranian, German Shepherd, Irish Setter, Chihuahua, Maltese and Yorkshire Terrier.

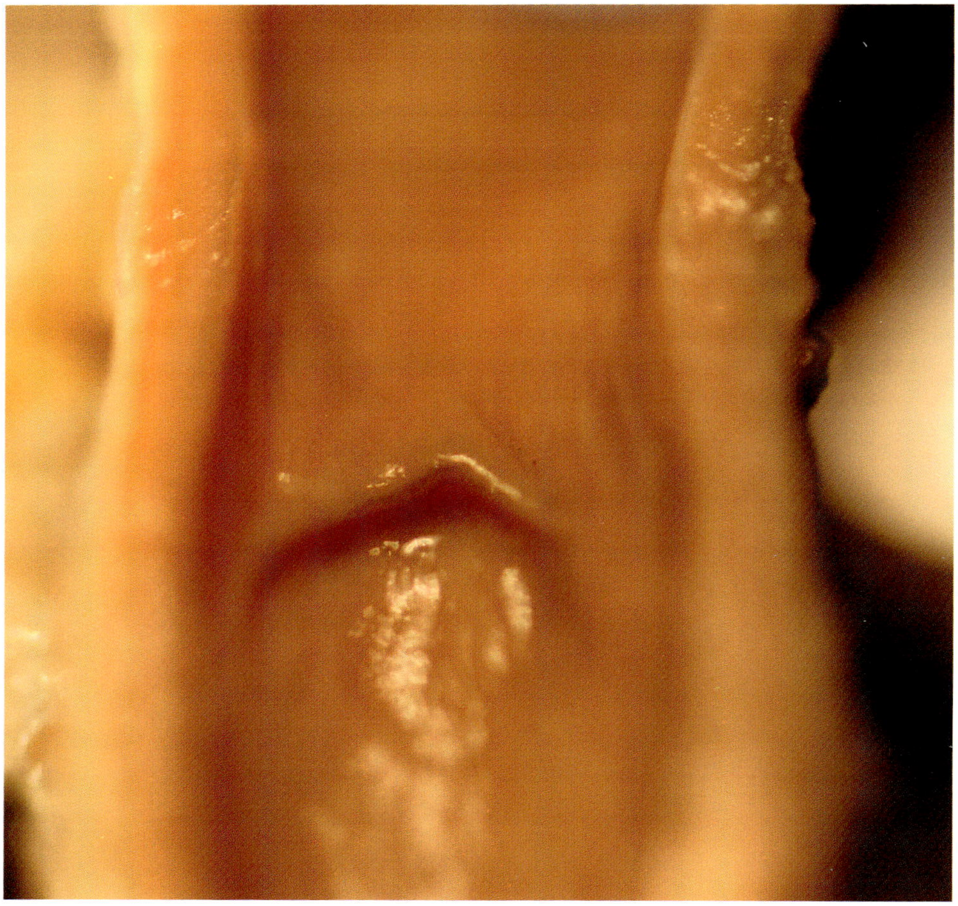

Figure 4. Ductal aneurysm. The absence of muscles in the aortic part of the duct leaves this diverticular area on the floor of the descending aorta, which corresponds to the "opening" of the ductus arteriosus.

The defect is based on the histological differentiation of the ductus arteriosus, with a hypoplastic and poorly distributed ductal smooth muscle and an increase in the number of elastic fibres. Depending on the extent and distribution of this hypoplastic muscle, these ducts are classified into various types:

- The first group includes those that lack sufficient muscle to close the aortic end, but have enough muscle at their pulmonary end, which leads to ductal closure, resulting in an aneurysmatic dilation of the aorta termed "ductal aneurysm".
- The second group includes small, medium and large-sized ducts. In this case, there is no muscle at the aortic end either, but there is a smaller or greater amount of muscle present along the ductus, which is sufficient to lead to partial closure. The more muscle there is, the more closed the ductus will be. This distribution of the ductal muscle causes the characteristic funnel shape of patent arterial ducts with a left-right shunt.
- In the last group, the absence of muscle along almost the whole course of the duct does not allow its constriction; the ductus arteriosus has, in these cases, nearly the same size as during the foetal period, resulting in a significant left-right shunt that may eventually reverse.

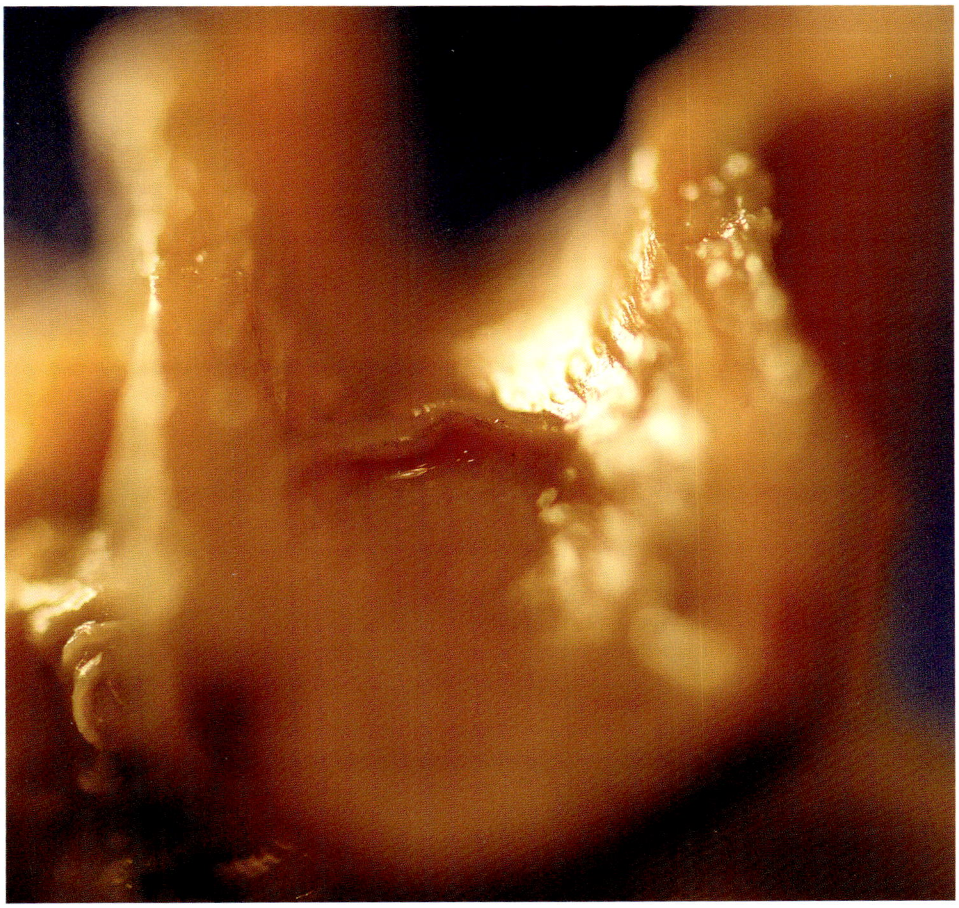

Figure 5. Ductal aneurysm. Cross-section. It is possible to see that there is no continuity in the duct as it is closed at its aortic end.

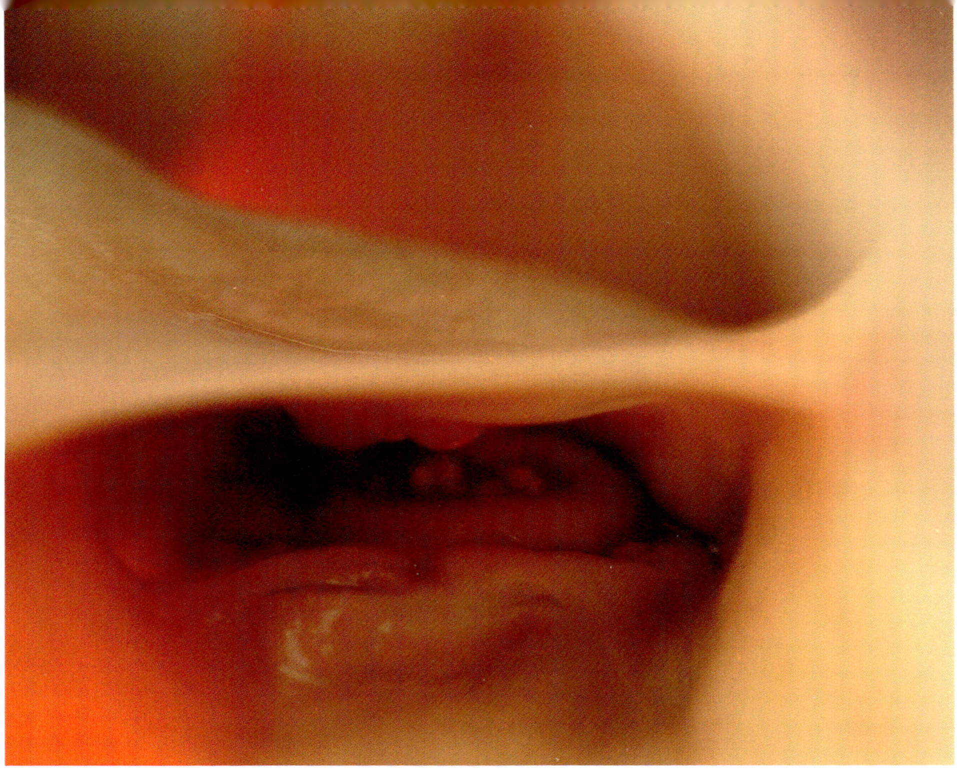

Figure 6. Ductus arteriosus, view from the aorta. The pulmonary area is nearly closed, while the aortic area is greatly dilated.

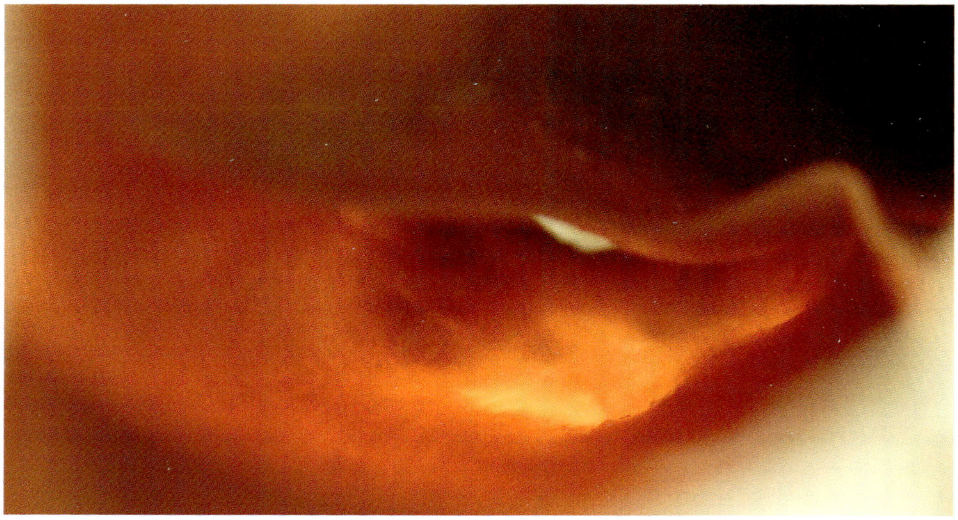

Figure 7. Ductus arteriosus, view from the inside of the aorta.

A patent ductus arteriosus with an aortopulmonary shunt will lead to volume overload in the pulmonary circulation. This will in turn cause significant diastolic overload of the left atrium and ventricle, which will lead to the dilation of both cavities and even of the mitral valve annulus, thus producing valvular insufficiency with regurgitation.

An excessive diastolic volume, the decrease of heart contractility due to chronic volume overload and possible arrhythmias due to atrioventricular dilation will contribute to congestive heart failure.

The turbulent flows that originate in the aorta and pulmonary artery due to the passage of blood through the duct may cause dilation of these structures.

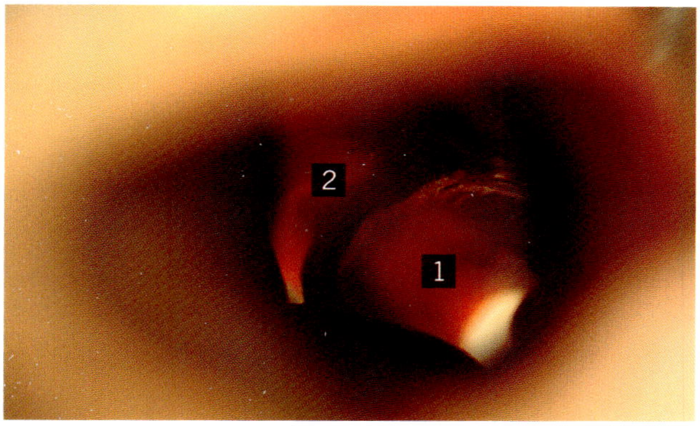

Figure 8. Ductus arteriosus, seen from the pulmonary trunk.

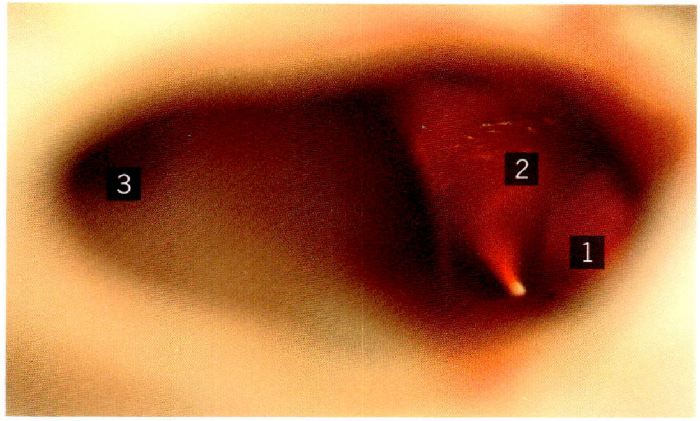

Figure 9. Ductus arteriosus, seen from the pulmonary trunk.

[1 Left pulmonary artery] [2 Ductus ateriosus] [3 Right pulmonary artery]

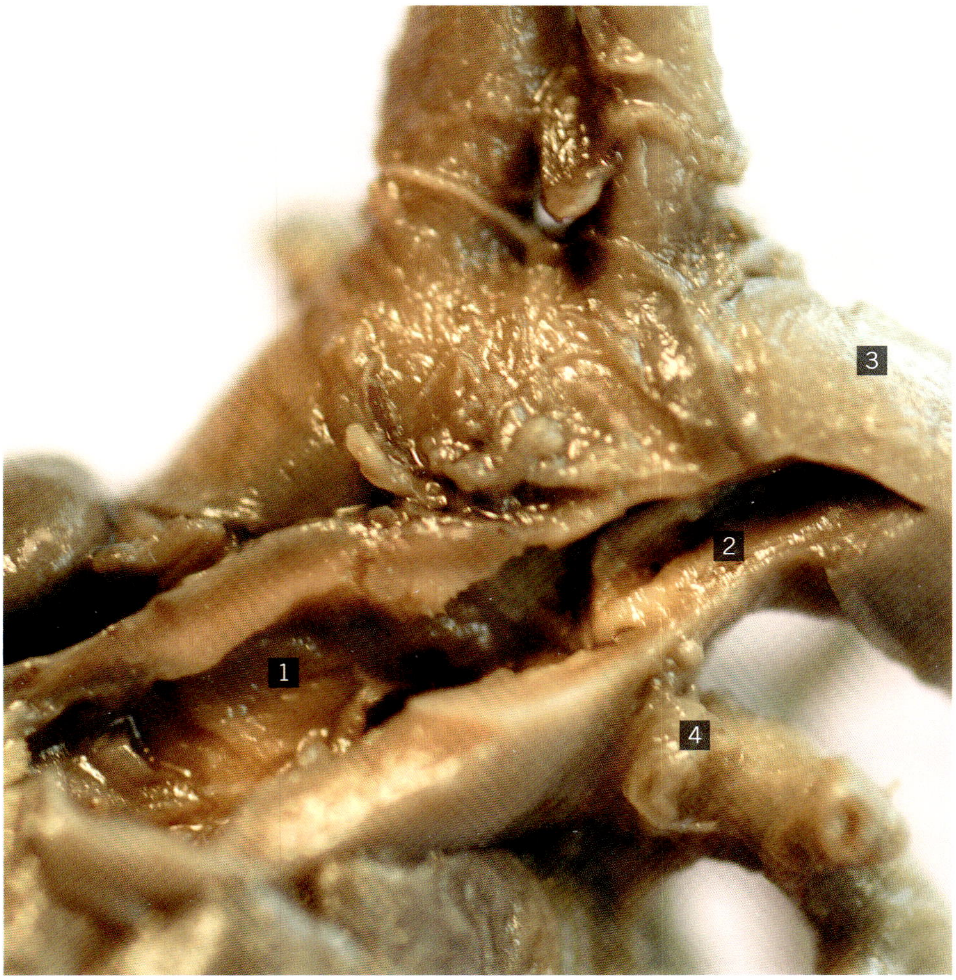

[1 Pulmonary trunk]

[2 Ductus arteriosus]

[3 Descending aorta]

[4 Left pulmonary artery]

Figure 10. Sagittal section of the pulmonary trunk and ductus arteriosus. In this case, the duct has the same diameter throughout its entire length. This type of duct is the one in which the flow can most easily be reversed.

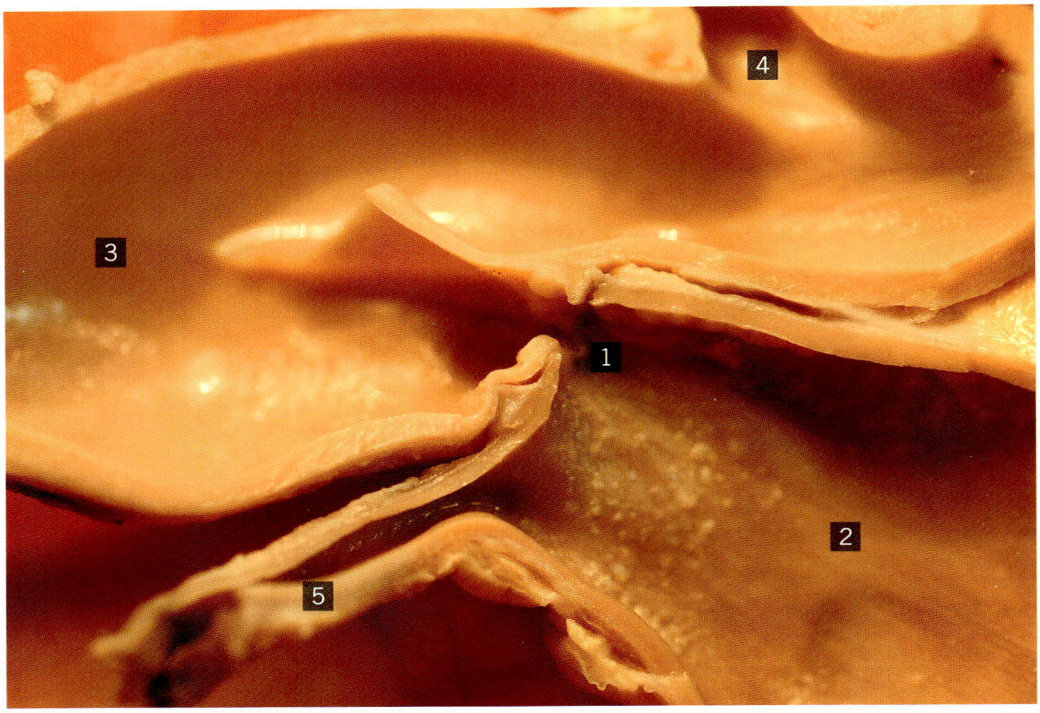

Figure 11. Sagittal section of a patent ductus arteriosus; inside view of the left lateral wall.

[1 Ductus arteriosus] [3 Descending aorta] [5 Left pulmonary artery]

[2 Pulmonary trunk] [4 Left subclavian artery] [6 Brachiocephalic trunk]

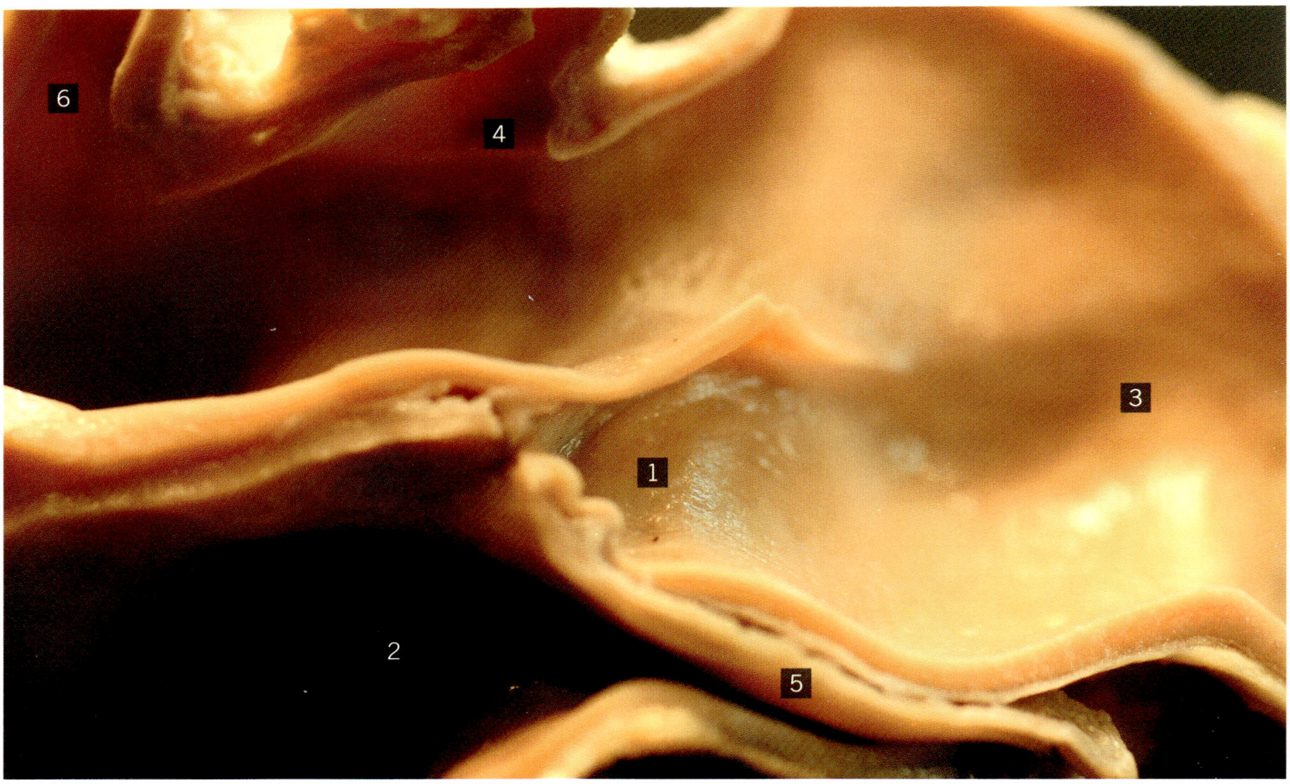

Figure 12. Sagittal section of a patent ductus arteriosus; inside view of the right lateral wall.

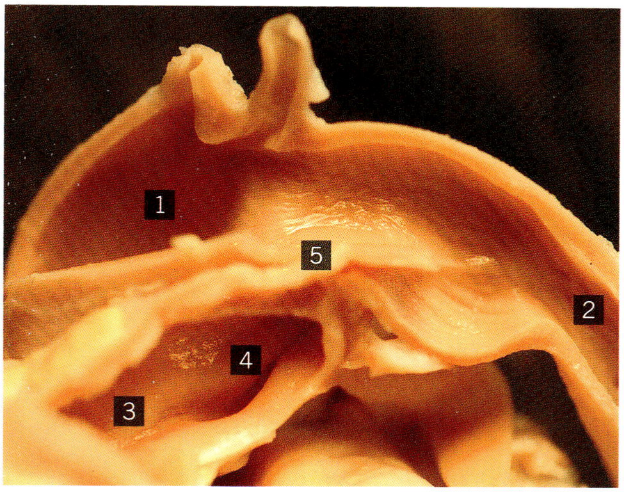

Figure 13. Sagittal section of the patent ductus arteriosus with central constriction and muscular hypoplasia at the aortic and pulmonary sides; inside view of the right lateral wall.

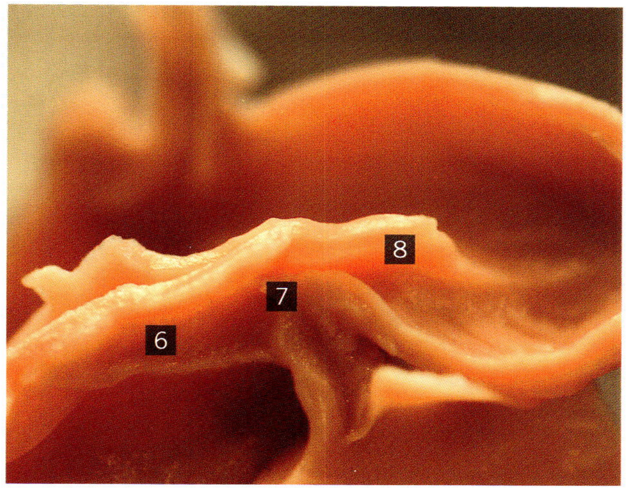

Figure 14. More detailed view of the ductus arteriosus of the previous image.

[1 Ascending aorta]
[2 Descending aorta]
[3 Pulmonary trunk]
[4 Origin of the right pulmonary artery]
[5 Ductus arteriosus]
[6 Pulmonary septum of the duct]
[7 Constriction area of the duct]
[8 Aortic septum of the duct]

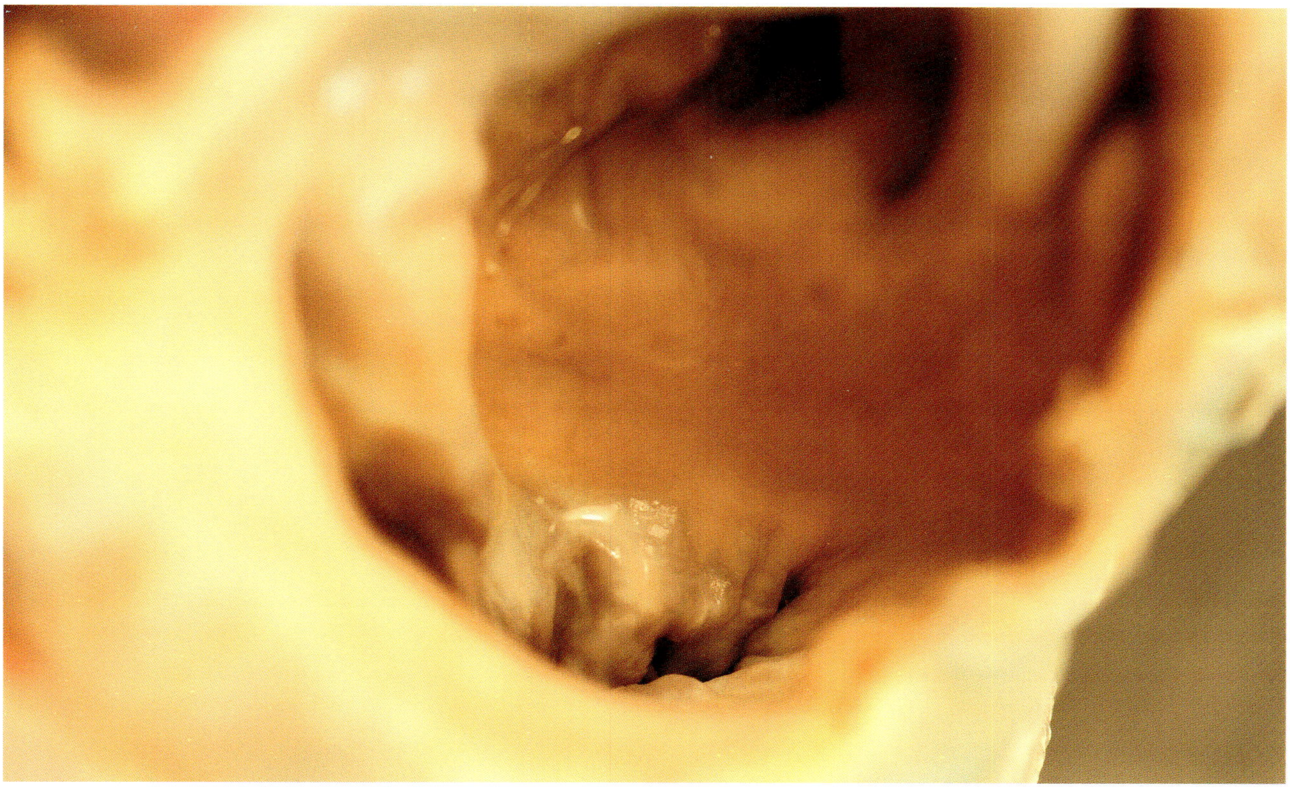

Figure 15. Dilation of the left atrium as a result of volume overload.

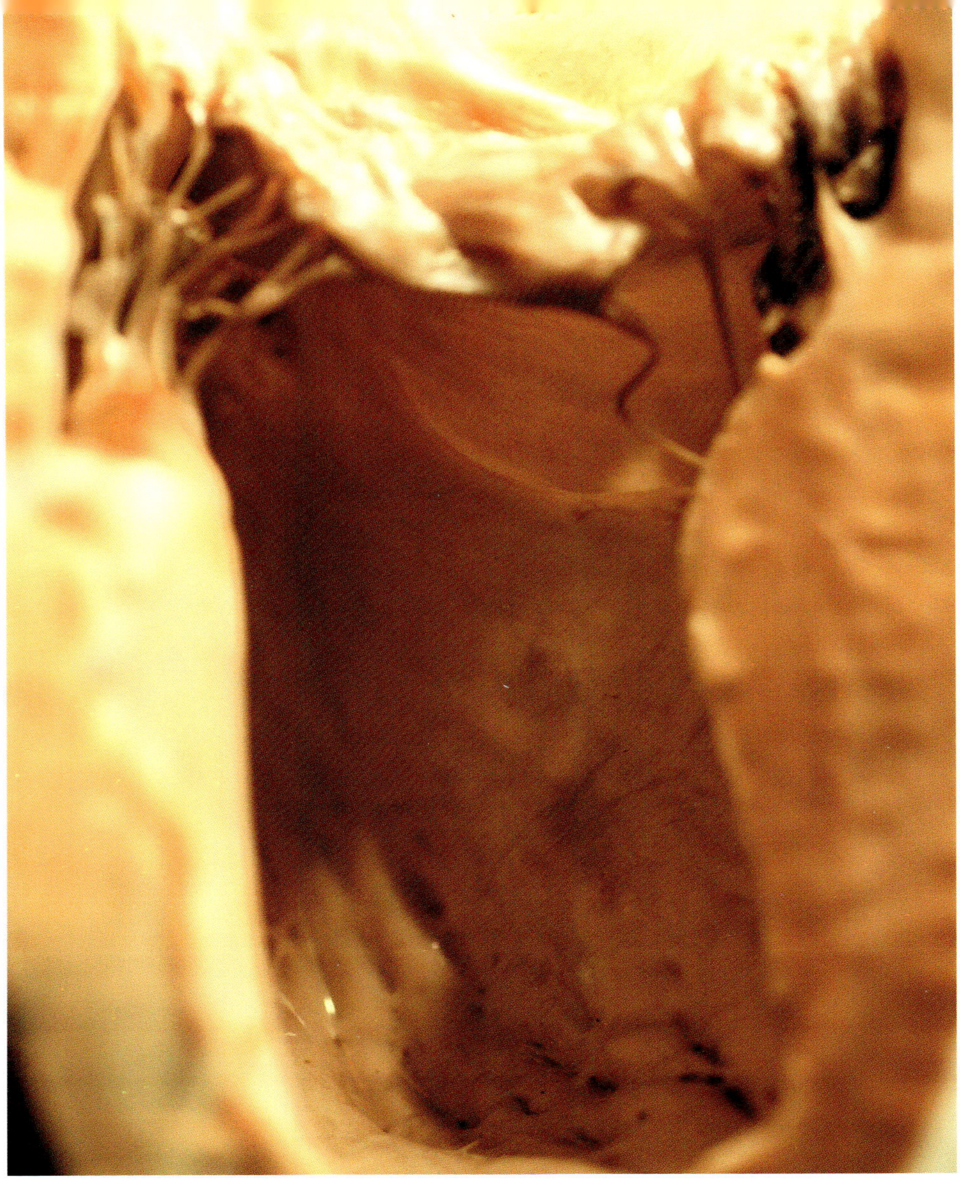

Figure 16. Dilation of the left ventricle as a result of volume overload, which will eventually lead to heart failure.

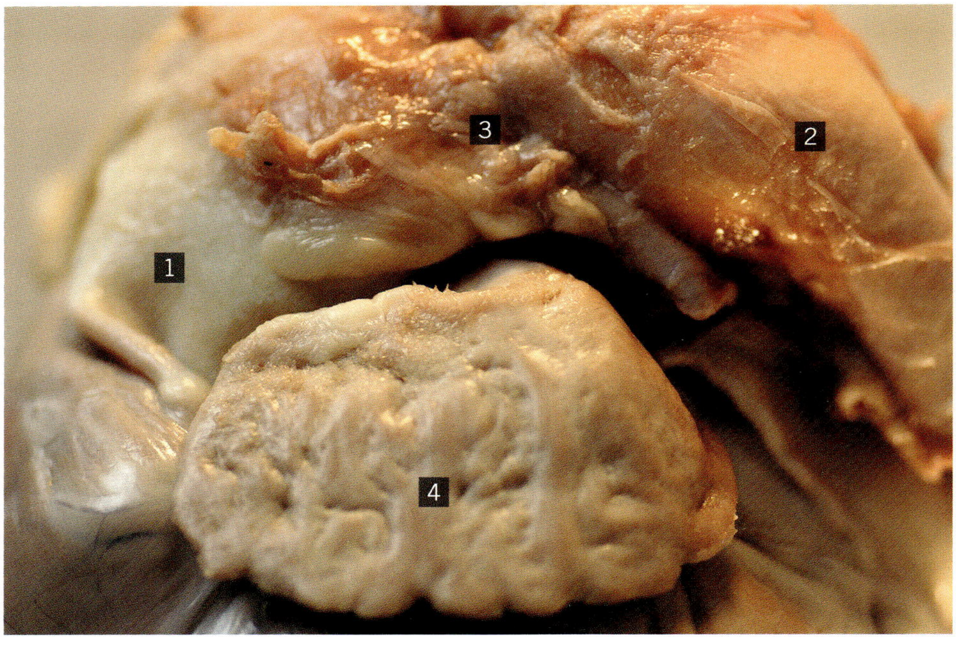

[1 Pulmonary trunk]

[2 Descending aorta]

[3 Ductus arteriosus]

[4 Dilated left atrial appendage as a result of volume overload]

Figure 17. Dilation of the pulmonary trunk and aorta as a result of turbulent flows.

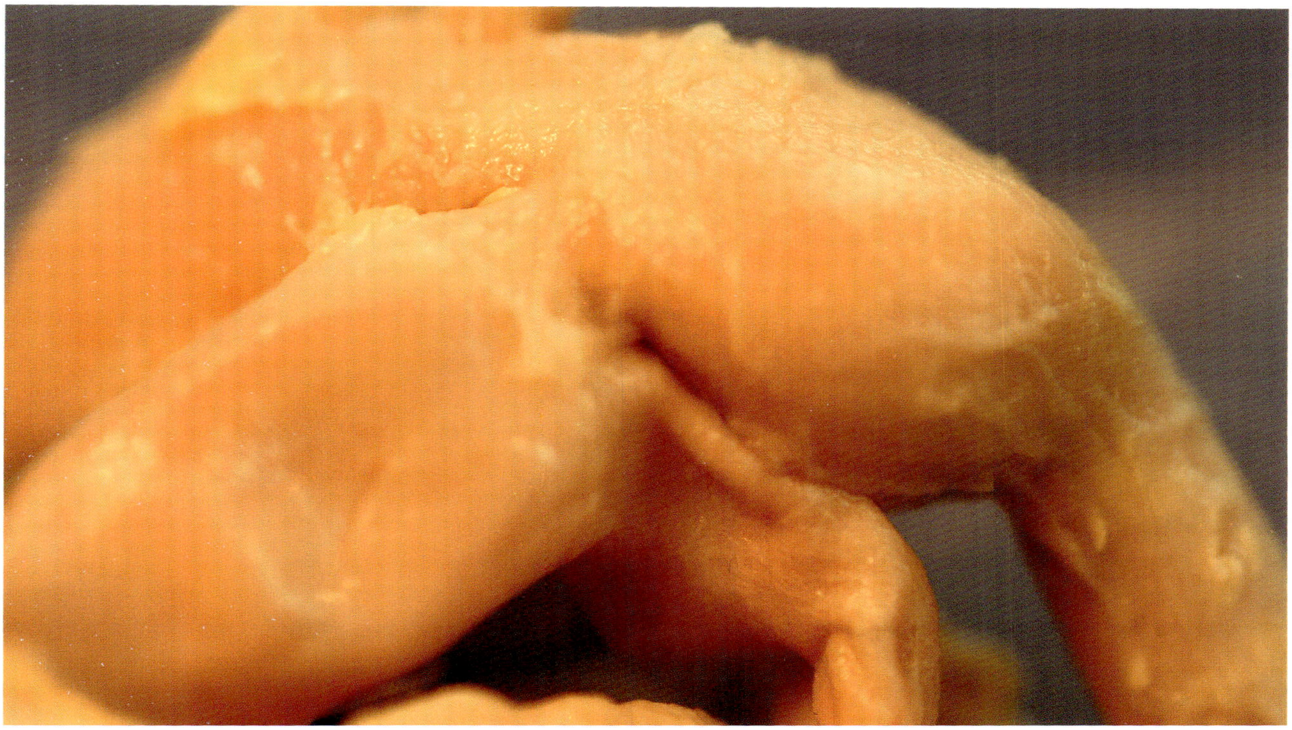

Figure 18. Dilation of the pulmonary trunk and of the descending aorta.

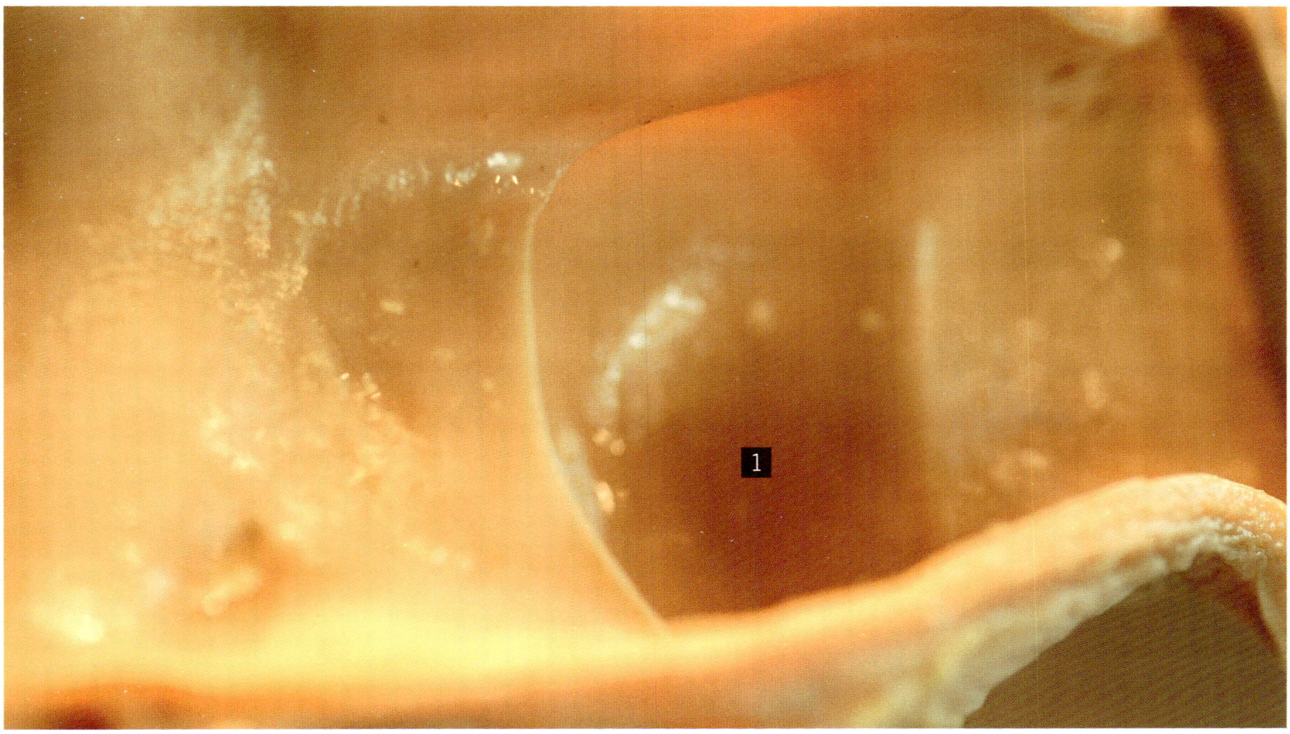

[1 Dilation of the posterior descending aorta at the opening of the duct]

Figure 19. Sagittal section of the descending aorta.

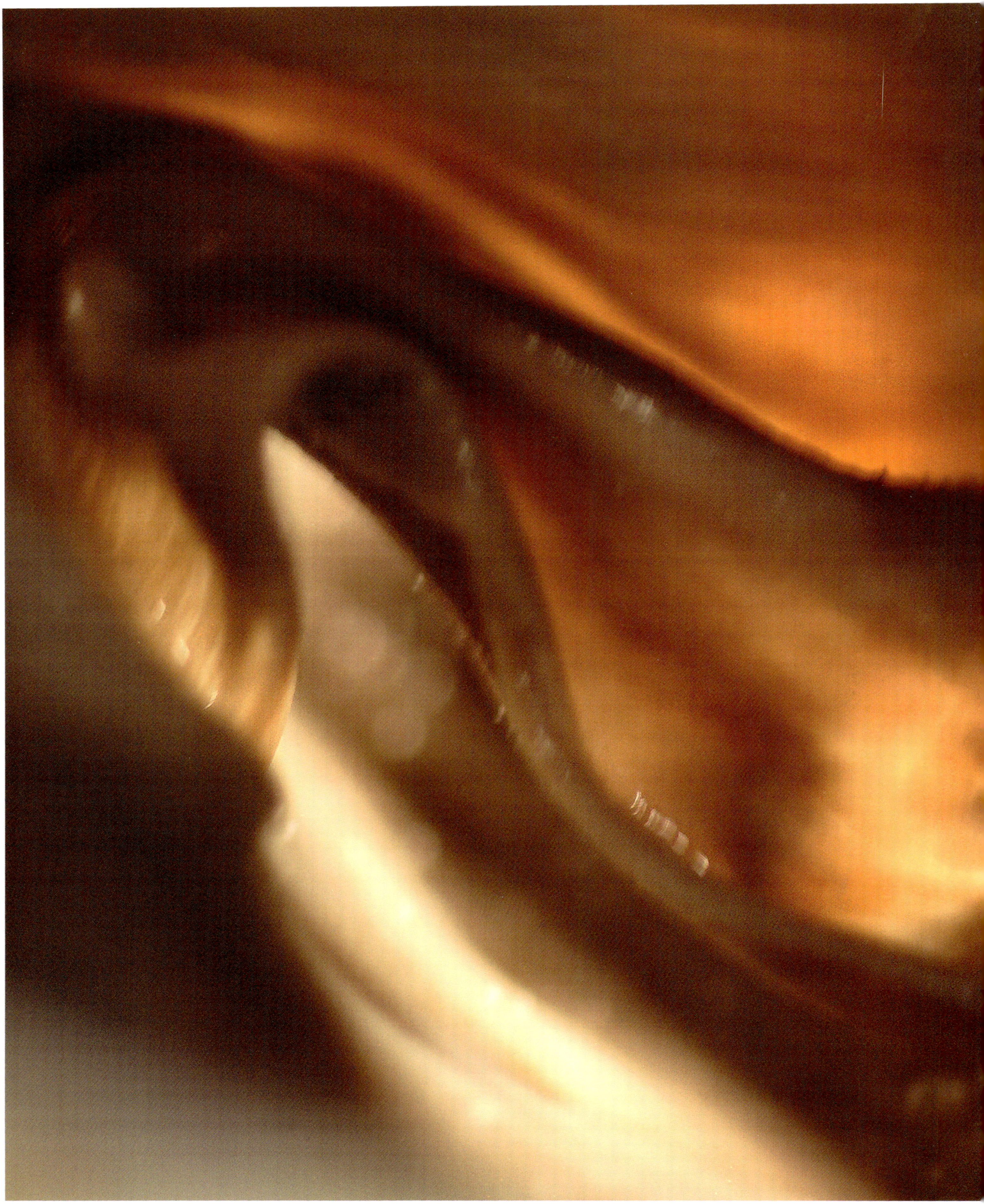

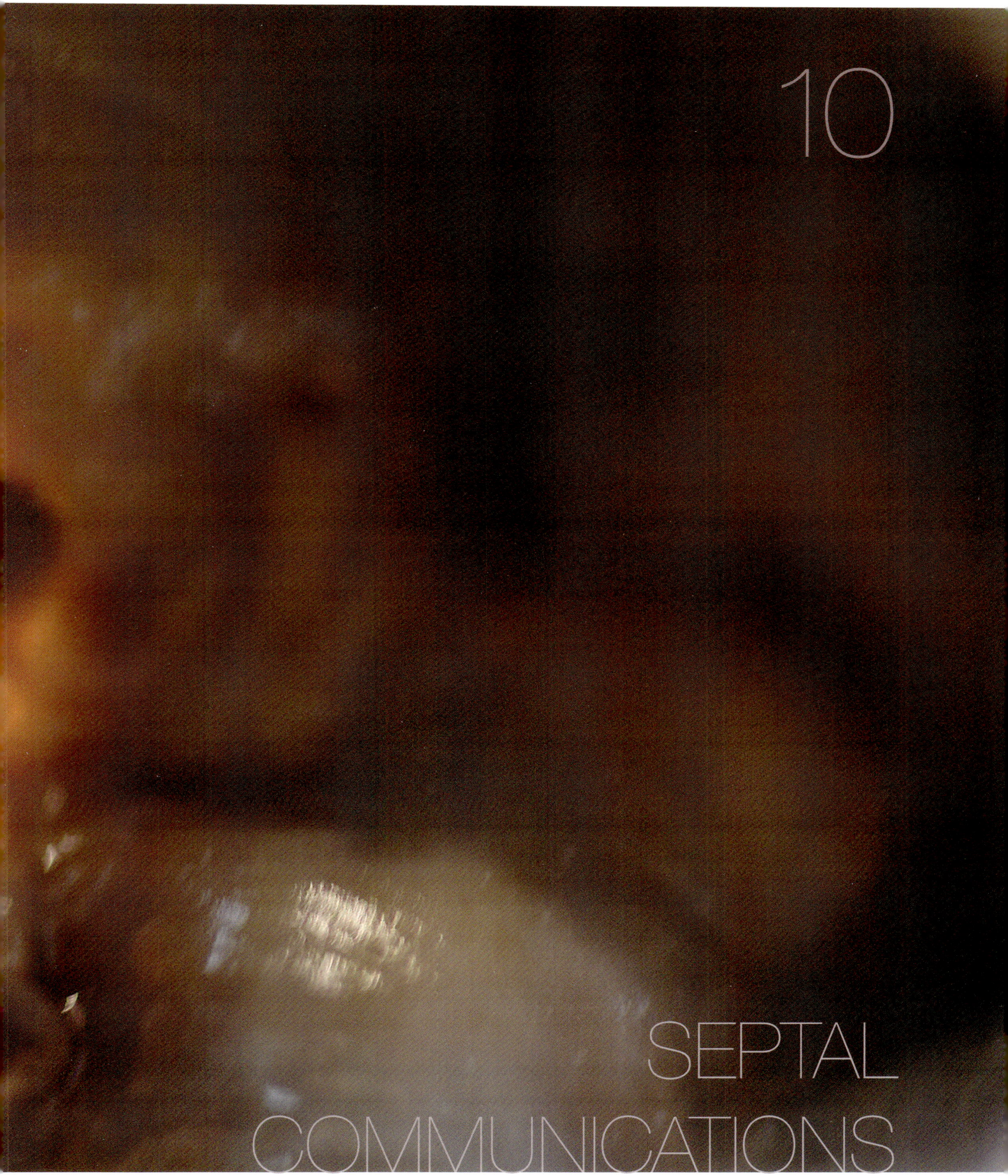

10

SEPTAL COMMUNICATIONS

During embryonic development, the atria and ventricles form a common chamber, the atrioventricular canal. The growth of the cardiac septa (atrial septum and ventricular septum) causes its division, thus originating the four-chambered heart.

ATRIAL COMMUNICATIONS

A proper knowledge of the embryonic development of the atrial septum is important in order to understand the different communications that may be found between the right and left atria.

We can talk about three types of defects: sinus venosus defects, ostium primum or secundum defects and patent foramen ovale.

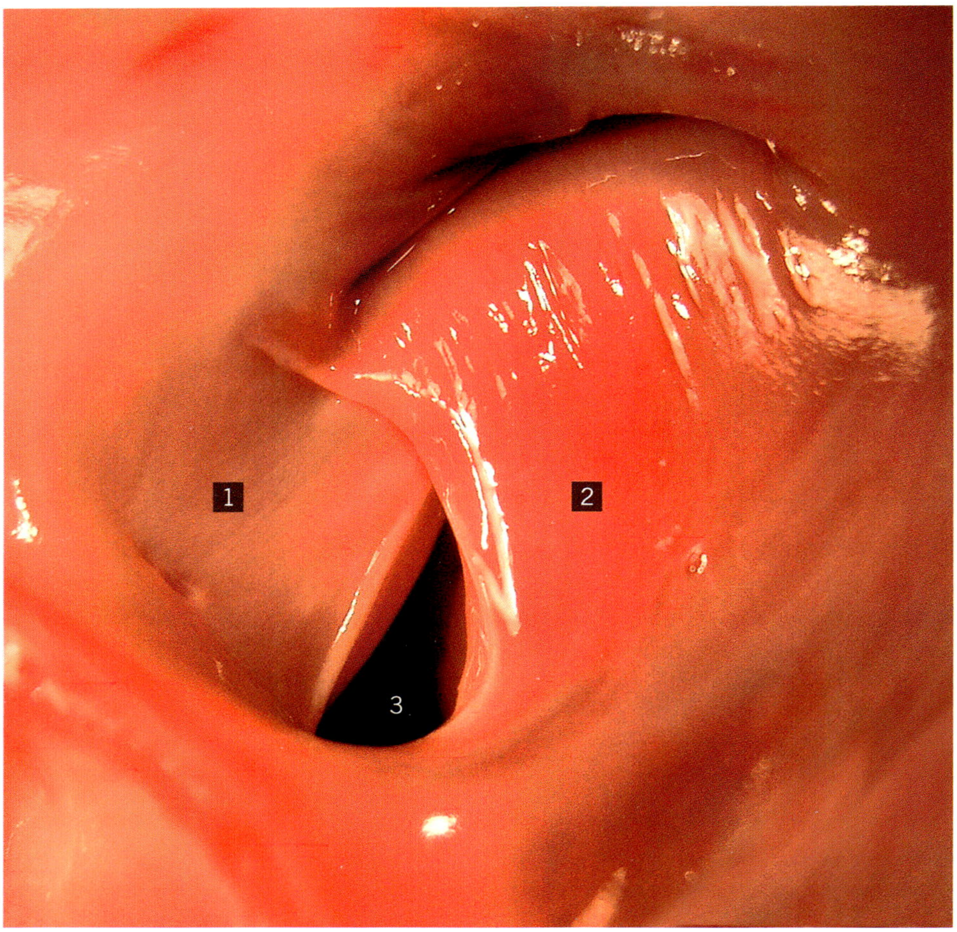

[1 Septum primum]

[2 Septum secundum]

[3 Foramen ovale]

Figure 1. Atrial septation.

ATRIAL SEPTATION PROCESS

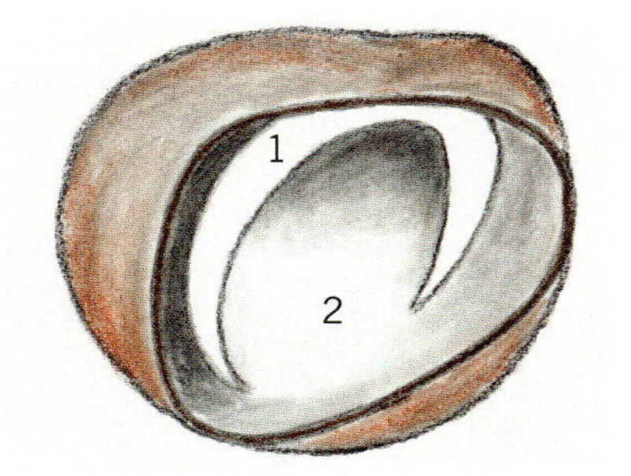

Figure 2. The septum primum starts to form, leaving an orifice of communication, the ostium primum, on the side of the growing edge. View of the illustrations from the right hand side.

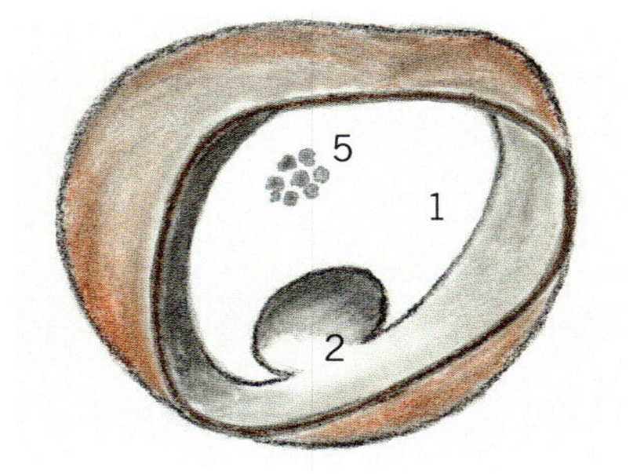

Figure 3. The septum primum keeps growing and the ostium primum progressively decreases in size. At the same time, due to a mechanism of apoptosis, the ostium secundum starts to form.

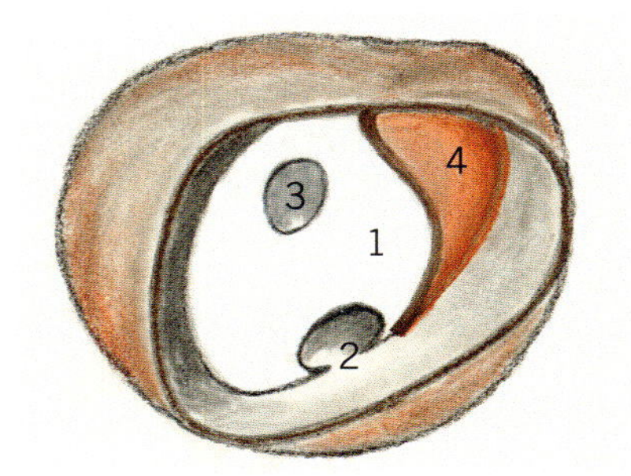

Figure 4. The septum primum keeps growing and the ostium primum decreases in size; the ostium secundum is now totally formed and the septum secundum starts to develop.

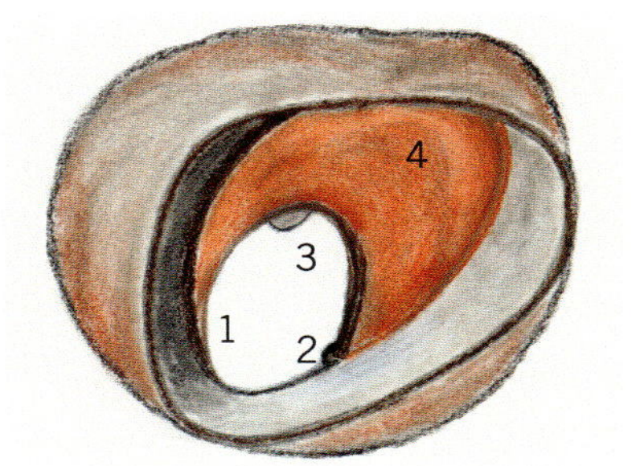

Figure 5. The ostium primum has practically disappeared; the septum secundum keeps developing and covers the ostium secundum.

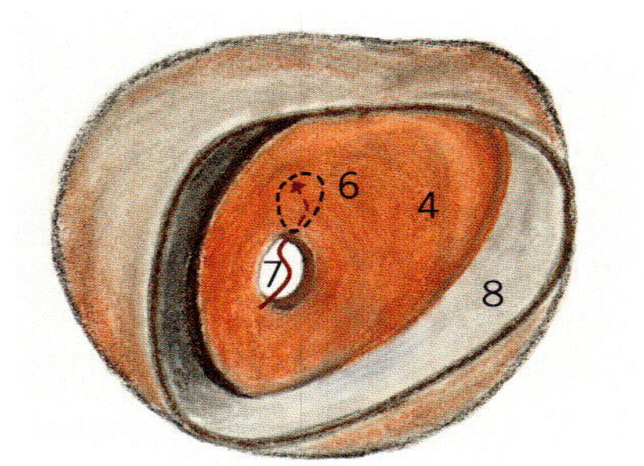

Figure 6. End of the atrial septation; the septum secundum has covered almost the whole septum primum, leaving only a small "defect" in the central area, the foramen ovale, which will facilitate the passage of blood towards the ostium secundum, thus maintaining the right-left flow until birth.

1 Septum primum

2 Ostium primum

3 Ostium secundum

4 Septum secundum

5 Start of formation of the ostium secundum

6 Area of the septum secundum that occludes the ostium secundum

7 Foramen ovale (blood will pass in the direction going from 7 to 6 until birth)

8 Right atrium

The division originates from the two septa. The first one, named septum primum, is a thin septum of mesenchymal nature that develops from the craniodorsal area to the endocardial cushions. As it grows, the lower free margin delimits the ostium primum, which maintains the communication between the two atria. The proliferation of the septum primum and endocardial cushions leads to their union, which closes the ostium primum. Before the closure of this ostium, resorption takes place in the dorsal part of the septum, which forms a second opening, the ostium secundum. This allows blood to continue passing from one cavity to another before the closure of the ostium primum.

At the same time as the previous events take place, a new septum, the septum secundum, starts to develop to the right side of the septum primum. This new septum is of muscular nature, with a thickness that is similar to that of the atrial wall. It grows in a semilunar shape from the craniodorsal area to the floor of the atrium, as well as caudally to close the ostium secundum and towards the caudal vena cava. This septum is incomplete and has an orifice in its centre, named the foramen ovale. The passage of blood is maintained between these two orifices –foramen ovale and ostium secundum– until birth, after which the differences of pressure are inverted and the thin septum primum is pushed against the thick septum secundum, thus closing the communication.

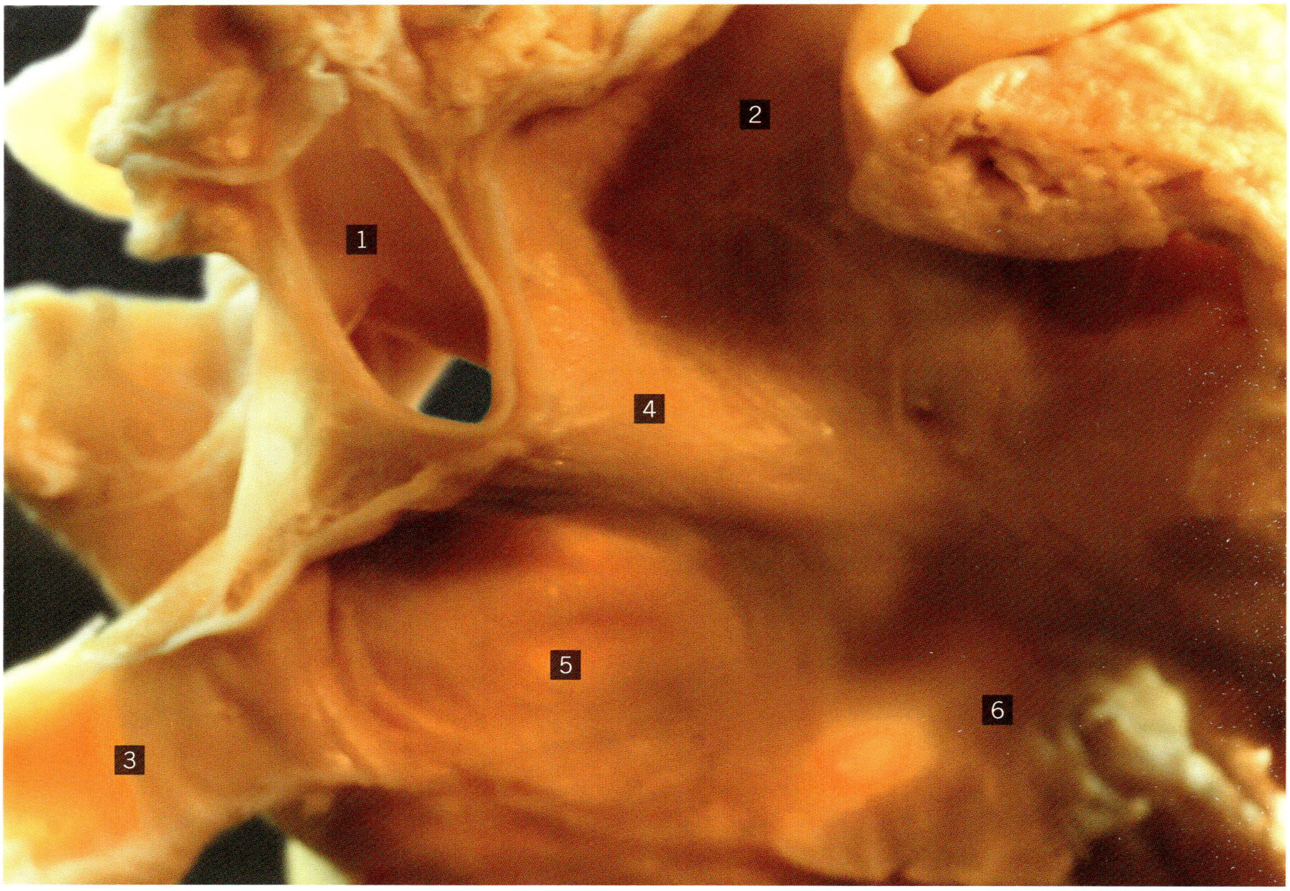

Figure 7. Sinus venosus atrial septal defect located in the area adjacent to the atrium, close to the cranial vena cava.

[1 Defect] [2 Cranial vena cava] [3 Caudal vena cava]

[4 Intervenous tubercle] [5 Fossa ovalis] [6 Septal leaflet of the tricuspid valve]

We can talk about three types of defects: sinus venosus defects, ostium primum or secundum defects and patent foramen ovale,

SINUS VENOSUS DEFECTS

They are located in the area adjacent to the atrium, usually close to the cranial vena cava, to the caudal vena cava, or, more rarely, at the opening of the coronary sinus.

[1 Defect]

[2 Mitral valve]

[3 Caudal vena cava]

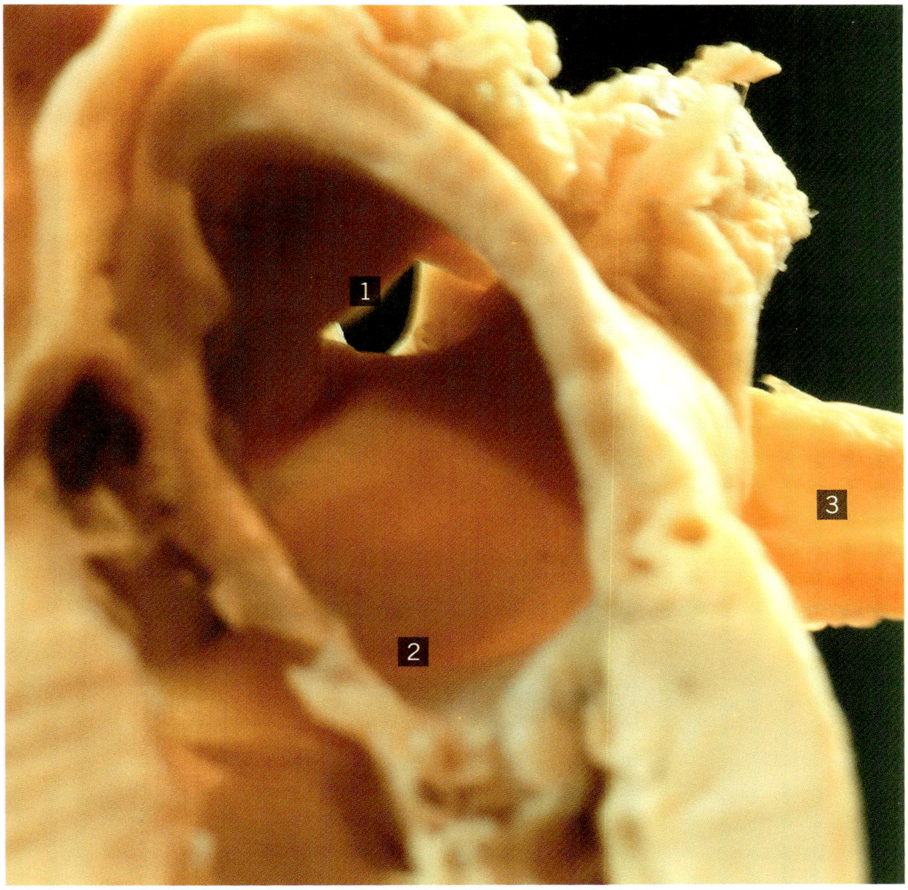

Figure 8. Same defect as in the previous image seen from the left atrium.

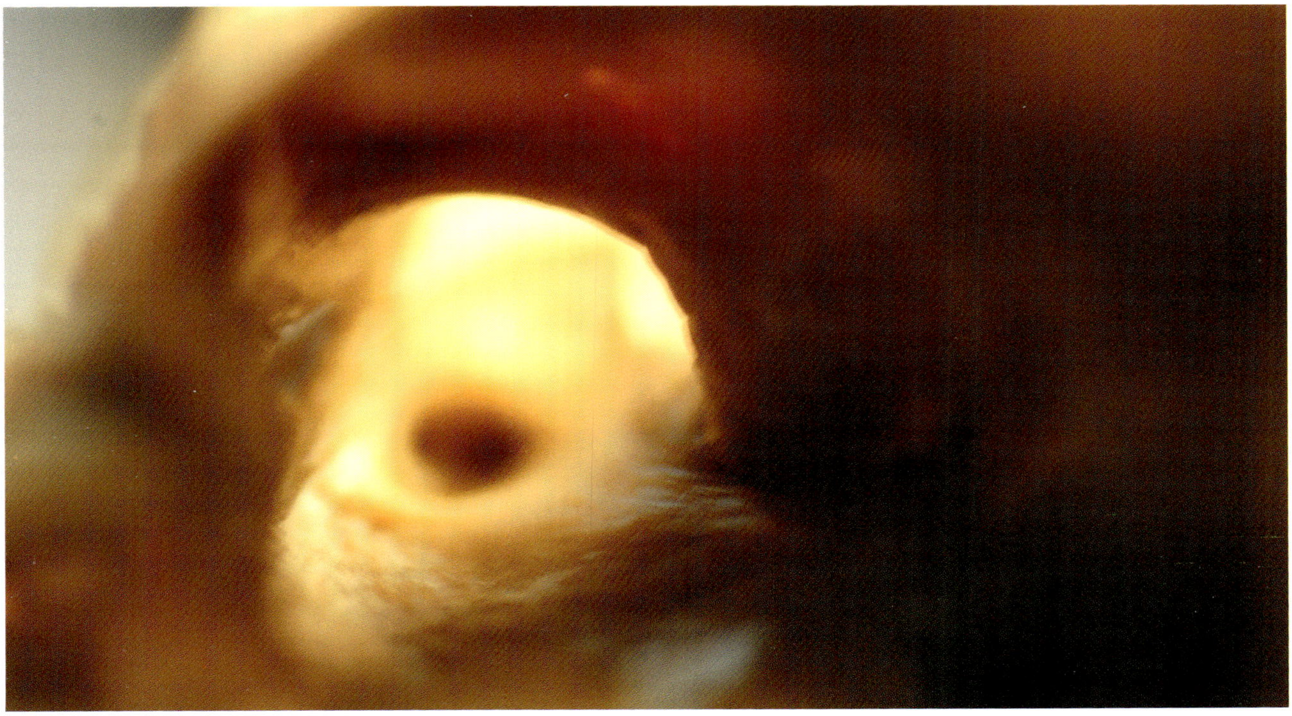

Figure 9. Sinus venosus defect located on the coronary sinus.

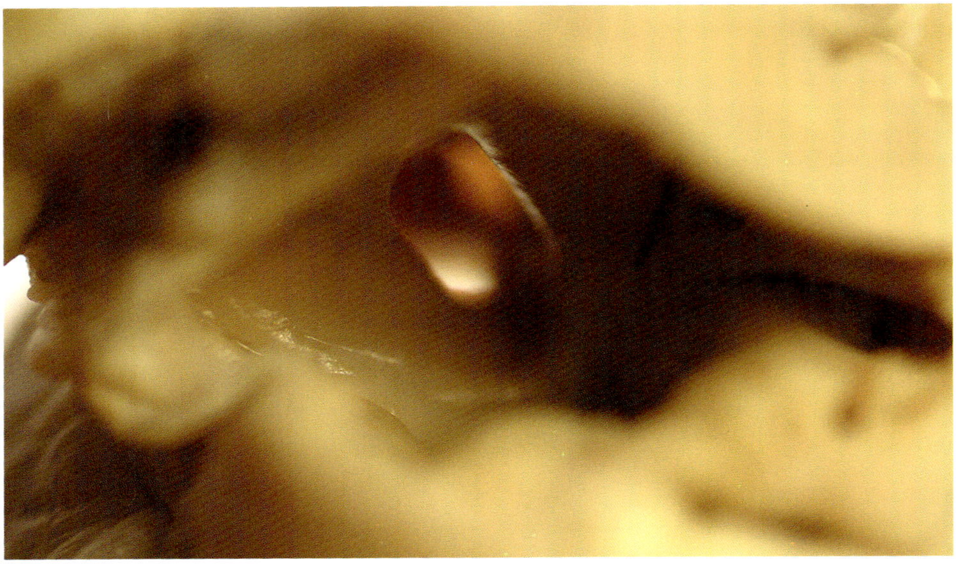

Figure 10. Ostium secundum defect located centrally in the right atrium, occupying nearly the whole fossa ovalis.

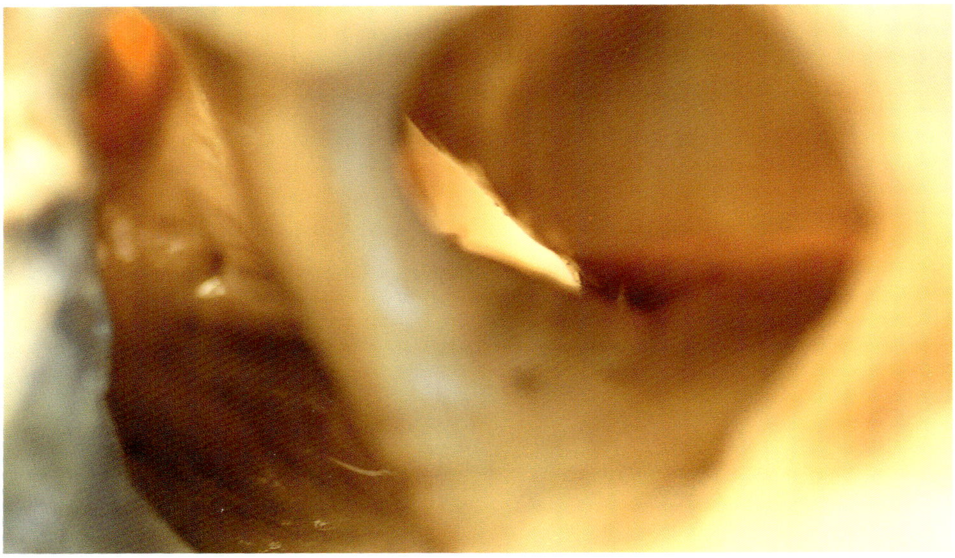

Figure 11. Ostium secundum defect located cranial to the intervenous tubercle. This location is more frequent in ostium primum defects but, in this case, the more central position of the defect seems to indicate that this is an ostium secundum defect.

OSTIUM PRIMUM OR SECUNDUM DEFECTS

They are located in the central area and are usually due to a too wide ostium secundum or to hypoplasia of the septum secundum, which does not completely cover the area of the orifice. This is usually the most frequent type of defect.

As regards ostium primum defects, they may be due to the persistence of this orifice or to a failure in the closing of the endocardial cushions, in which case the atrioventricular valves may be involved.

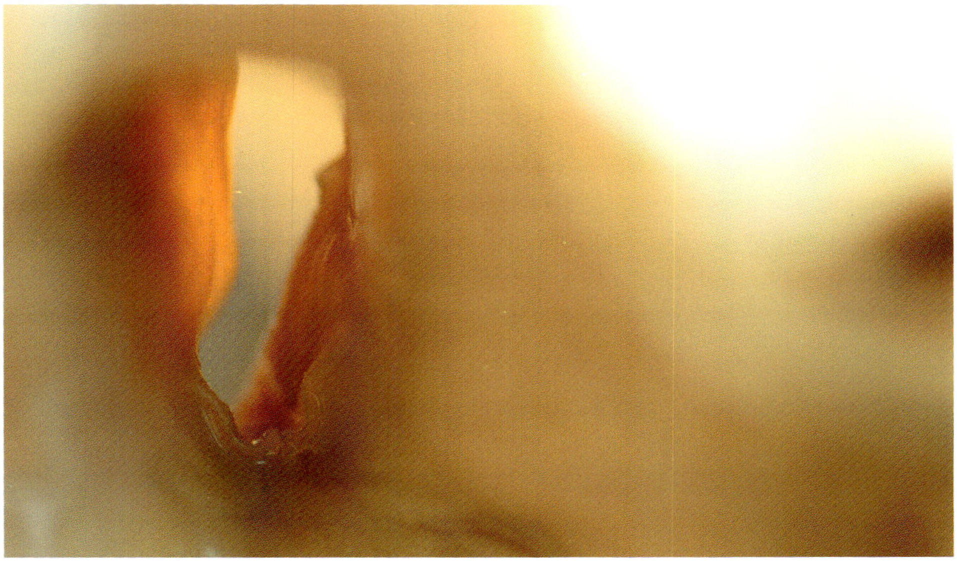

Figure 12. Same defect as in the previous image seen from the left atrium. Remnants of the thin septum primum can be observed.

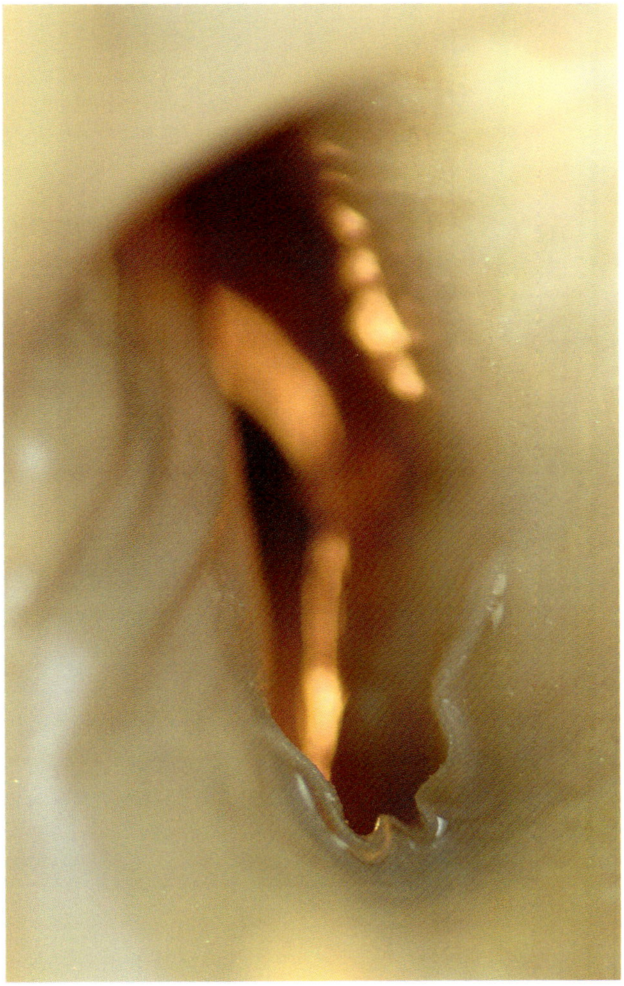

Figure 13 . Detail of the same defect as in the previous images, where the remnants of the septum primum may be observed. View from the left atrium.

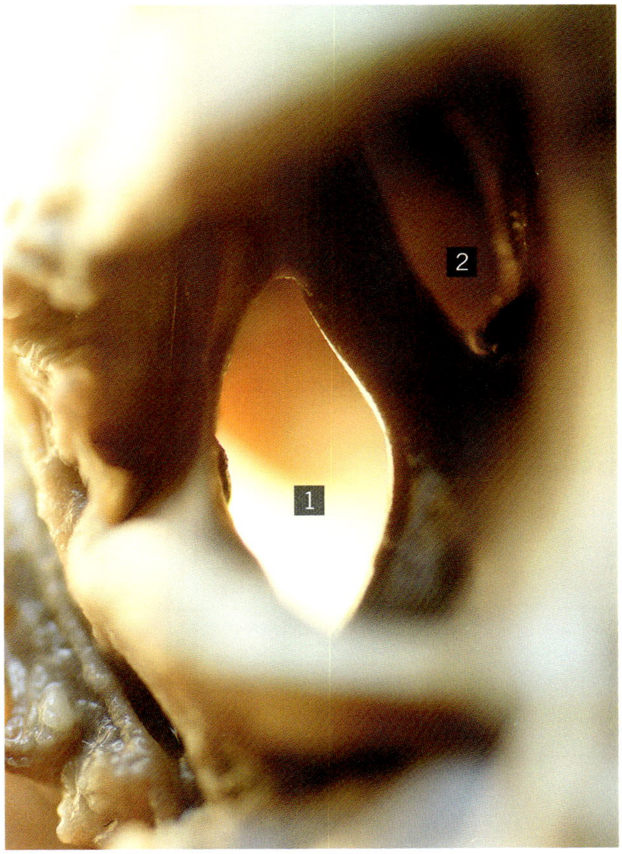

Figure 14. View from the left atrium of a double interatrial defect. No description of this type of double defect has been found in the literature.

[1 Cranial ostium primum defect]

[2 Caudal ostium secundum defect]

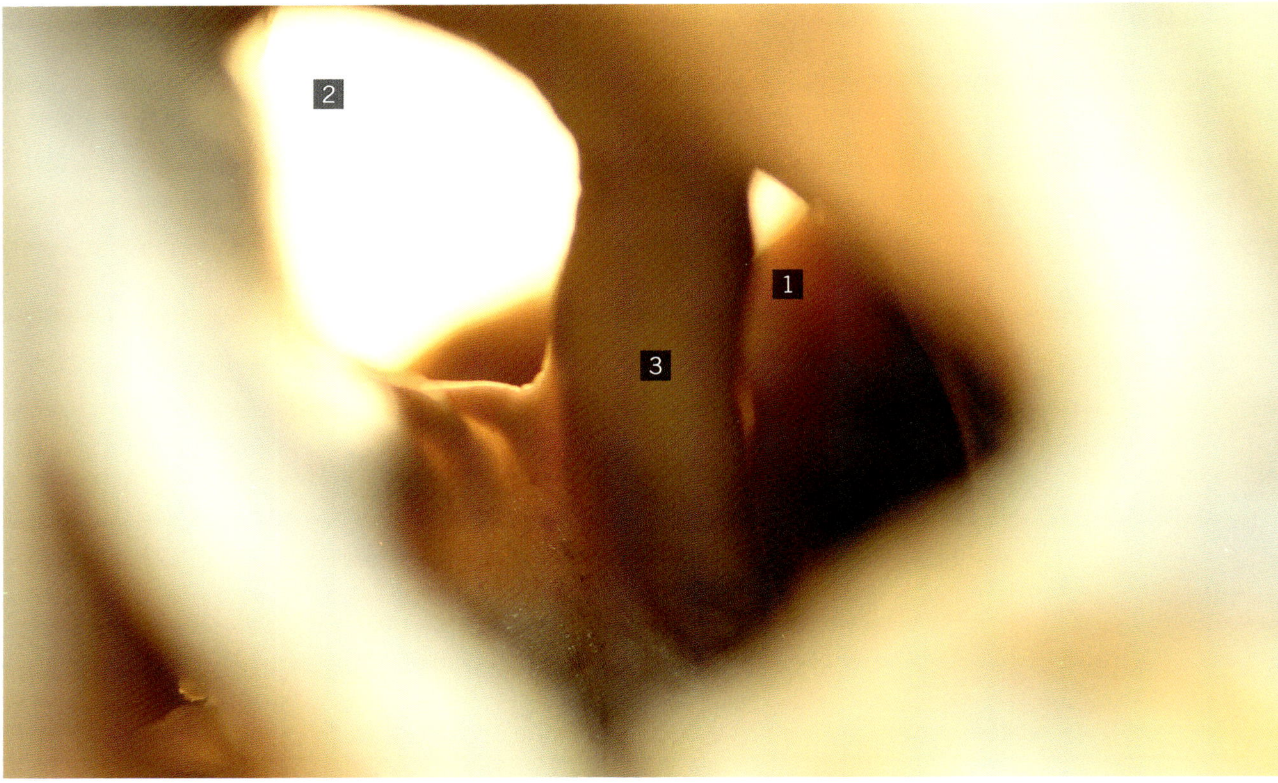

Figure 15. View of the double communication from the right atrium.

[1 Cranial ostium primum defect]

[2 Caudal ostium secundum defect]

[3 Remnant of interatrial septum corresponding to the area of location of the intervenous tubercle]

[4 Coronary sinus]

[5 Dyplastic mitral valve]

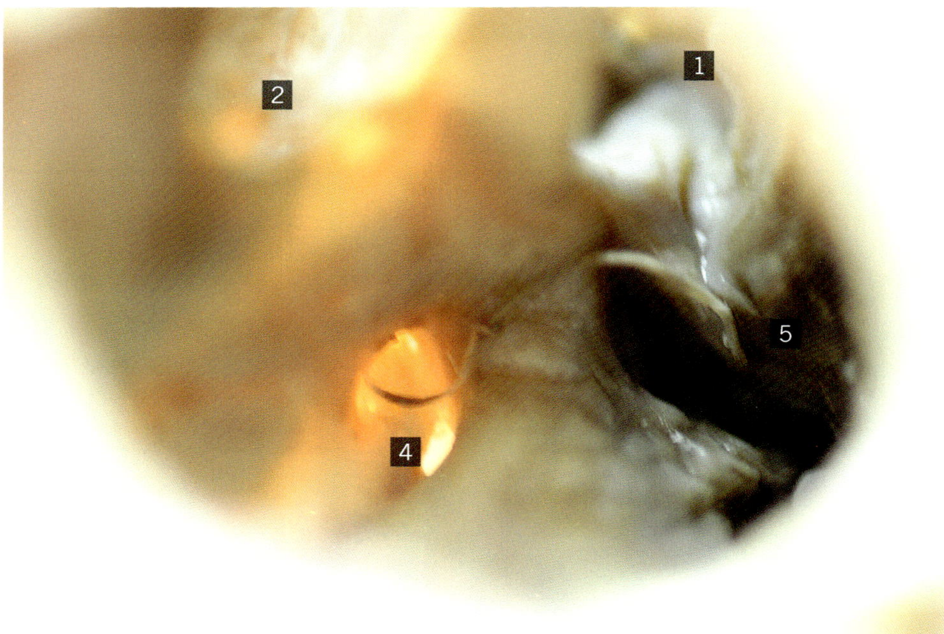

Figure 16. Same lesion as in the previous image with a view of the atrial floor.

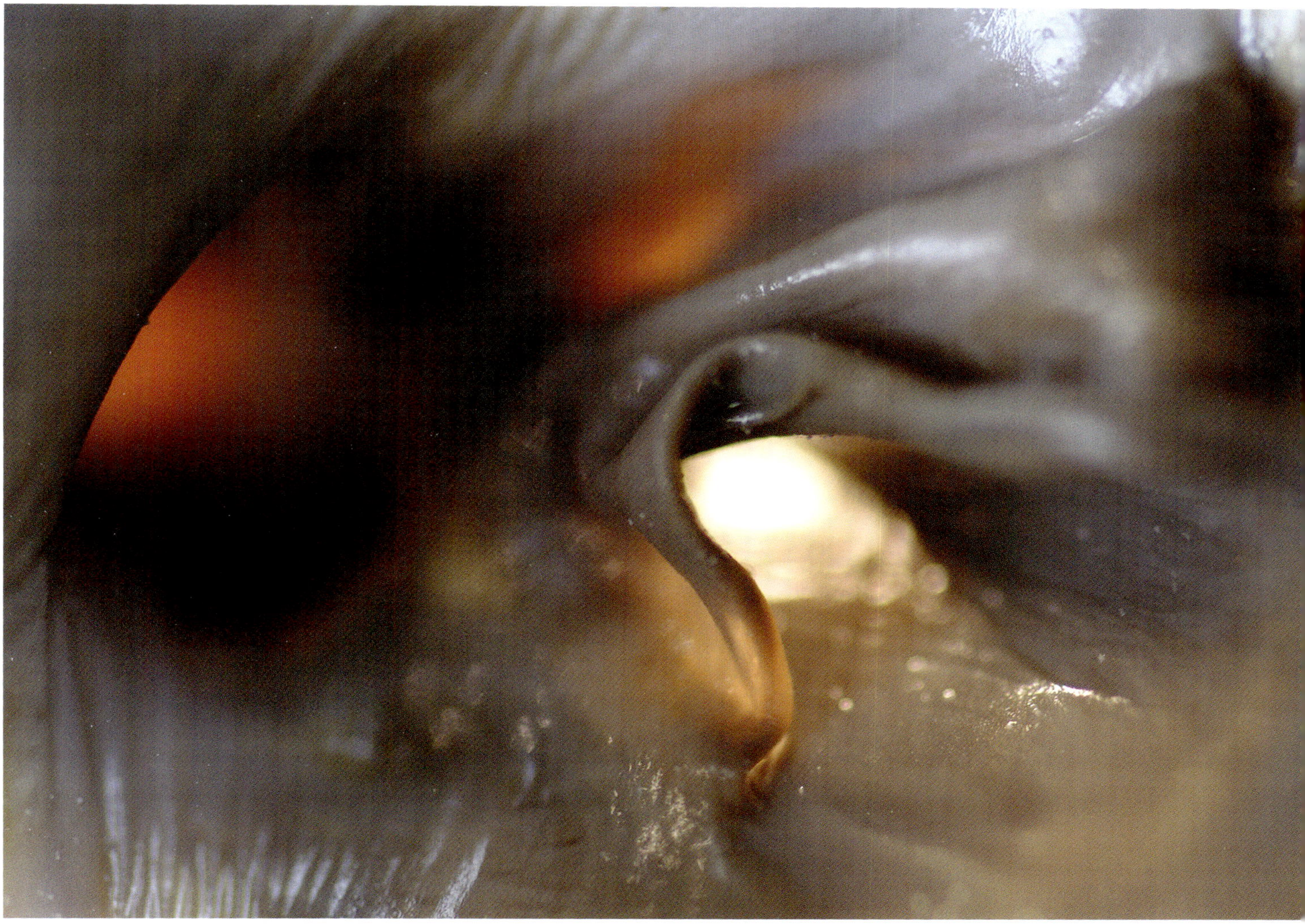

Figure 17. Patent foramen ovale. View from the left atrium. The so-called valve of the foramen ovale is formed by the remnants of the thin septum primum.

PATENT FORAMEN OVALE

In this case we cannot talk about a congenital defect as such, since the persistence of this communication is due, in general, to failures in the normal inversion of the pressure gradients that occurs after birth. Such failures are usually associated with other defects such as pulmonary stenosis or mitral dysplasia.

These defects, especially if they are small, can easily go unnoticed and may not be diagnosed as they do not usually cause any clinical signs and are often haemodinamically silent.

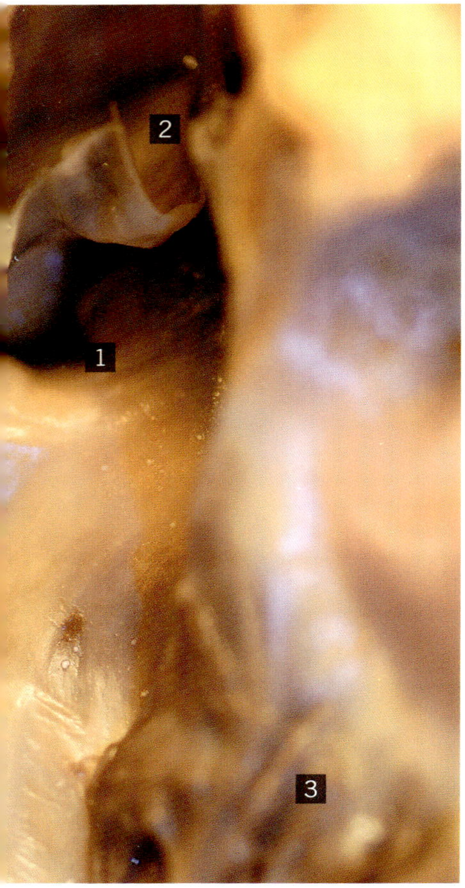

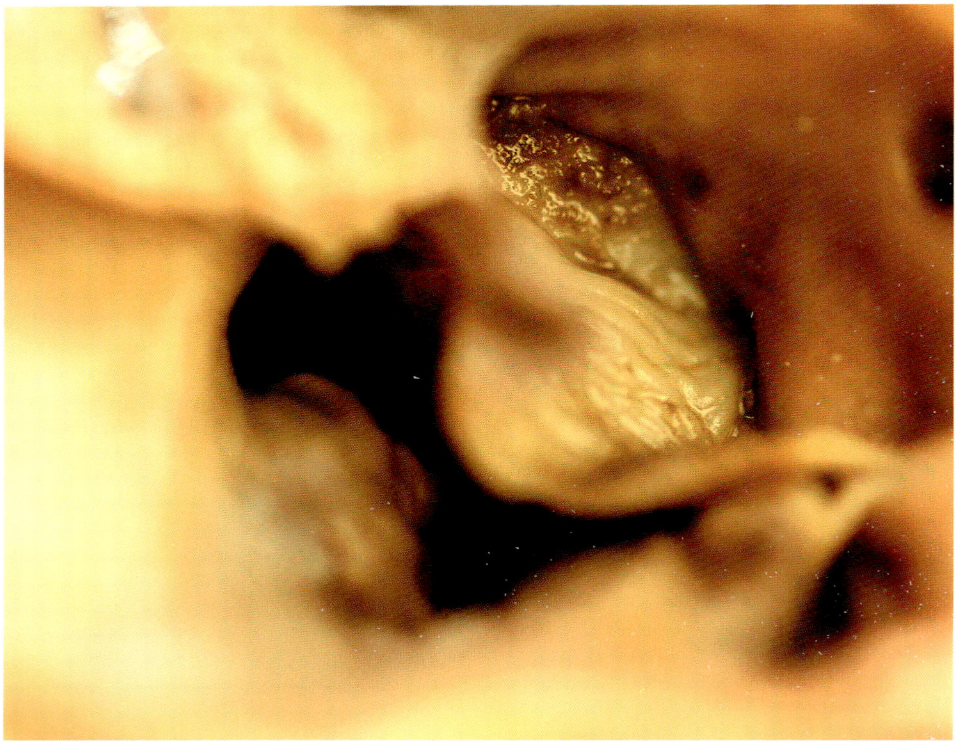

Figure 19. Interventricular communication and left coronary cusp.

Figure 18. Interventricular communication.

[1 Communication]

[2 Non-coronary aortic cusp]

[3 Cranial leaflet of the mitral valve]

VENTRICULAR COMMUNICATIONS

The interventricular septum may be divided in several parts:

- The **inlet septum**, which extends from the orifice of the tricuspid valve to the papillary muscles.
- The **trabecular septum**, which occupies the apical part of the septum and is characterised by numerous trabeculae.
- The **outlet septum**, which extends from the supraventricular crest to the pulmonary valve.
- The **membranous septum**, which is a small region defined by the lower part of the aortic valve on the left side and by the area that goes from the septal leaflet of the tricuspid valve to the pulmonary valve on the right side.

Interventricular septal defects are generally perimembranous, since defects in other areas are extremely rare in dogs and cats.

[1 Communication close to the valvular commissure]

[2 Mural leaflet of the tricuspid valve]

[3 Papillary muscles]

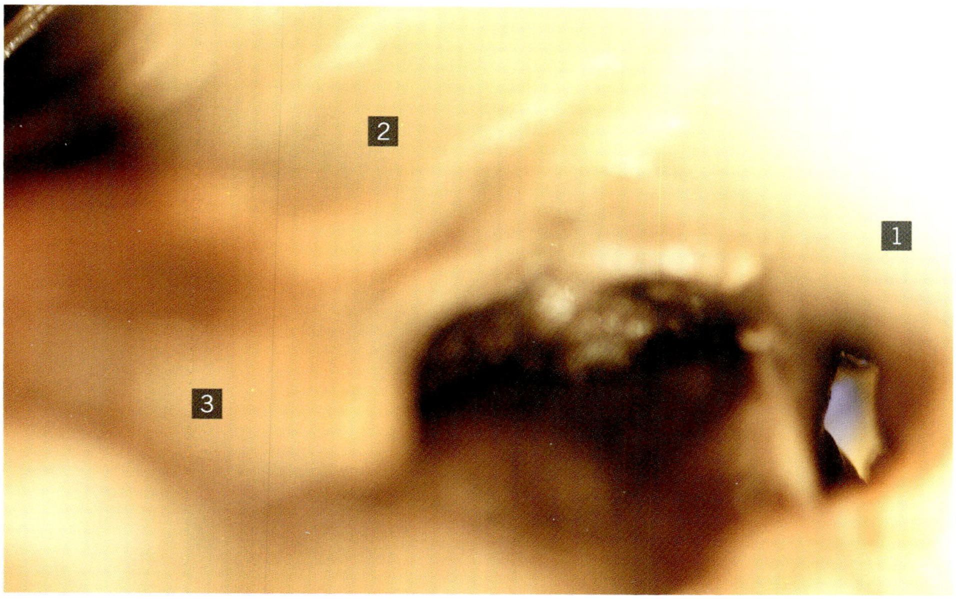

Figure 20. Interventricular communication. View from the right ventricle.

[1 Communication]

[2 Tricuspid valve]

[3 Infundibulum]

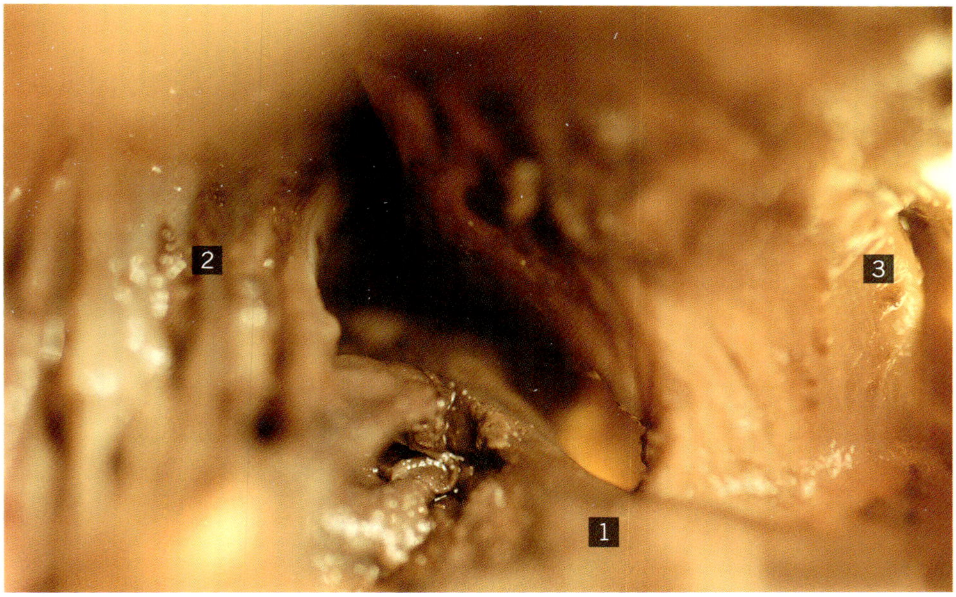

Figure 21. Interventricular communication. View from the right ventricle.

These perimembranous defects can be located, on the right side, in the part of the septum that is located in the cranial area of the septal leaflet, close to its commissure and, on the left side, below the right coronary and non-coronary cusps of the aortic valve.

Except in the case of the English Springer Spaniel breed, in which some cases of hereditary transmission of interventricular communication have been documented, there does not seem to be any predisposition to septal defects in any dog or cat breed.

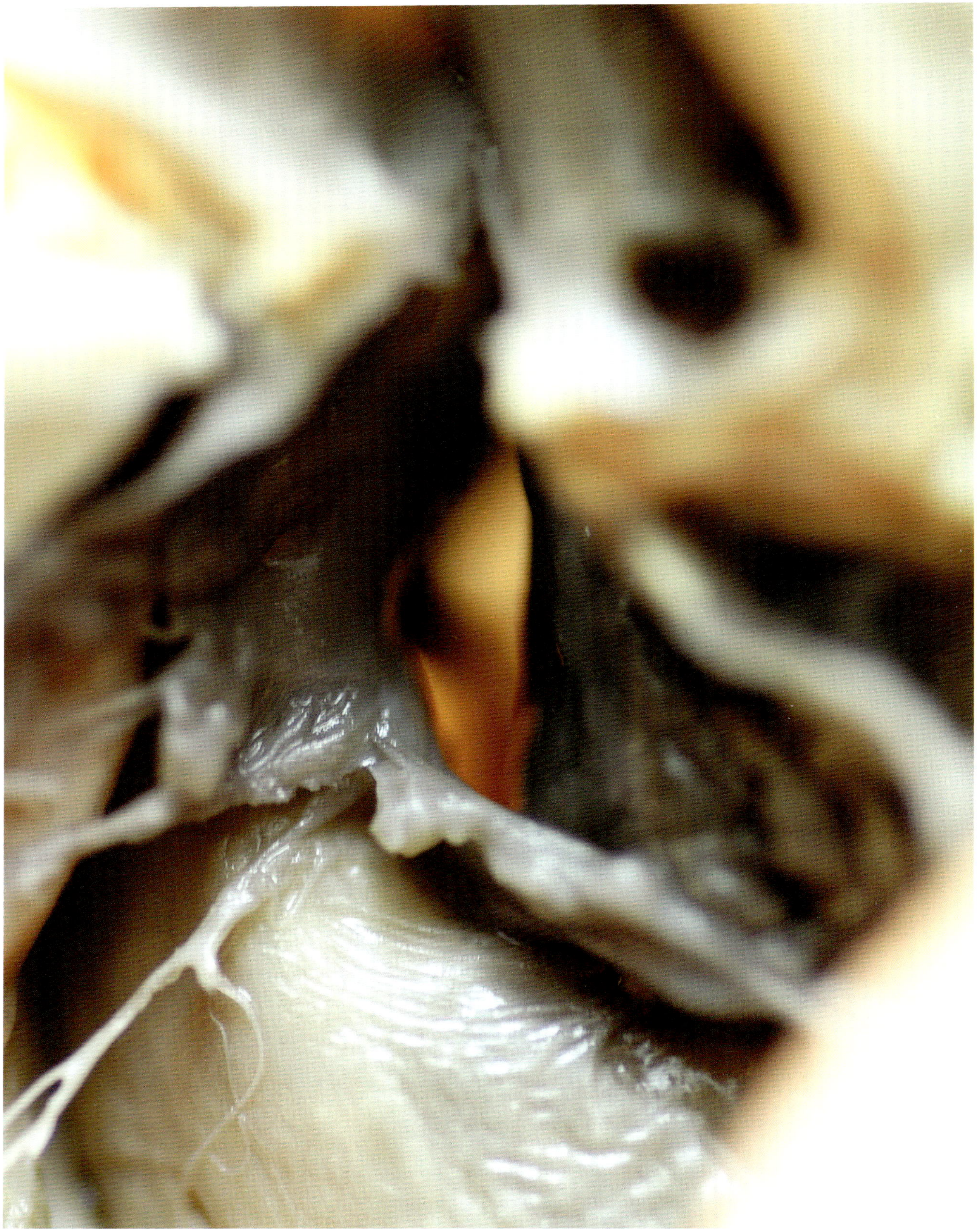

Figure 22. Interventricular communication. The defect is located in the muscular area of the septum. Aplasia of the mitral valve can also be observed.

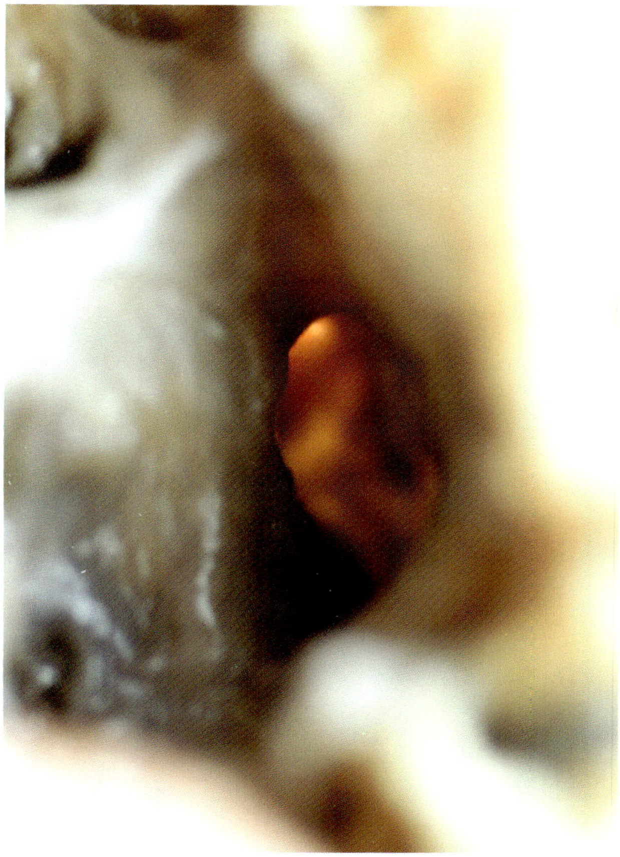

Figure 23. Interventricular communication. Same defect as in the previous image seen from the right side.

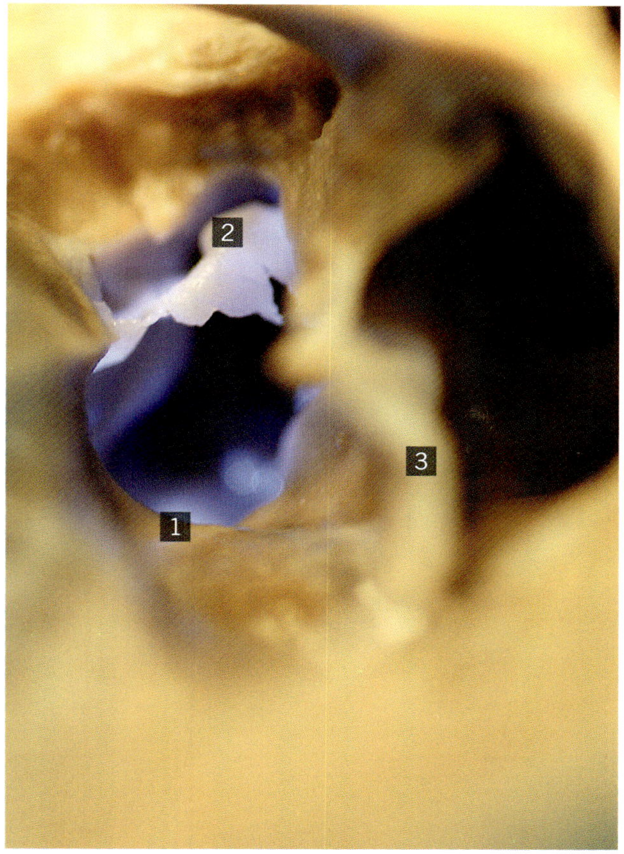

Figure 24. Interventricular communication in a tetralogy of Fallot.

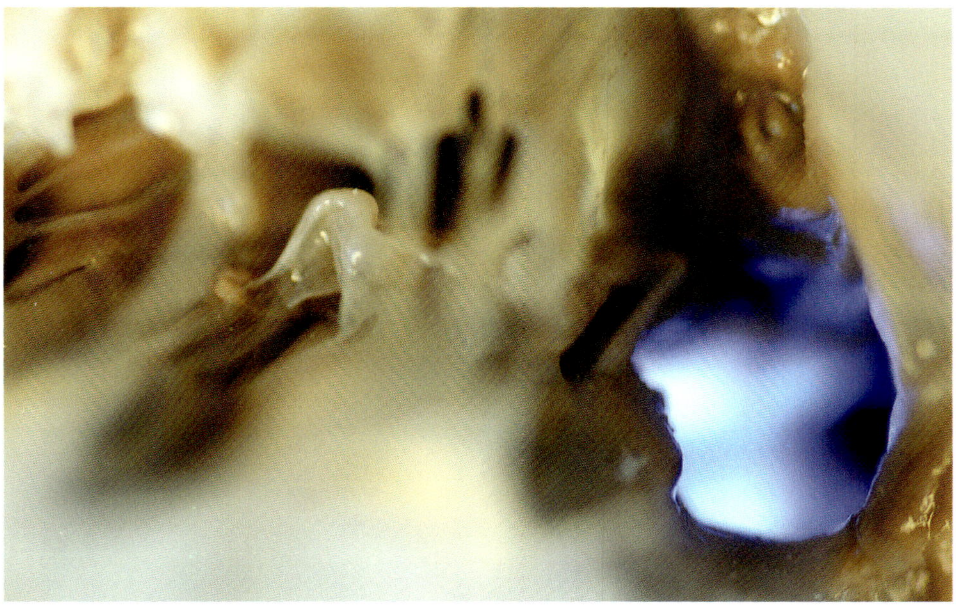

Figure 25. Interventricular communication. Infundibular defect. The tricuspid valve can be seen on the left.

[1 Communication]

[2 Aortic cusp]

[3 Cranial leaflet of the mitral valve]

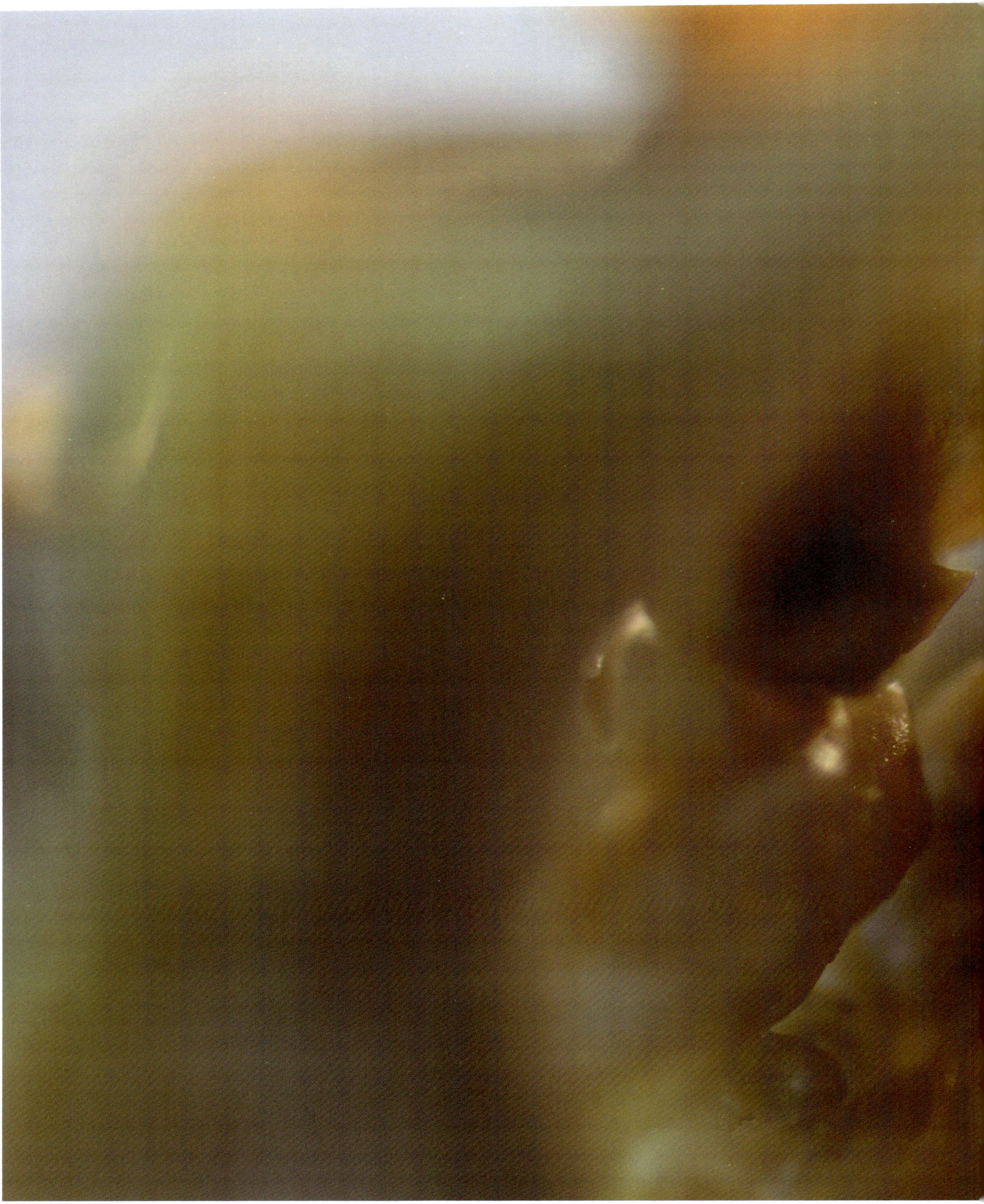

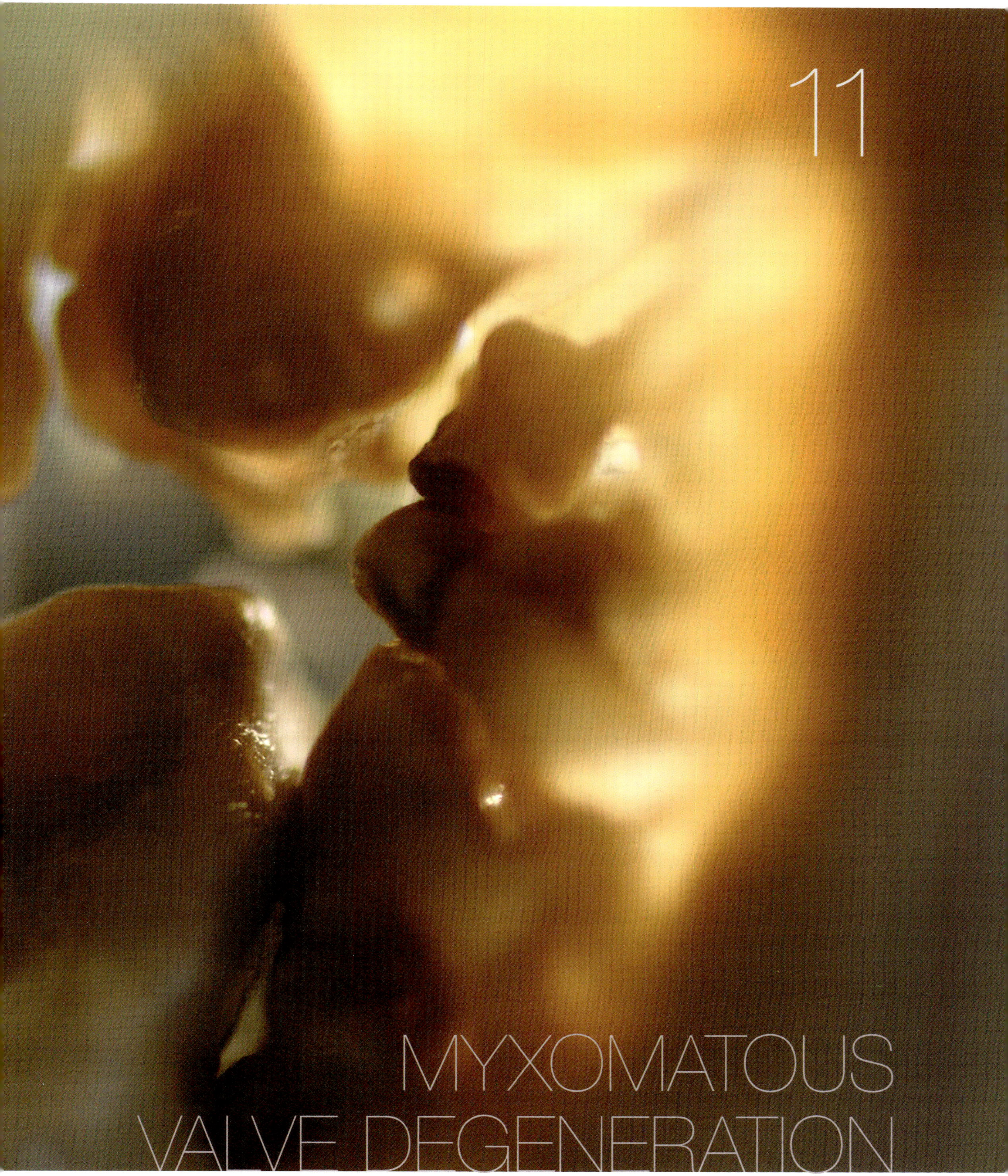

11

MYXOMATOUS VALVE DEGENERATION

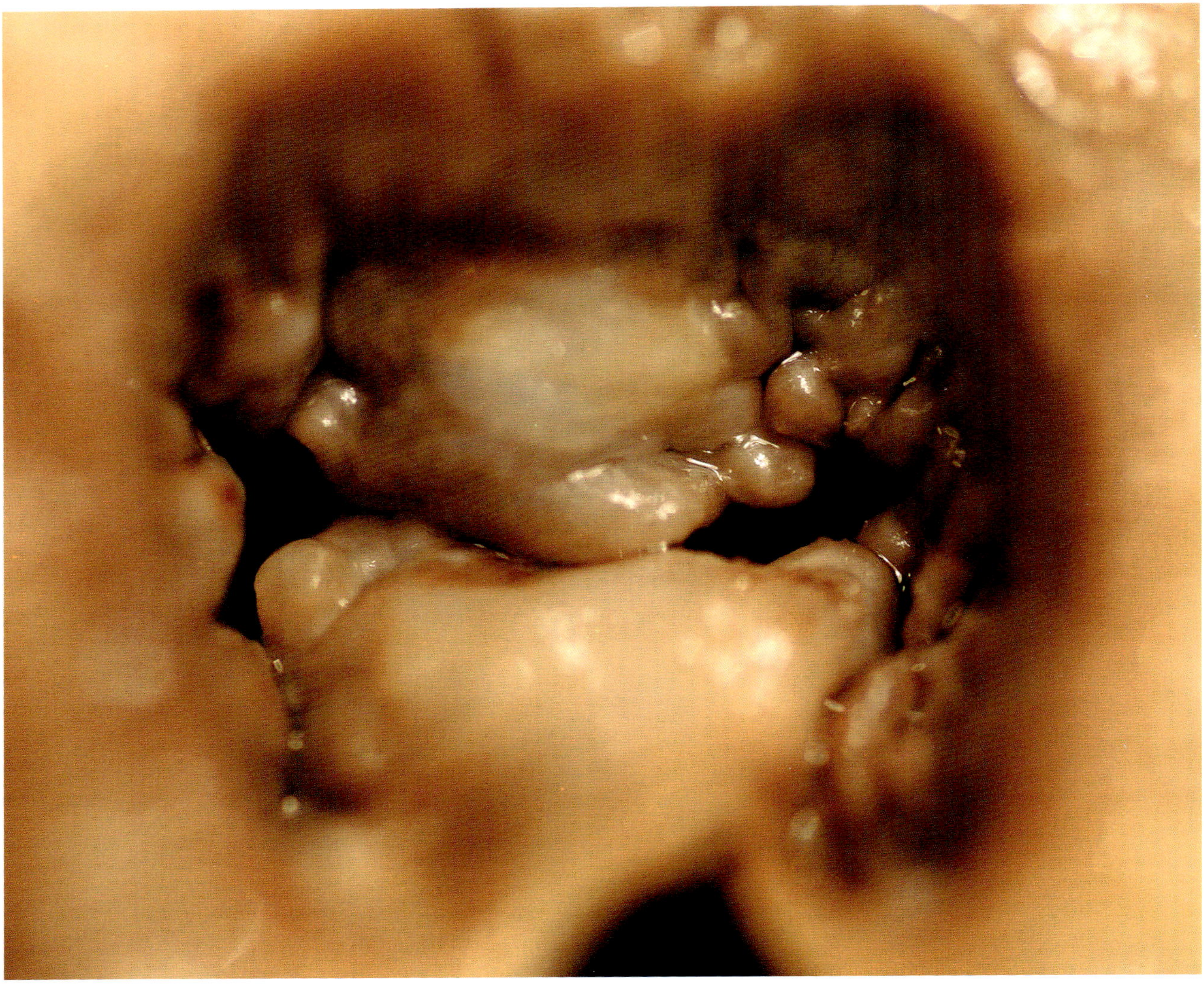

Figure 1. The main characteristic of myxomatous valve degeneration is the development of valvular insufficiency. In the image, seen from the left atrium, the incompetent coaptation of the leaflets of the mitral valve may be observed. This is going to result in regurgitation from the ventricle to the atrium, with the production of a turbulent flow, which (systolic ejection murmur).

Myxomatous valve degeneration is also known as acquired chronic valvular disease or valvular encocardiosis. It is a degenerative alteration of unknown origin that affects the leaflets and chordae tendineae of the atrioventricular valves. The mitral valve is the most frequently affected valve (60 %). On many occasions both the mitral and tricuspid valves are affected (30 %), while the tricuspid valve is the only affected valve on very rare occasions (10 %). It is the most important cause of heart disease in the veterinary practice and makes up about 75 % of these diseases in dogs.

Small-sized breeds and dogs of more than 8 years of age are the most predisposed to this disease. It is uncommon to find the disease in dogs under 5 years of age, except in Cavalier King Charles Spaniels, as signs may be observed with only one year of age in this breed.

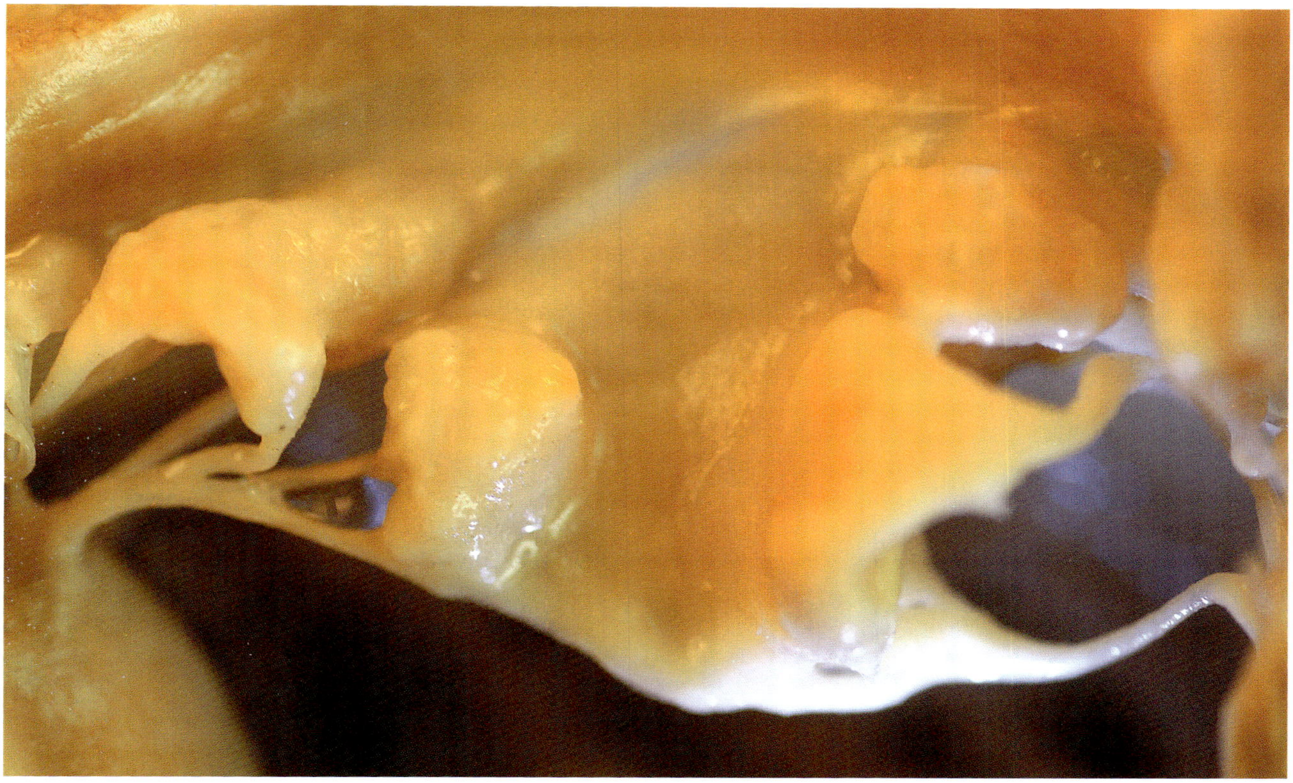

Figure 2. The mitral valve is the most affected valve. Cranial leaflet with endocardiosis.

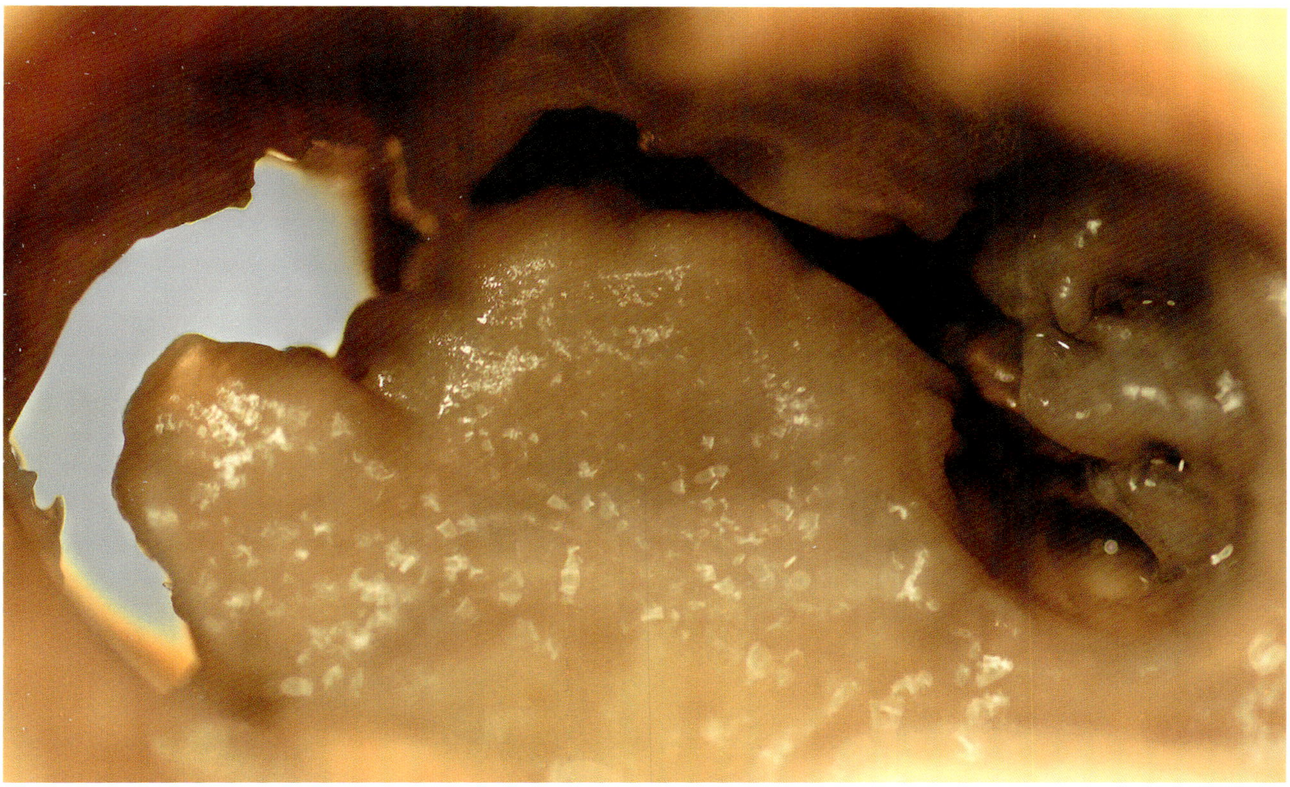

Figure 3. The tricuspid valve may also be affected, although it is the only one to be affected in less than 10 % of the cases. View from the right atrium.

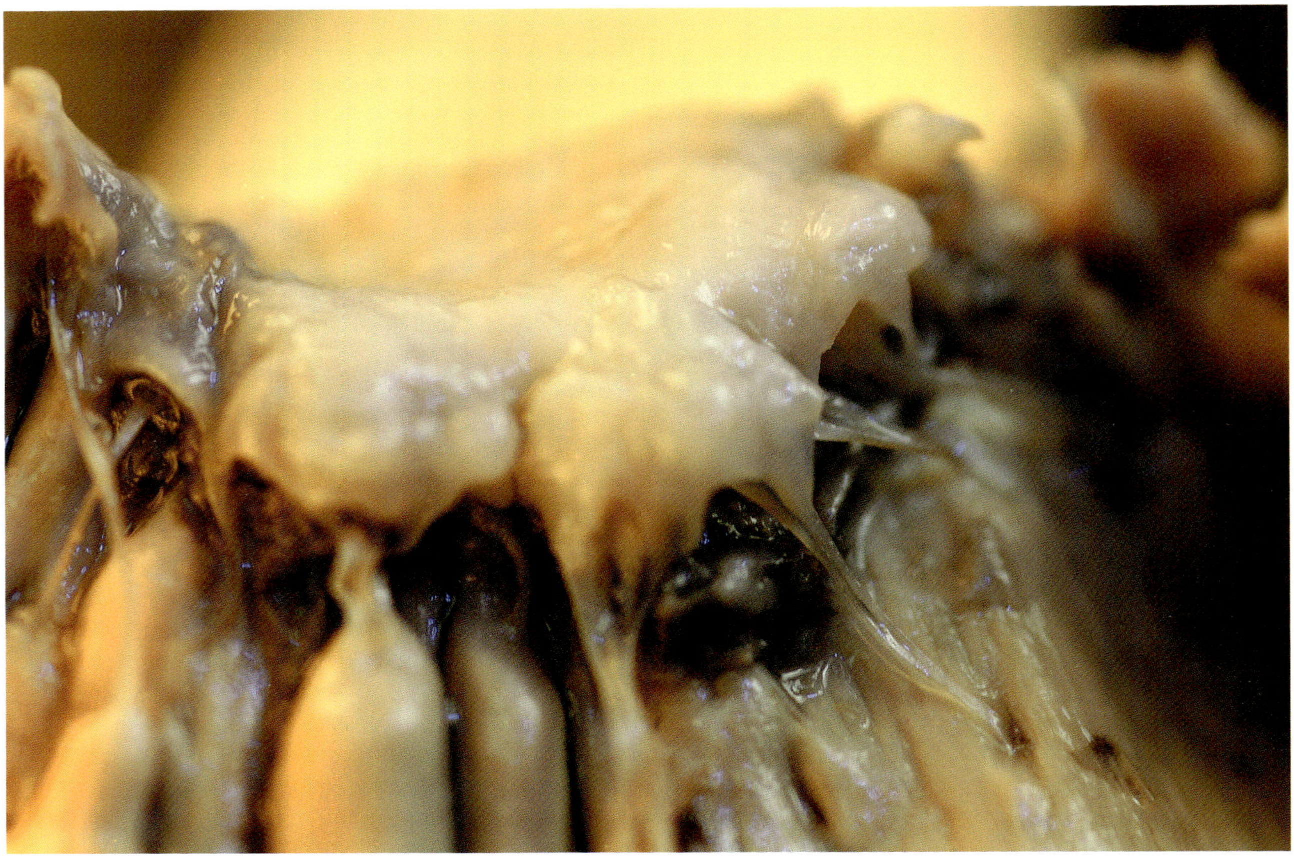

Figure 4. Septal leaflet of the tricuspid valve affected by myxomatous valve degeneration.

HISTOPATHOLOGY

The histopathological changes consist in the proliferation of the endothelium, although in some cases there may be localised losses of endothelium and an increase in the number of subendothelial fibroblasts. The elastic fibres between the atrial endothelium and the spongy layer tear apart while the spongy layer is thickened, with the presence of star-shaped and spindle-shaped cells in the middle of an extracellular matrix mainly formed by glycosaminoglycans (hyaluronic acid and chondroitin sulphate), and thus acquires an aspect that is similar to embryonic mesenchymal –myxomatous– tissue. The fibrous layer –skeleton of the valve apparatus– degenerates and collagen bundles eventually disappear.

These histological changes do not only affect the valves but also the chordae tendineae with a similar structure.

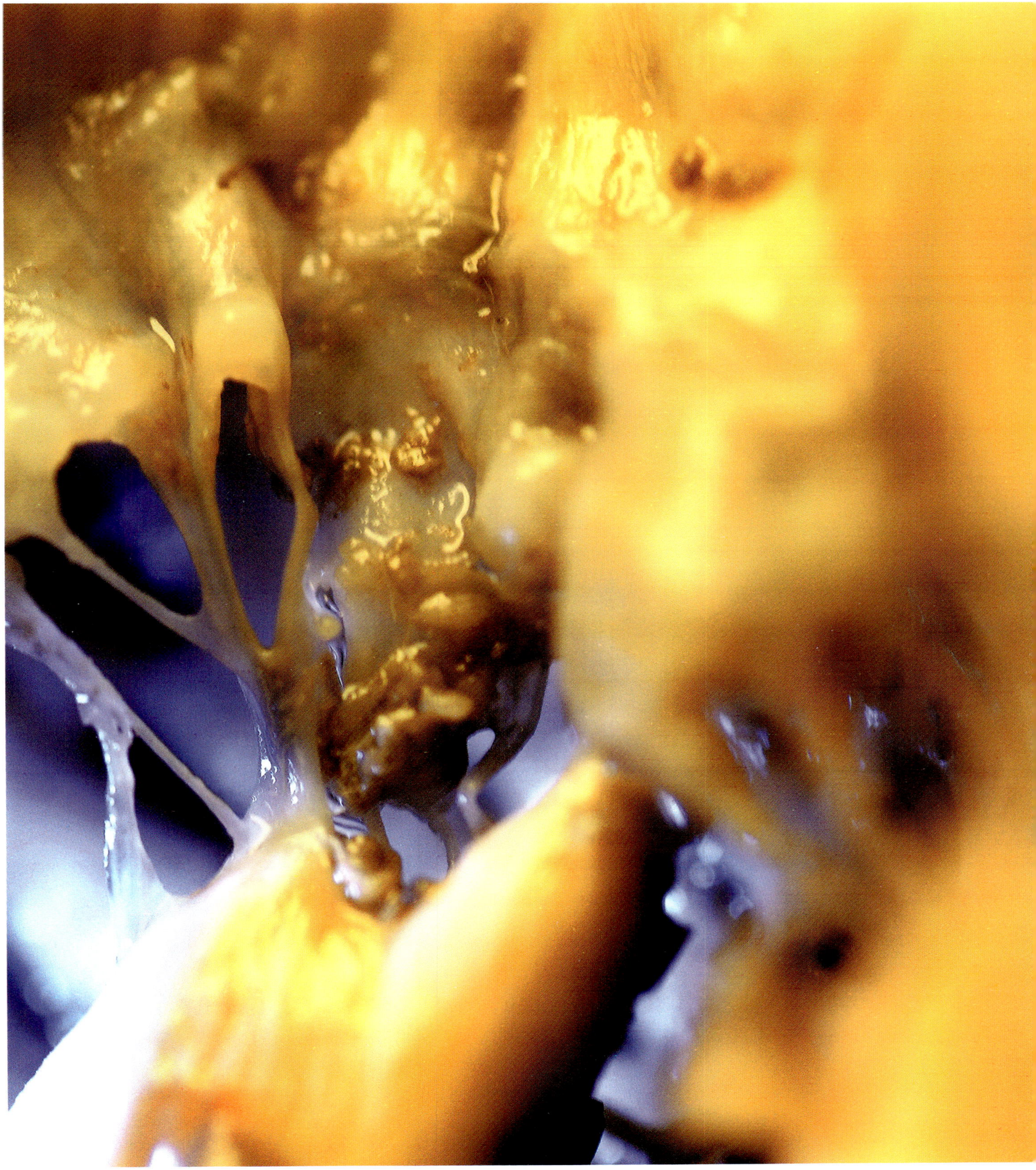

Figure 5. Mural leaflet of the tricuspid valve affected by myxomatous valve degeneration.

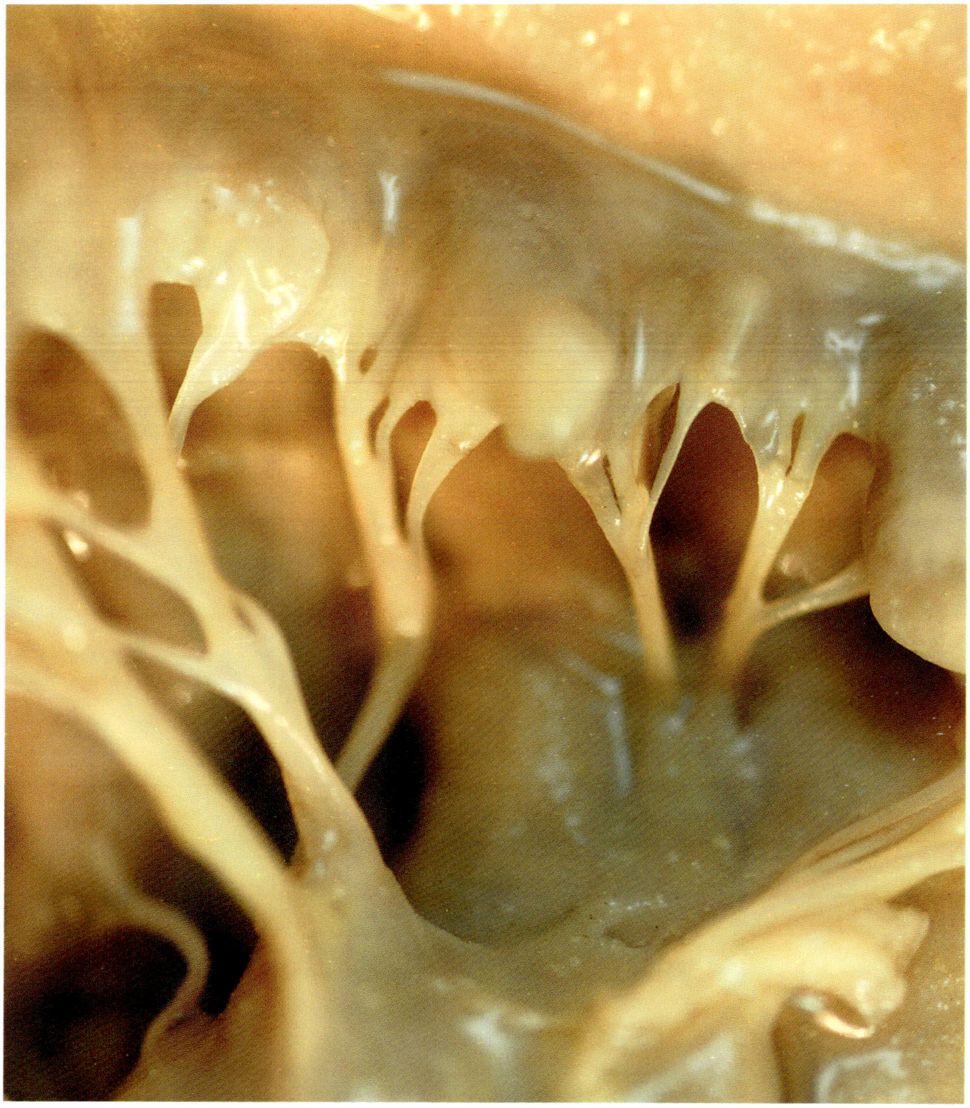

Figure 6. Type I lesion, presence of small isolated nodules in the margins of the valve leaflets.

PATHOLOGICAL CHANGES

The histopathological changes that take place are going to facilitate the stretching of the leaflets and chordae tendineae under normal pressures (valve prolapse) and the subsequent thickening and retraction of the valve leaflets.

Valvular changes can be classified into four groups:

I. Small unremarkable nodules in the free margins of the leaflets, which are sometimes associated with small areas of diffuse opacity.
II. The nodules increase in size and fuse together; the areas of opacity may increase.

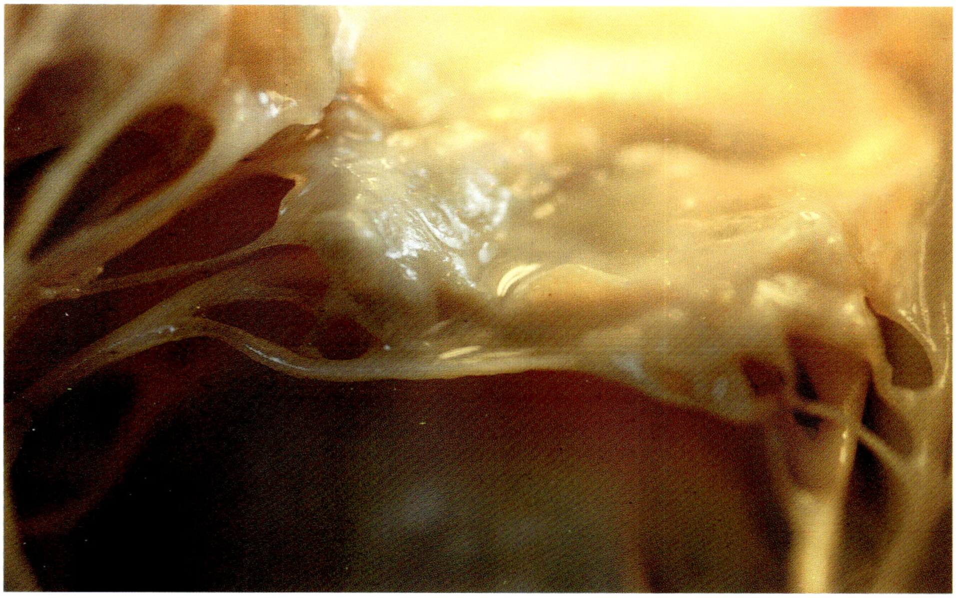

Figure 7. Type II lesion, the nodules increase in size and fuse together; the areas of opacity of the leaflets increase.

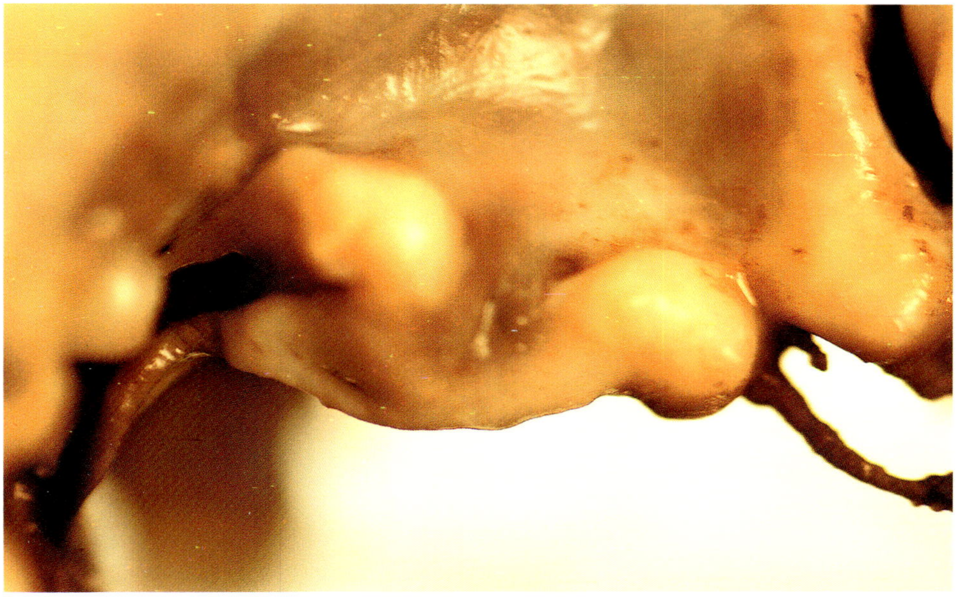

Figure 8. Type III lesion, the nodules cause irregularities in the valvular surface; these are almost completely opaque.

III. Large nodules causing irregularities in the valvular surface are observed. We may find thickenings in the rough area at the site of attachment of the chordae tendineae.
IV. The valve leaflets are thickened and wrinkled, and there may be a prolapse of part of the thickened tissue towards the atrium. There may be a rupture of the chordae tendineae.

In every group, it is possible to find sections that appear relatively normal with other adjacent areas that are mildly or severely affected.

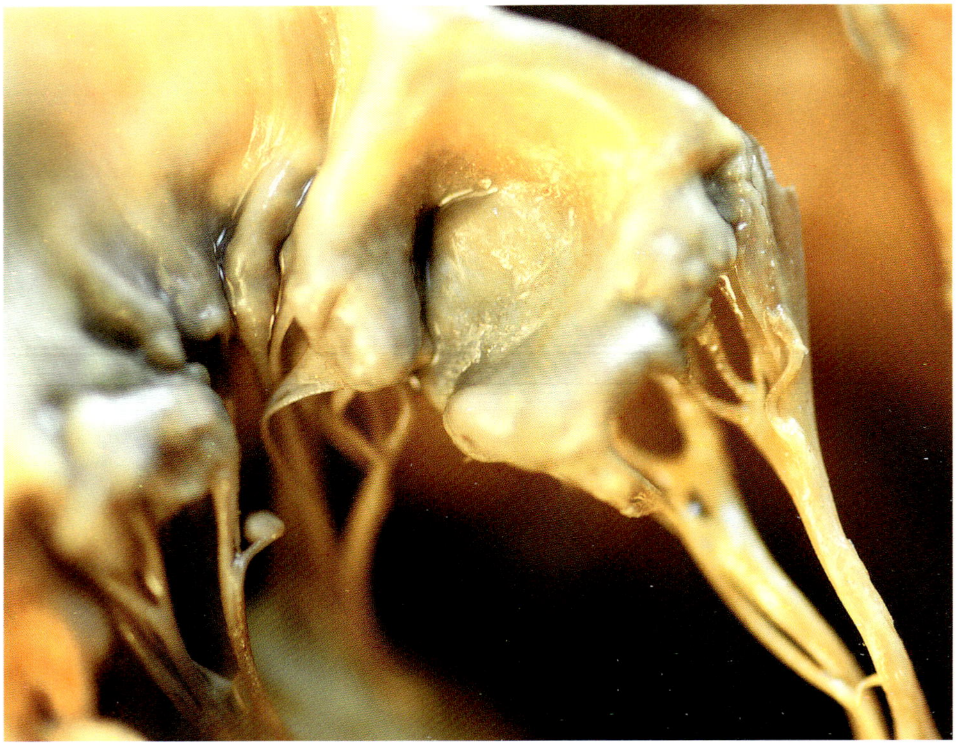

Figure 9. Type III lesion.

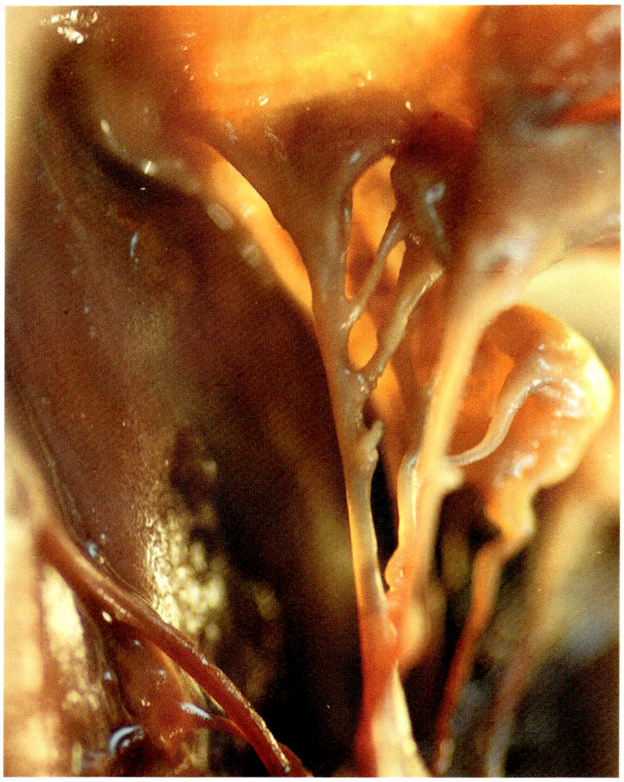

Figure 10. Type III lesion. Thickenings are usually found at the site of insertion of the chordae tendineae into the rough area.

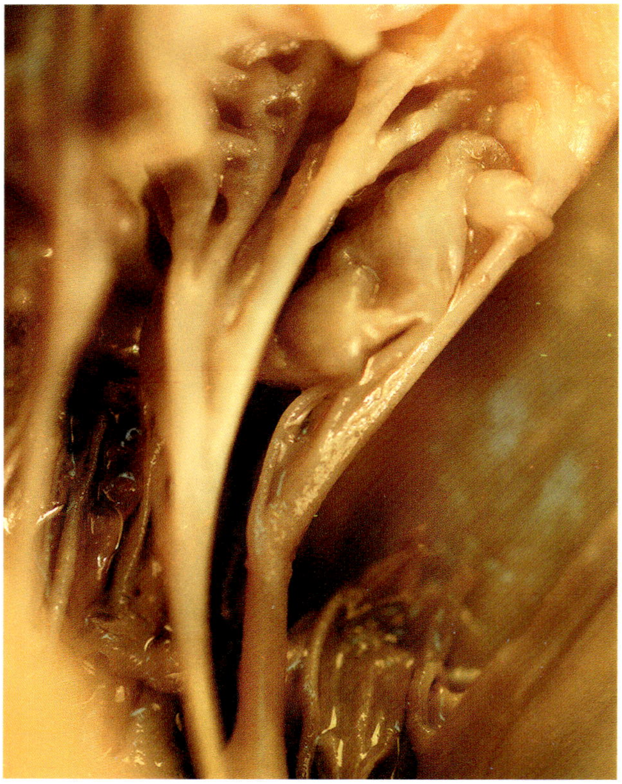

Figure 11. Type III lesion. Thickenings in the rough area.

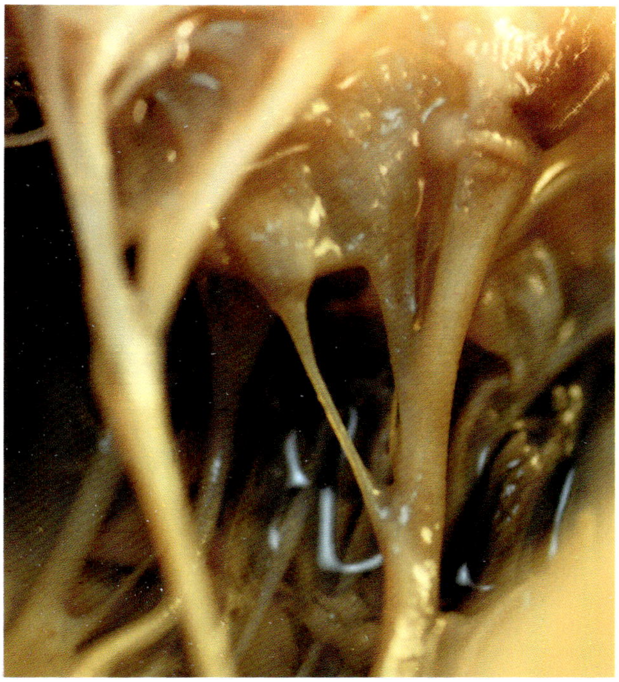

Figure 12. Thickenings at the site of attachment of the chordae tendineae predispose to their rupture.

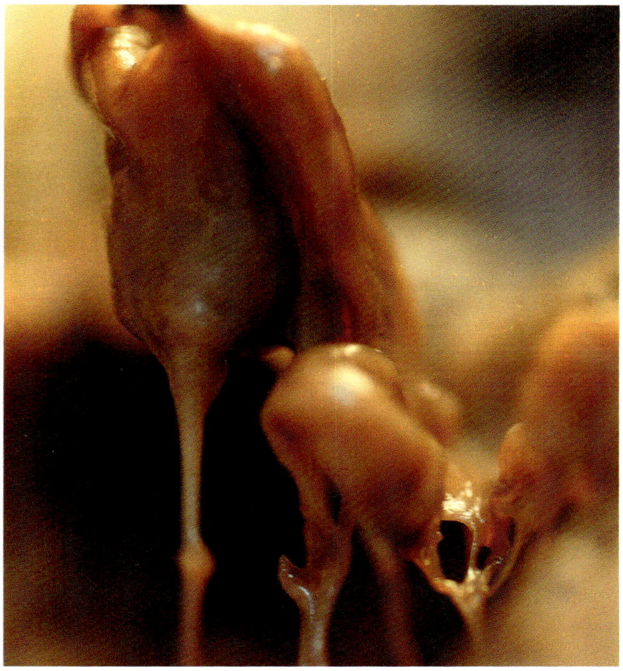

Figure 13. Important thickening of the site of insertion of the chorda tendinea with the leaflet. A thickened area may also be observed in the medial area of the chorda tendinea.

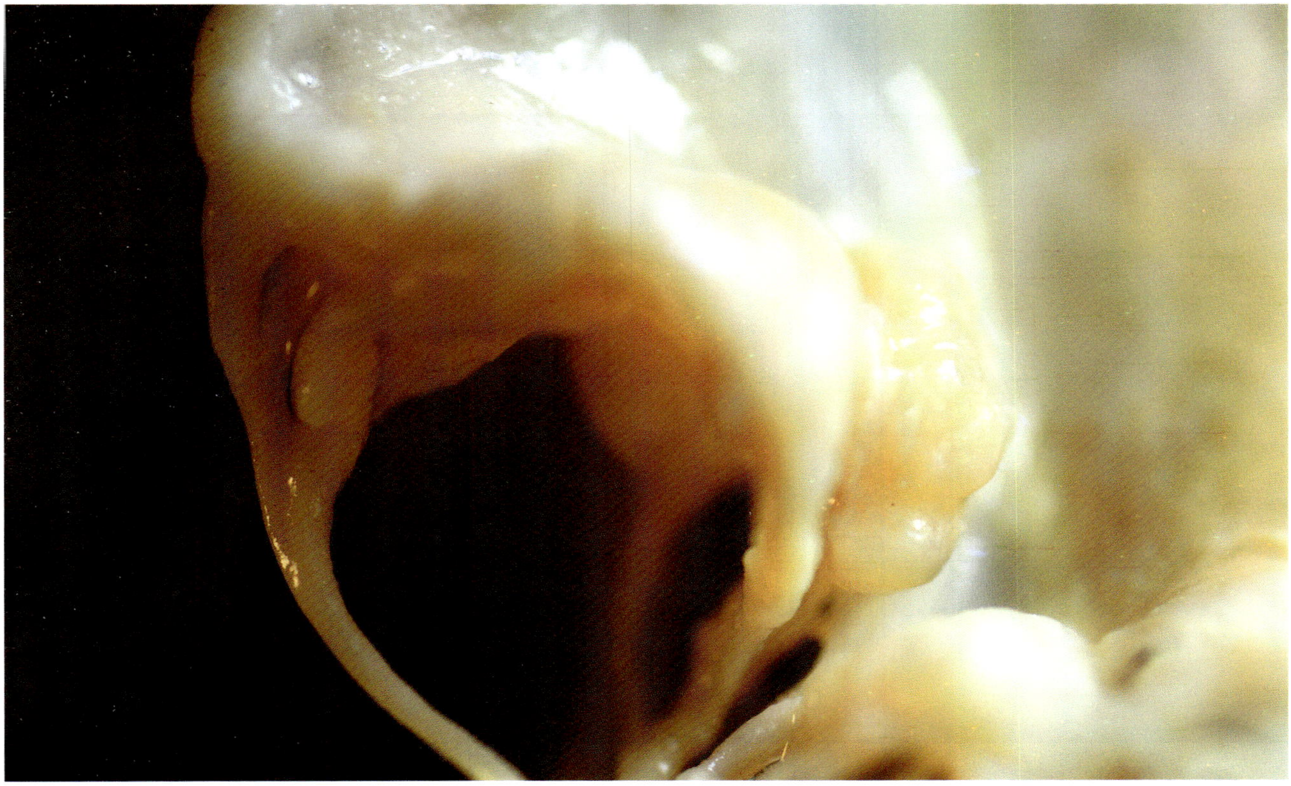

Figure 14. Type IV lesion. The leaflets are thickened and wrinkled and there may be a prolapse of thickened tissue towards the atrial surface.

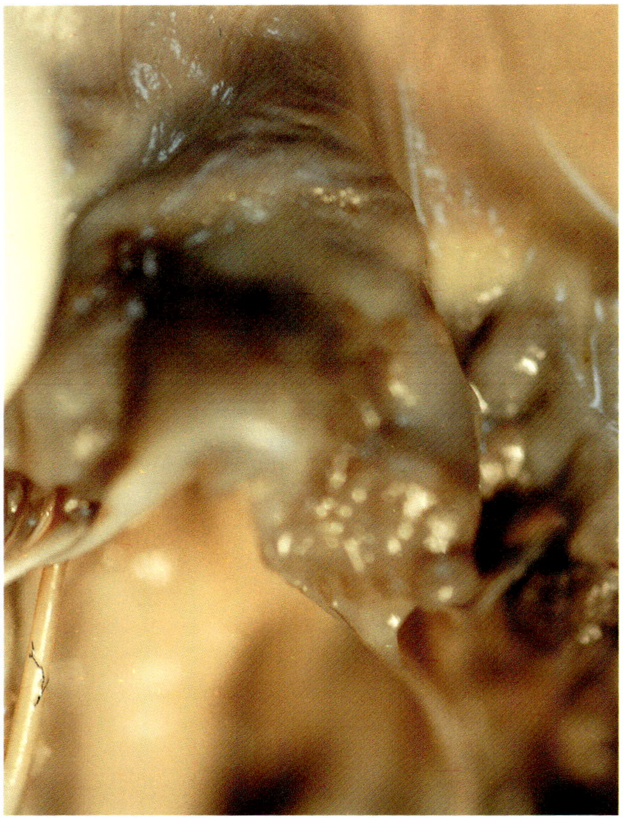

Figure 15. Type IV lesion, at this stage the lesion also affects the area of the valve annulus and rough and thickened areas appear.

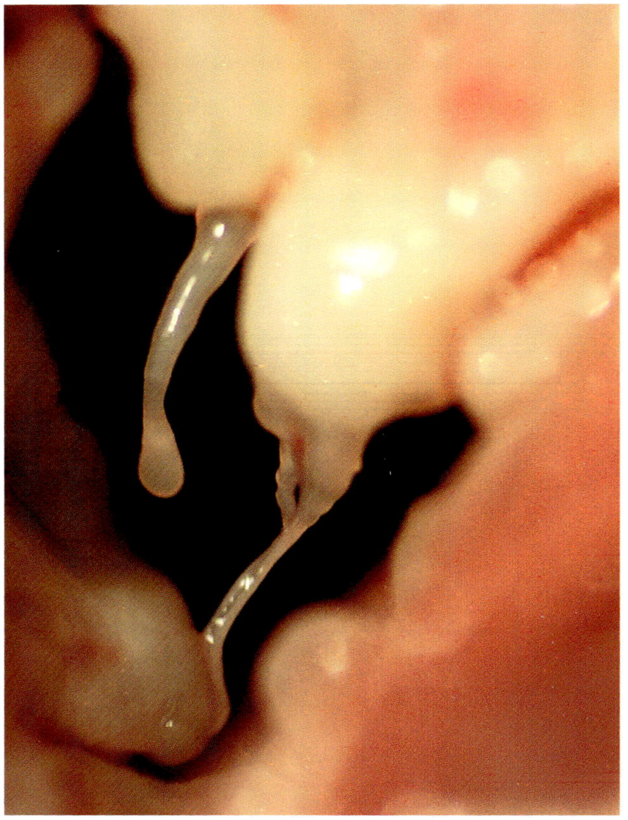

Figure 16. Chordae tendineae may also rupture at this stage.

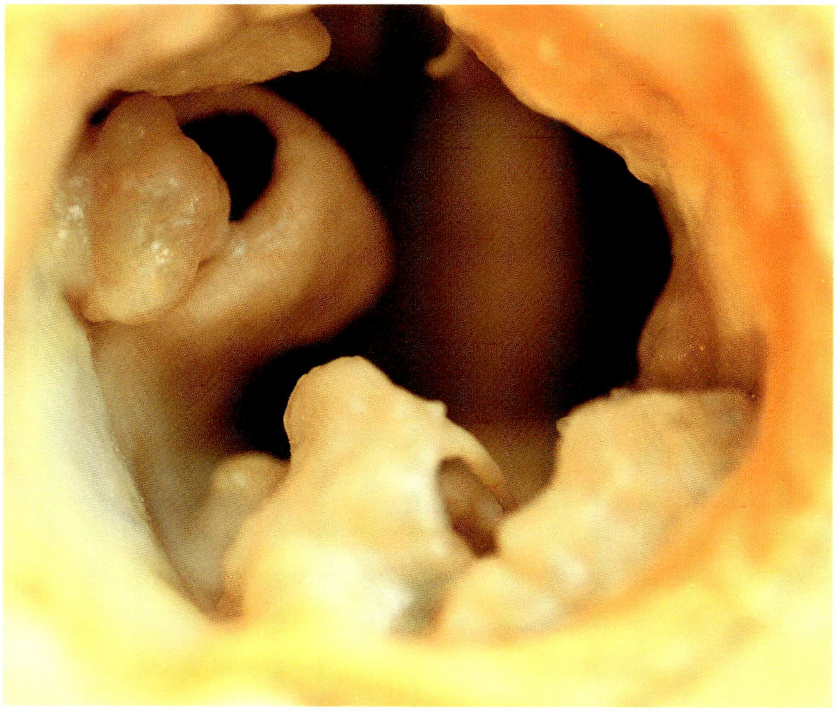

Figure 17. Type IV lesion, view from the atrial surface. The valve has lost much of its structure and the leaflets appear twisted, thickened and have prominent nodules.

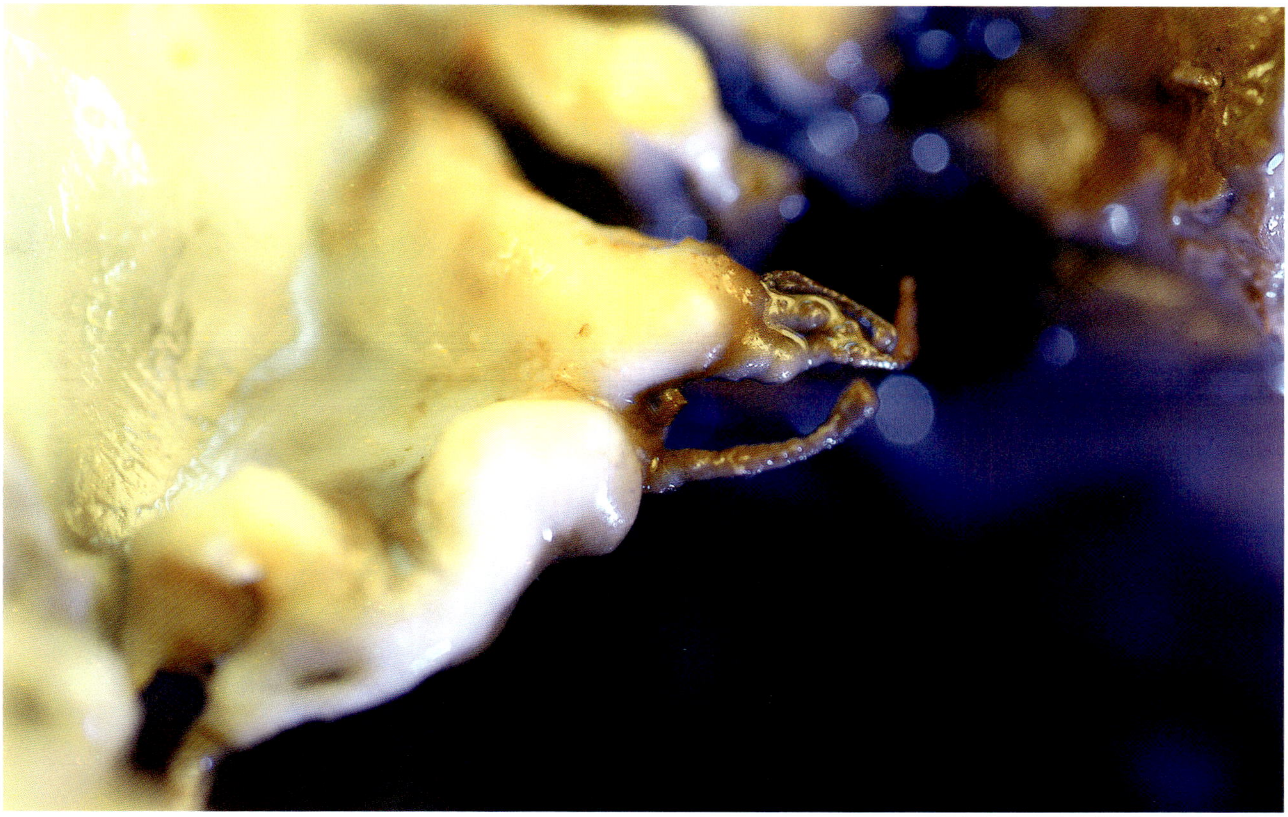

Figure 18. Ruptured chordae tendineae.

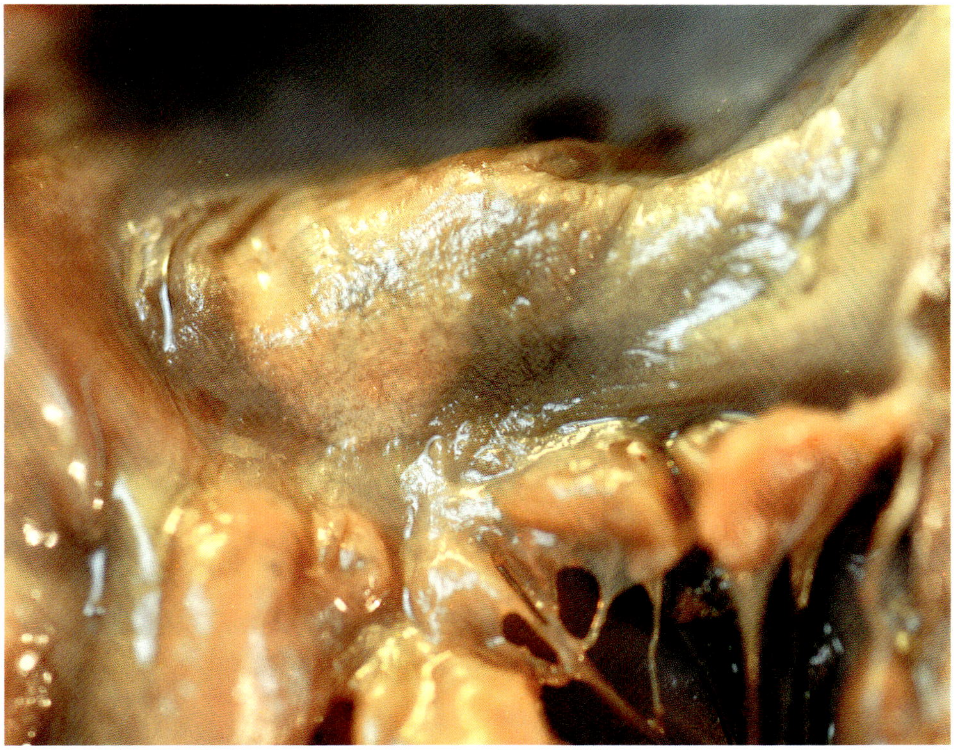

Figure 19. A fibrous plate in the area subject to high-velocity regurgitation may sometimes be observed in the atrium.

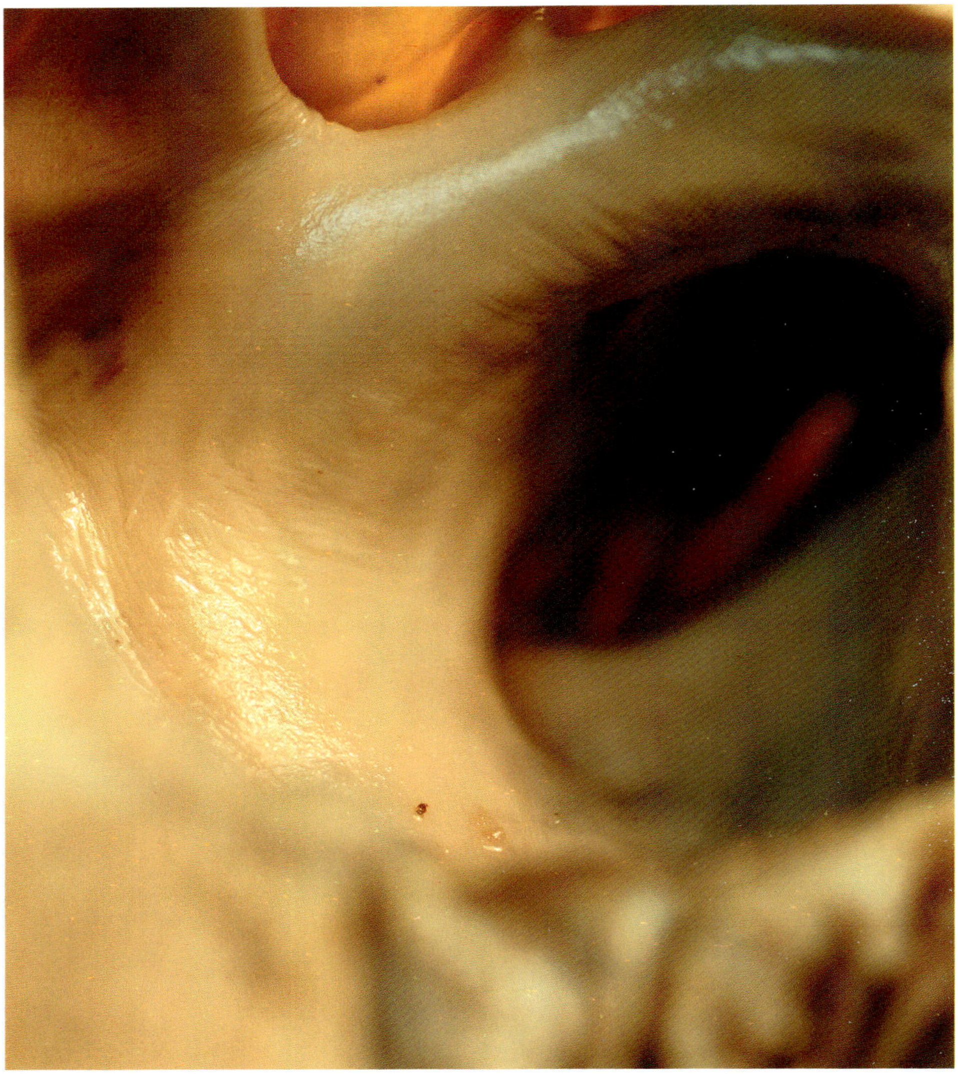

Figure 20. The dilation of the left atrium is the logical consequence of mitral valve insufficiency and one of the most important characteristics of this disease.

The valvular insufficiency produced is going to lead to the dilation of the atrium. If the volume of regurgitation gradually increases and the atrium responds by dilating proportionally, there may be small changes in intraatrial pressure. These are well tolerated; this explains why we may see dogs with severe cardiomegalies and few clinical signs. The opposite occurs when the volume of regurgitation increases in a sudden manner, due to lesions that develop rapidly and worsen the degree of valvular insufficiency, or to the rupture of a chorda tendinea. In this case, atrial distensibility is not sufficient and interatrial pressure rapidly increases with the appearance of pulmonary oedema. We may sometimes find dilation of the valve annulus caused by ventricular enlargement in response to a volume overload. It is also frequent to find concentric hypertrophy of the left ventricle.

The atrial area that is subject to high-velocity regurgitation may have fibrous plates and even endomyocardial tears.

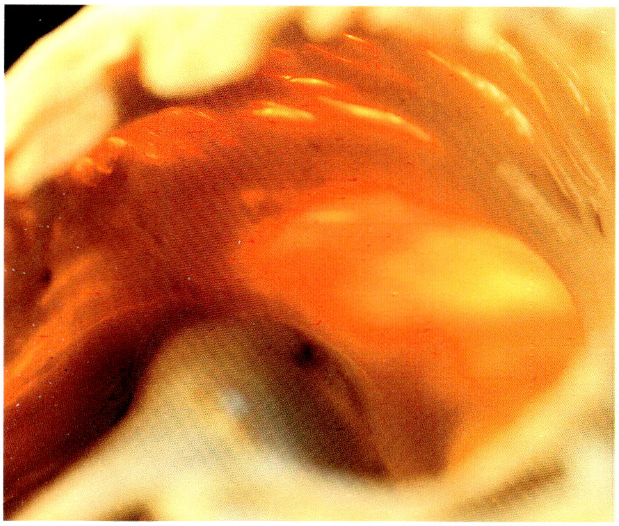

Figure 21. The left atrial appendage also appears markedly dilated.

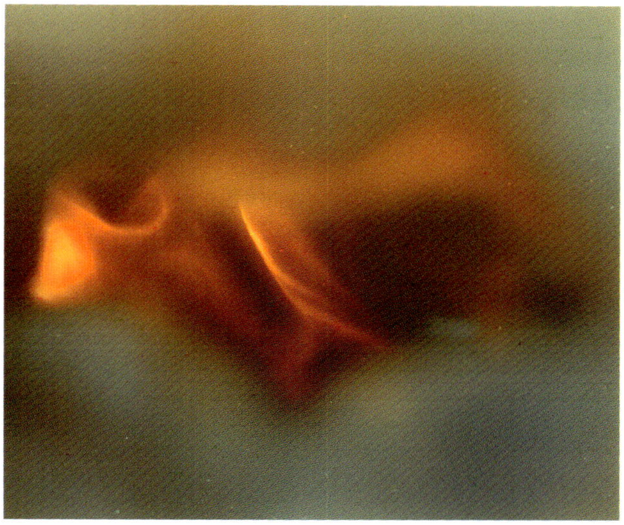

Figure 22. The openings of the pulmonary veins are also dilated.

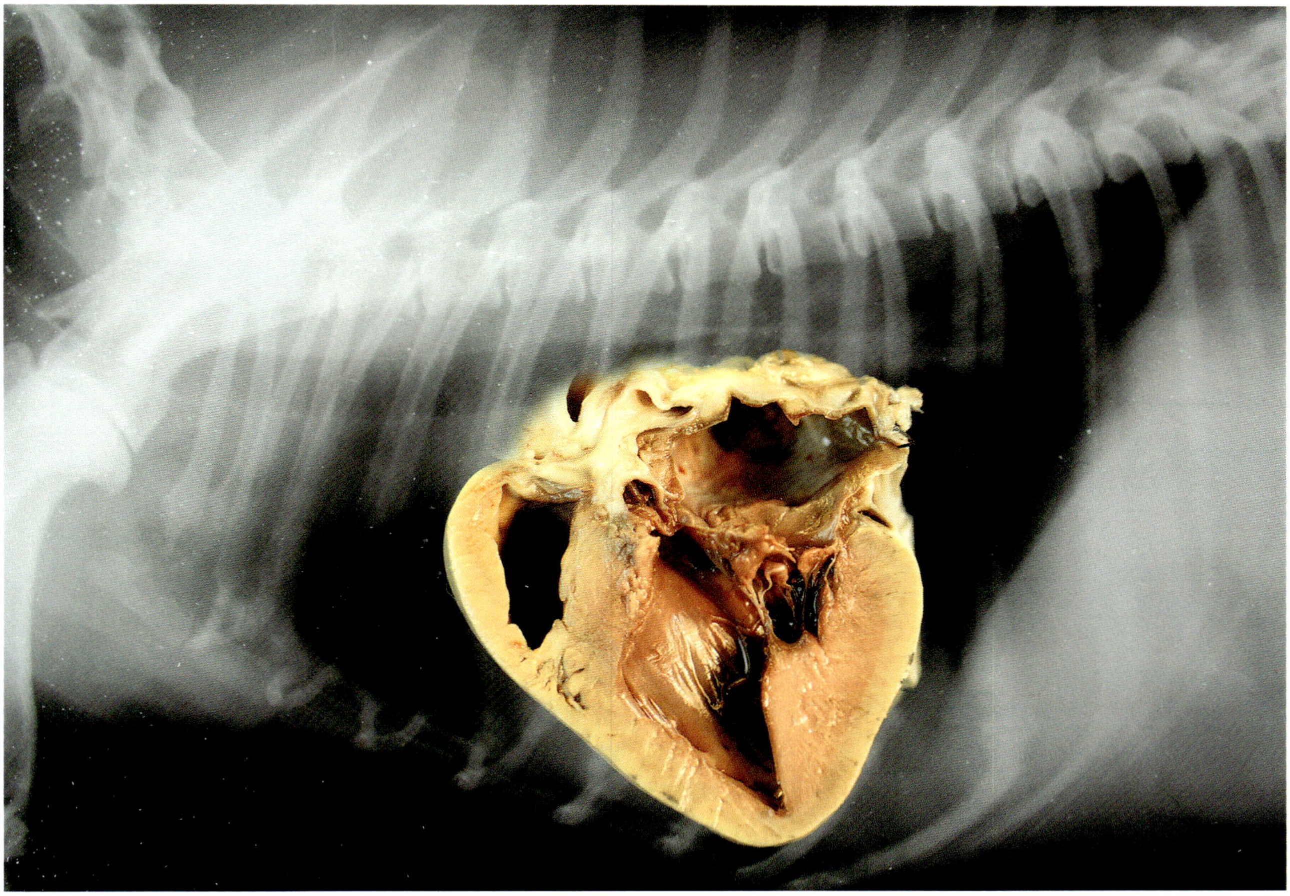

Figure 23. Cardiomegaly and marked dilation of the left atrium will be observed on radiographs. In this laterolateral projection, on which the heart anatomical image has been superimposed, it is possible to see how the enlargement of the left atrium is the main responsible factor for the elevation of the trachea and left bronchus.

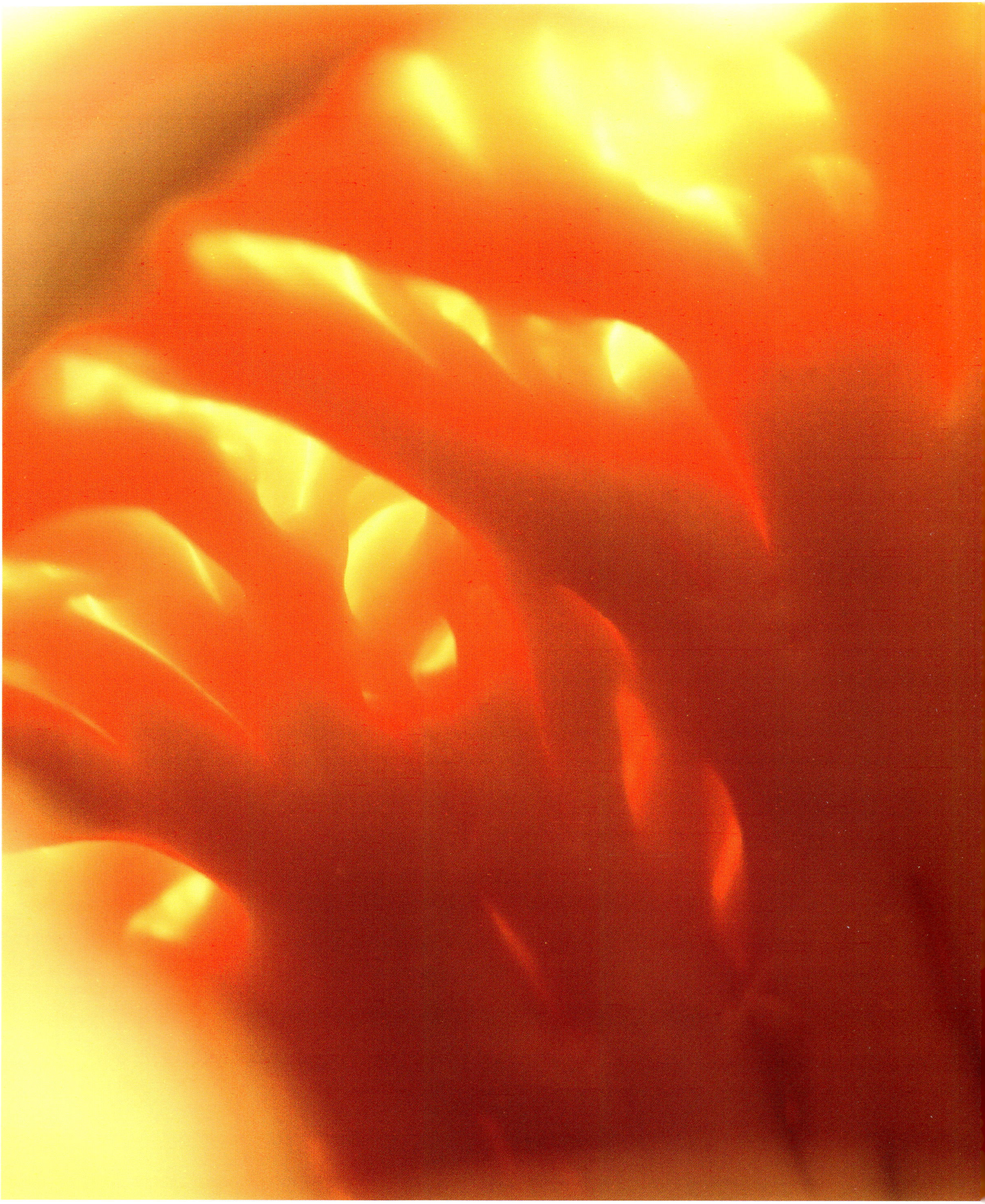

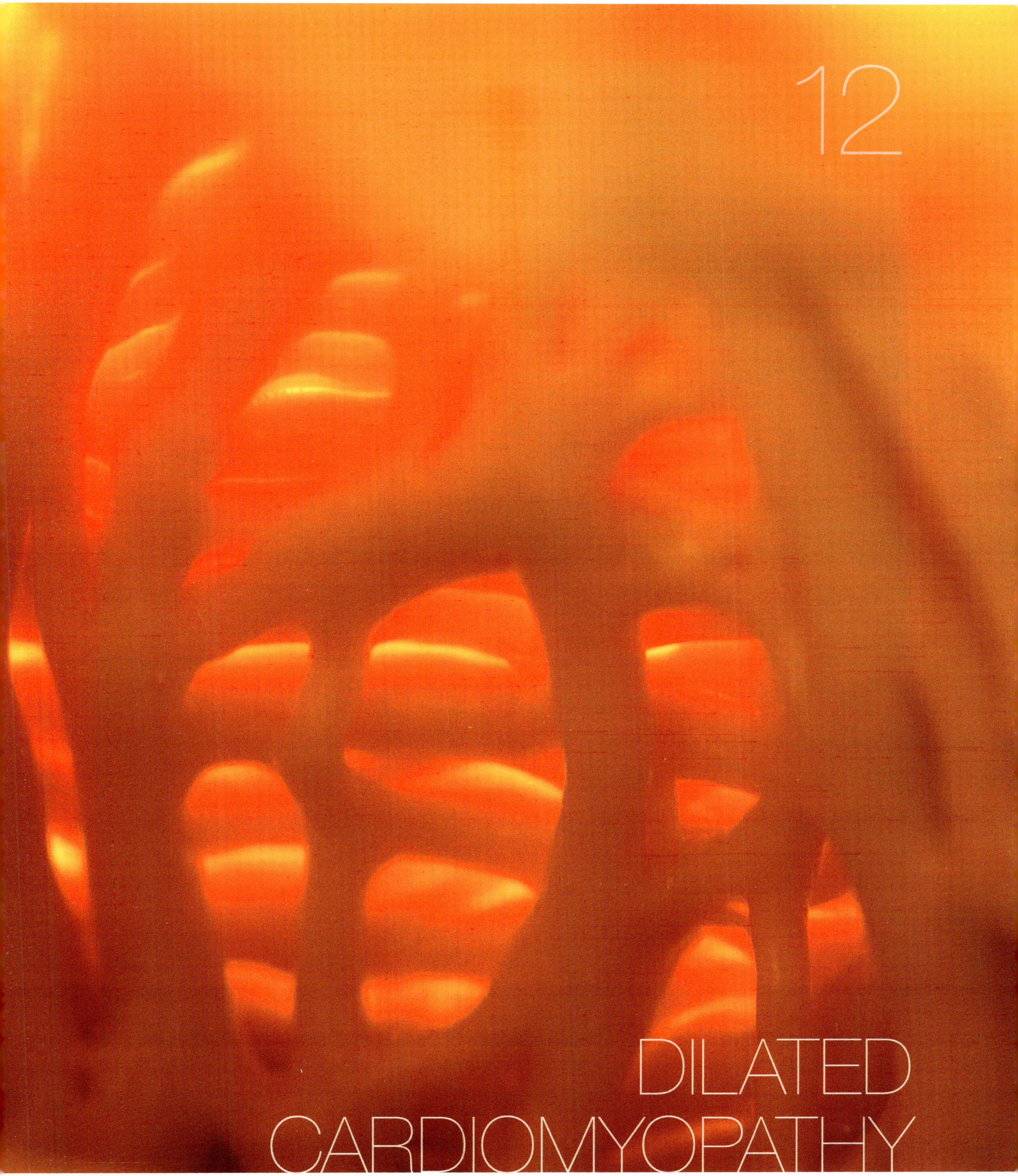

12

DILATED CARDIOMYOPATHY

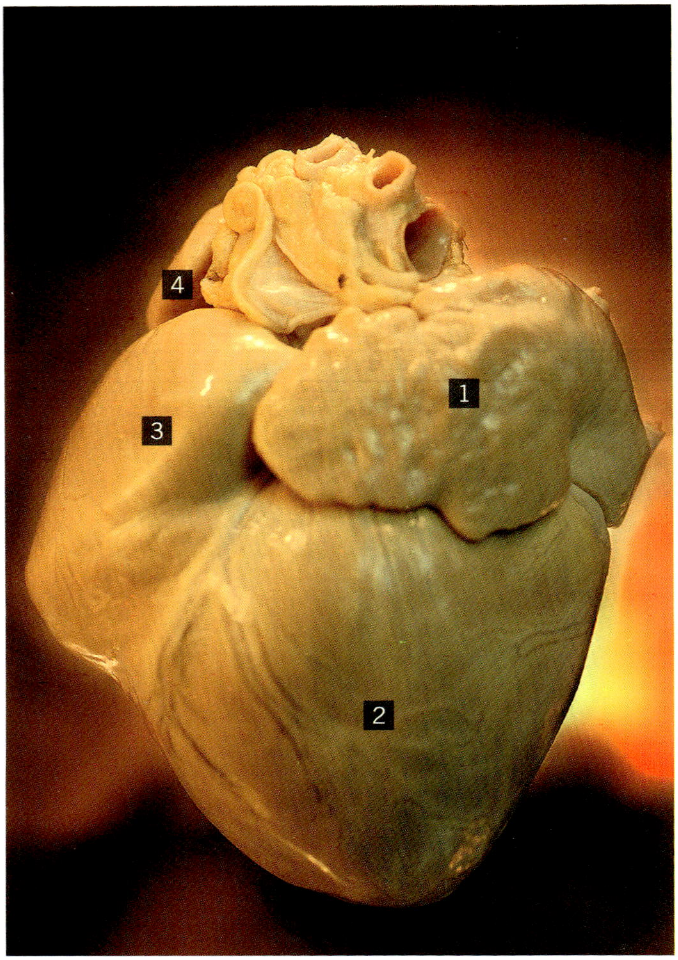

Figure 1. Dilation of the cardiac chambers is the main anatomical characteristic of dilated cardiomyopathy.

[1 Left atrial appendage] [3 Right ventricle]

[2 Left ventricle] [4 Right atrial appendage]

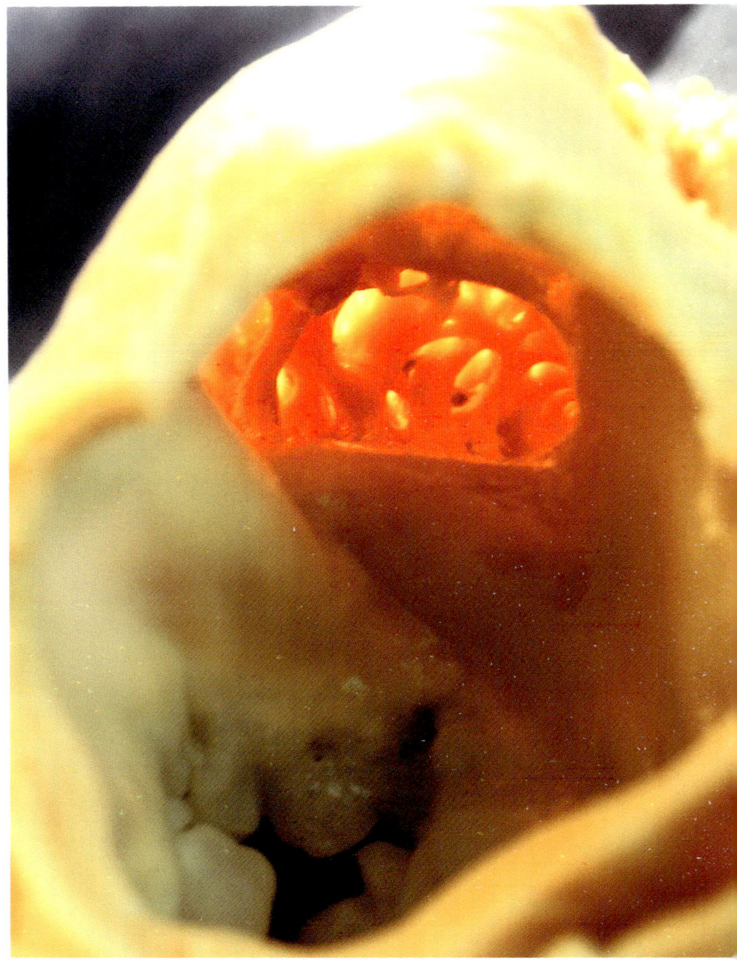

Figure 2. The pectinate muscles of a dilated atrial appendage sometimes acquire a spectacular aspect. Here we can see, at the back, the dilated left atrial appendage and pectinate muscles; in the forefront, the left atrium and mitral valve.

Dilated cardiomyopathy is literally defined as a disease of the cardiac muscle that causes the dilation of the heart.

One of the main characteristics of this disease is the reduction of myocardial contractility. The term "dilated" may be defined as compensatory, since it is related to the volume overload caused by this reduced contractility, to which the heart responds with eccentric hypertrophy. The term "hypertrophy" is used because the weight of the organ is increased in relation to the weight of the body, as a result of an increase in the size of the cells but not in their number; sarcomers, in this case, are increased in series, not in parallel as occurs in concentric hypertrophy.

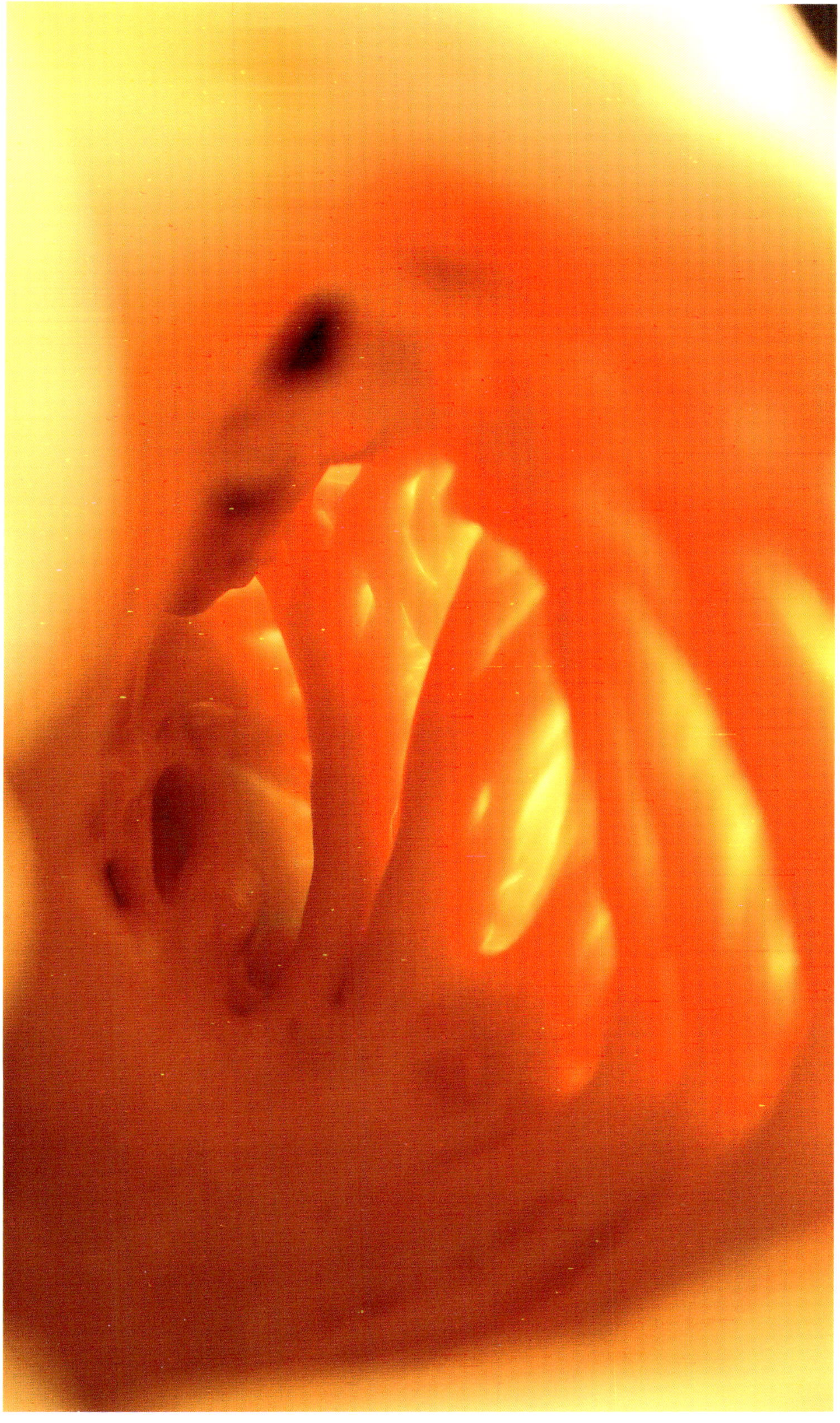

Figure 3. The pectinate muscles, which are usually much more numerous, may also have a remarkable appearance in the right atrial appendage when this latter is dilated.

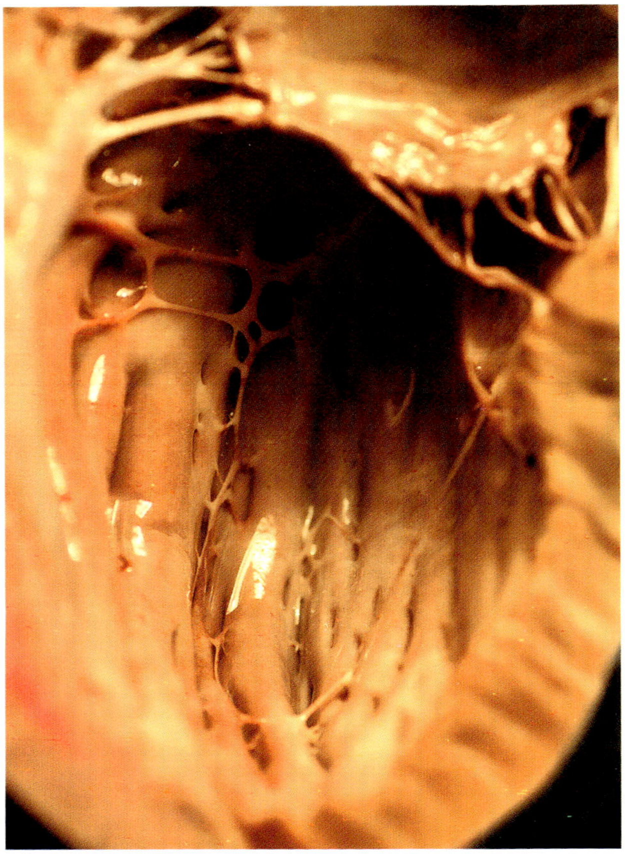

Figure 4. Enlargement of the left ventricular cavity.

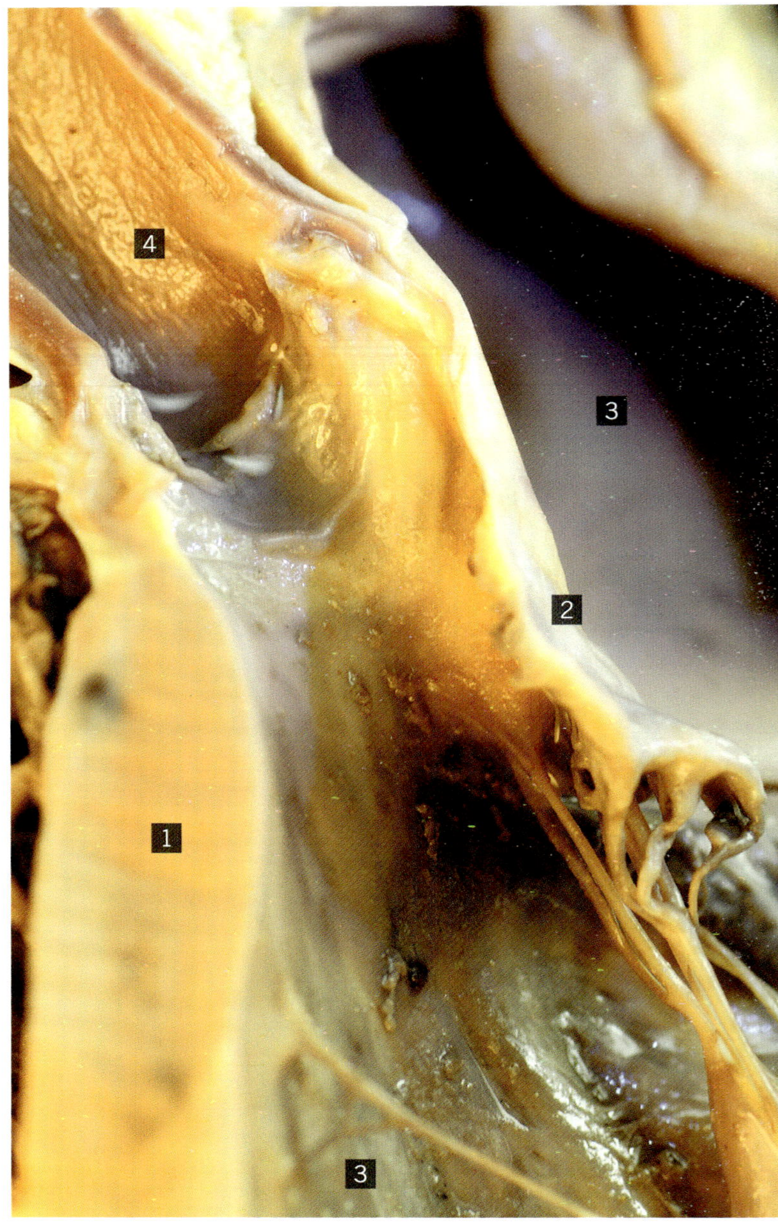

Figure 5. The enlargement of the left ventricular cavity leads to the cranial leaflet of the mitral valve, when it is opened at the maximum, being located farther away from the interventricular septum.

[1 Interventricular septum]

[2 Cranial leaflet of the mitral valve]

[3 Ventricular cavity]

[4 Aorta]

[5 Left atrium]

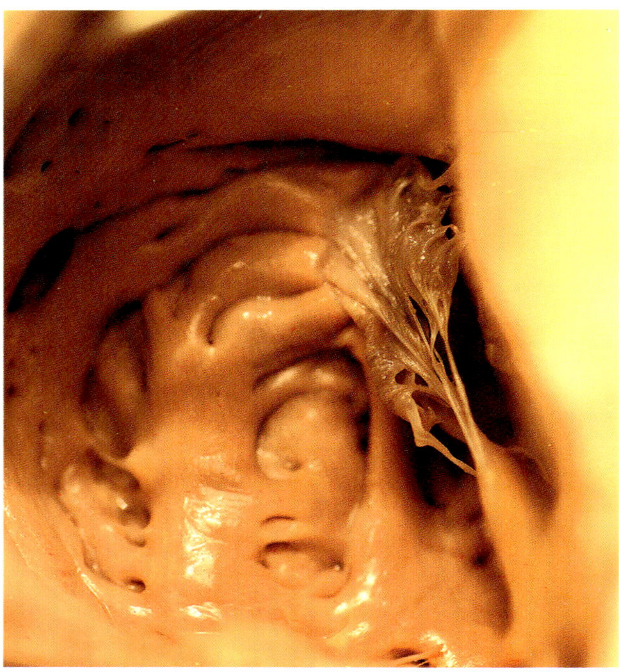

Figure 6. Enlargement of the right ventricular cavity.

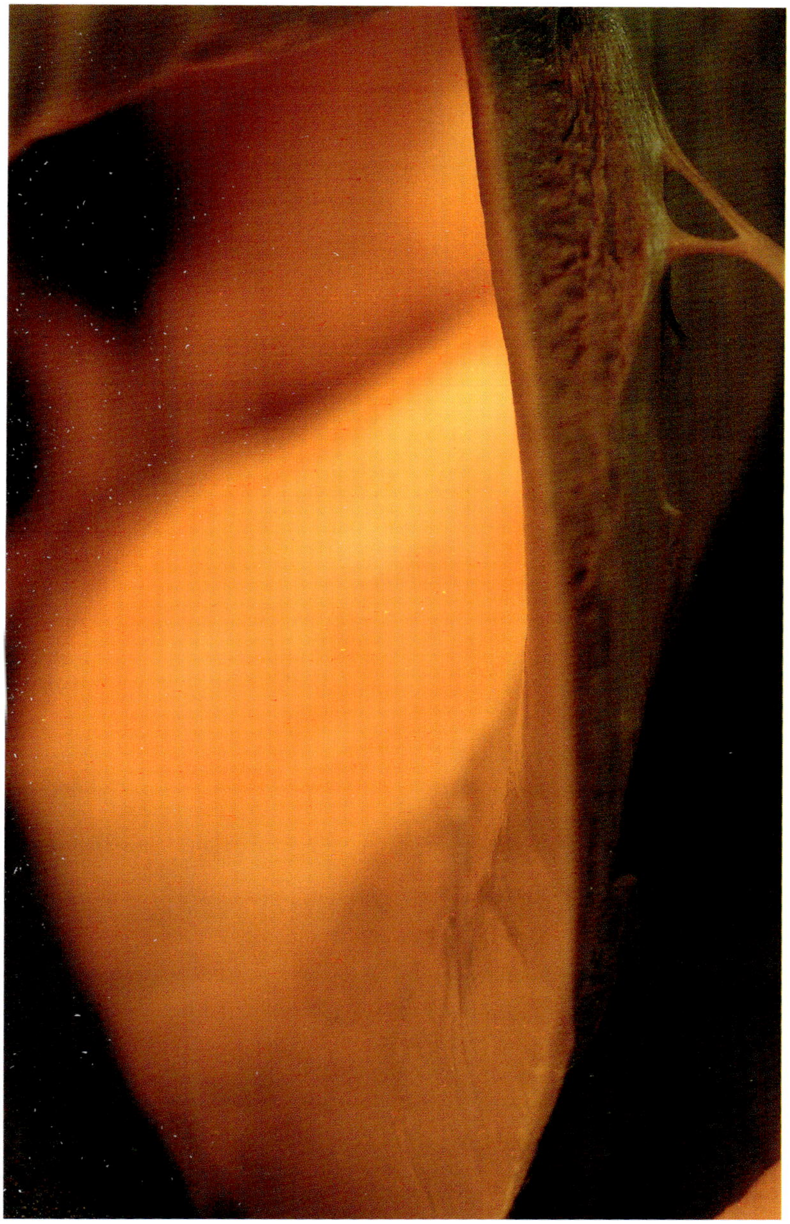

Figure 7. Thinning of the free wall of the right ventricle.

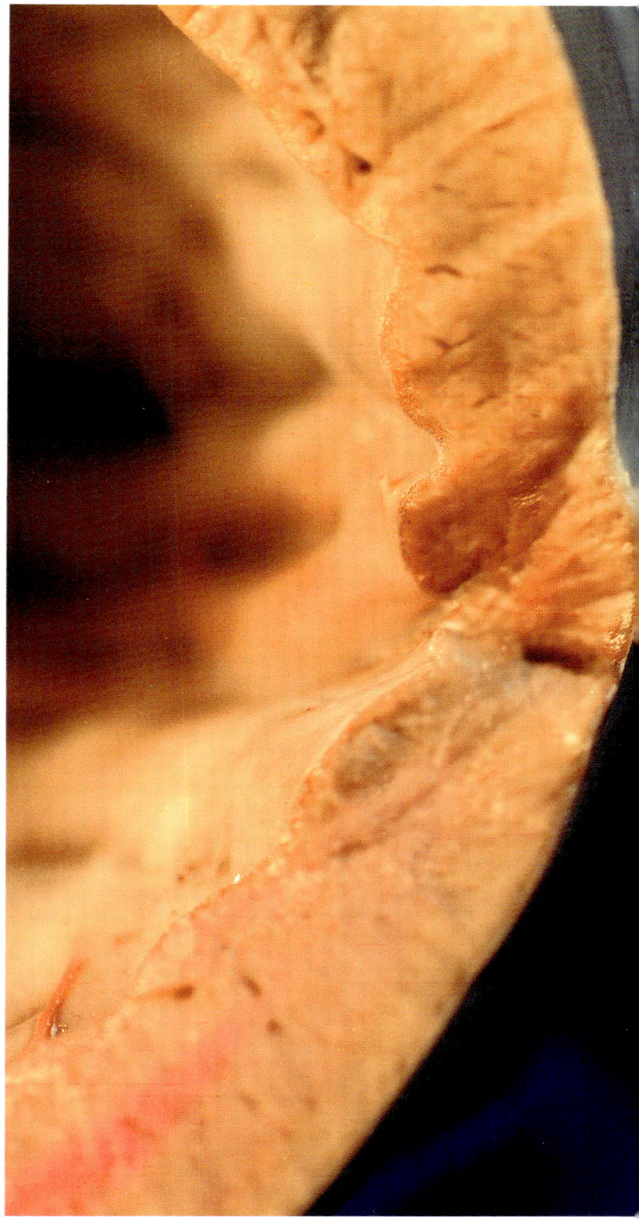

Figure 8. Thinning of the free wall of the left ventricle.

Taking into account what has just been said, the most accurate definition of dilated cardiomyopathy is a disease of the cardiac muscle that causes dilation of the cardiac chambers as a consequence of systolic dysfunction and, to a lesser extent, of diastolic dysfunction.

The aetiology of the disease is unknown, which is why it is also often named "idiopathic dilated cardiomyopathy". When the origin of the myocardial failure is known –less than 10 % of the total cases–, the name changes (cardiomyopathy due to parvovirus, to doxorubicin, etc.).

Dilated cardiomyopathy has a long period during which, although there is established myocardial failure, no clinical signs of the disease can be observed due to compensatory mechanisms. It can only be revealed by echocardiographic or electrocardiographic signs. This is called the "occult" stage of the disease. The duration of the occult stage, from the establishment of the disease to the appearance of symptoms, is much longer than the clinical stage.

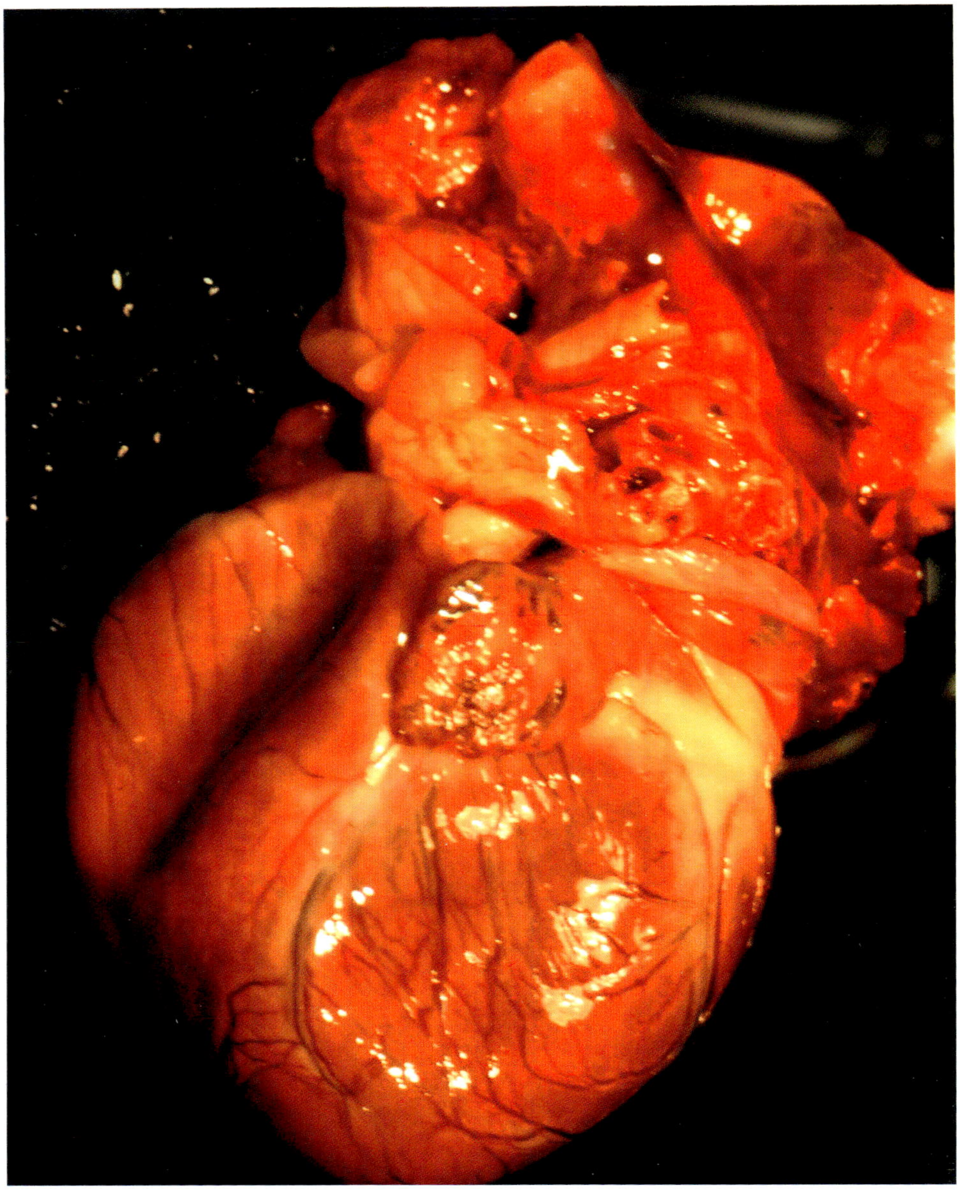

Figure 9. The ventricular walls have a flaccid aspect as can be seen in this unfixed specimen.

Dilated cardiomyopathy is more frequent in dogs of specific breeds than in crossbred dogs. The Doberman, followed by the Great Dane and the Cocker Spaniel are the breeds that accumulate the greater numbers of diagnosed cases. It is also common in other breeds such as the Golden and Labrador Retriever, the Saint Bernard, the Mastiff and the Greyhound.

The most commonly found anatomical alteration in this disease is the dilation of the four cardiac chambers (in 85 % of the cases), although those of the left side sometimes appear more affected than those of the right side. In unfixed specimens, the aspect of the heart is flaccid; it does not maintain its shape.

The ventricular walls may be thinner or have a normal thickness; in fact, they sometimes appear thinner because they are compared with the size of the dilated cavity. The dilation of the left ventricular cavity also leads to the dilation of the mitral valve annulus on the one hand, and on the other hand, to the papillary muscles, which have already become flat due to the myocardial disease, being laterally and apically displaced, the chordae tendineae being more elongated than normal. This results in incompetent closure of the valve and the presence of mitral regurgitation.

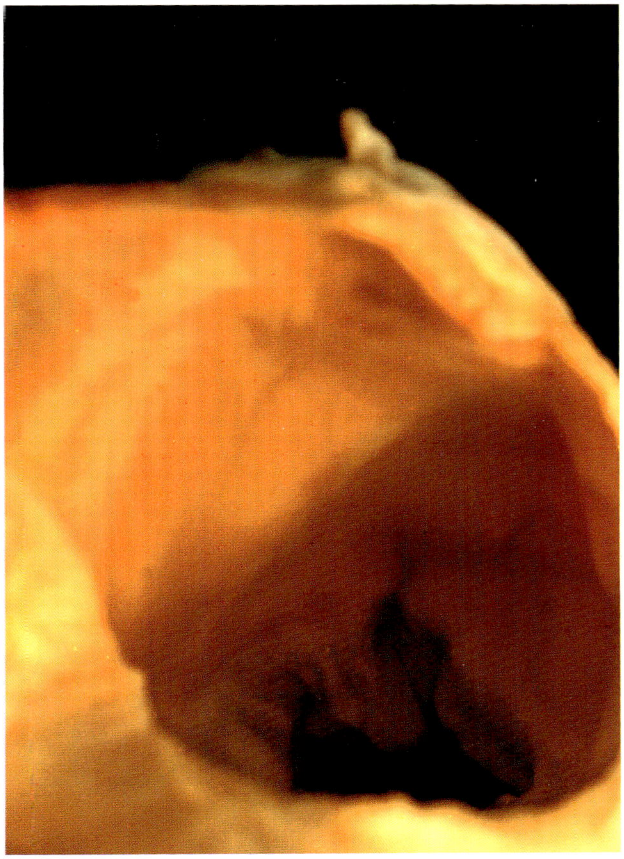

Figure 10. Dilation of the left atrium. A certain degree of dilation of the mitral valve annulus may also be observed.

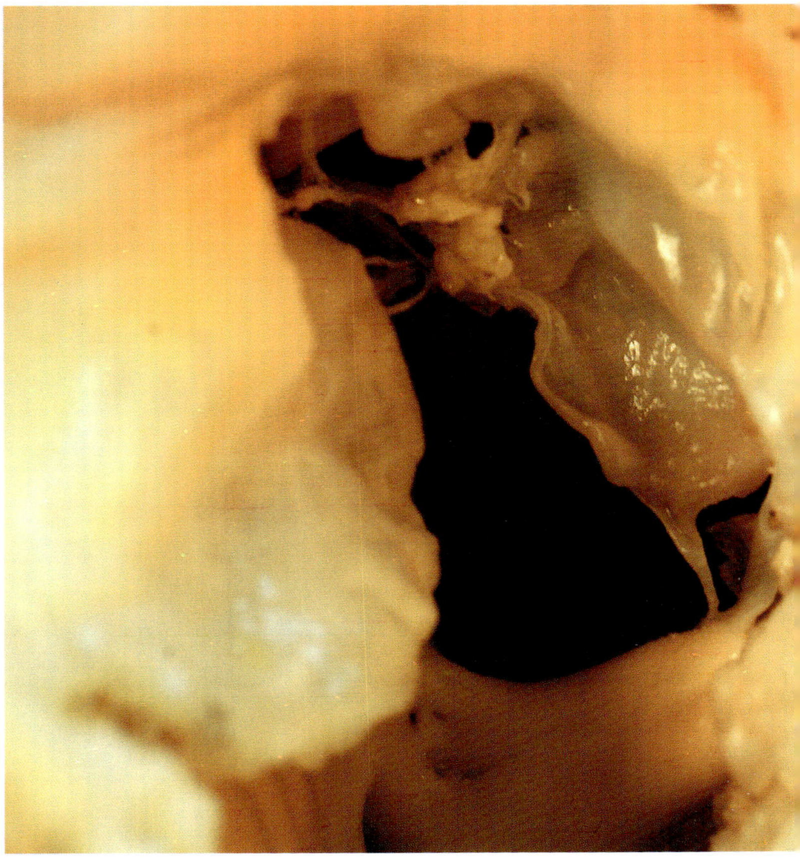

Figure 11. Although it is less frequent, the dilation of the tricuspid valve annulus may also sometimes be observed.

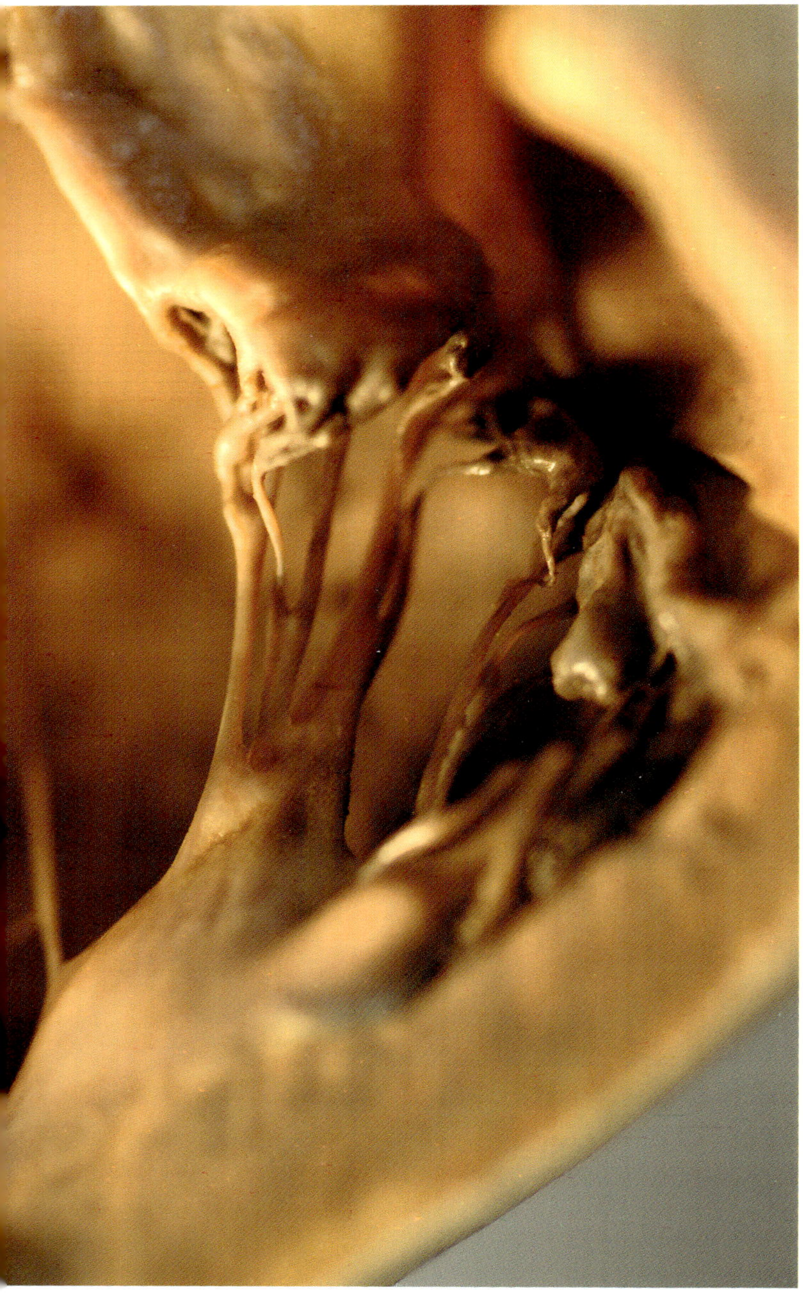

Figure 12. The papillary muscles become flat and reduced in size; in addition, the enlargement of the cavity makes them be farther apart, thus causing valvular insufficiency.

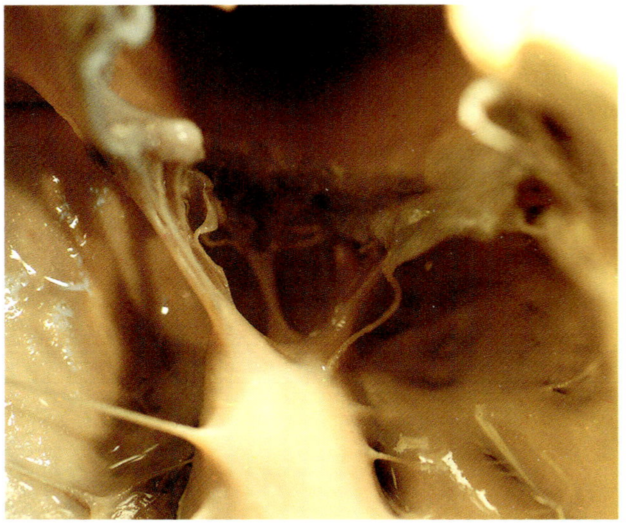

Figure 13. Papillary muscles in the left ventricle.

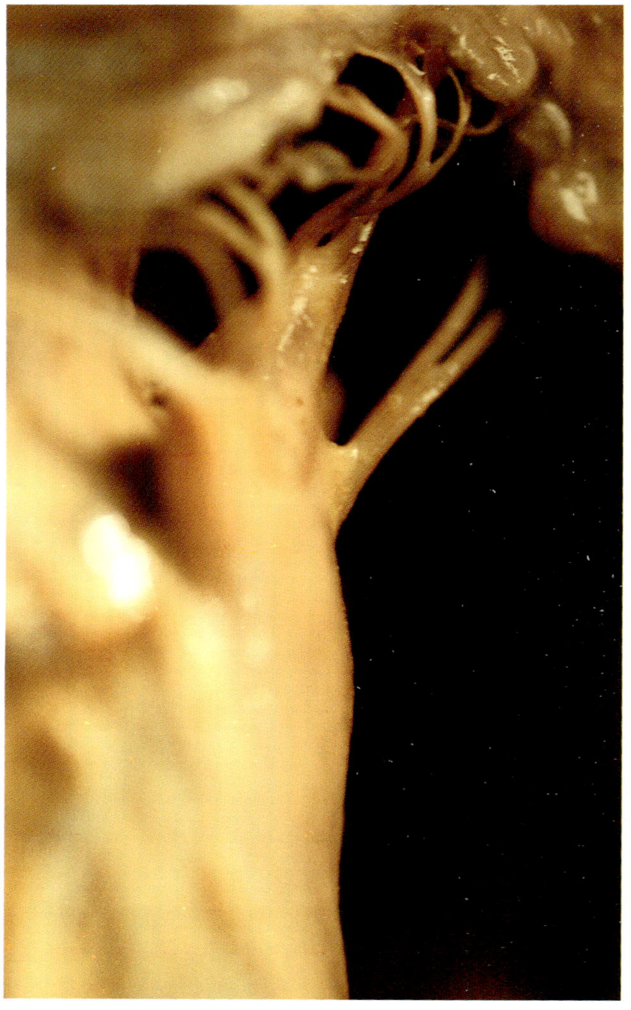

Figure 14. Flattened papillary muscle in the left ventricular cavity.

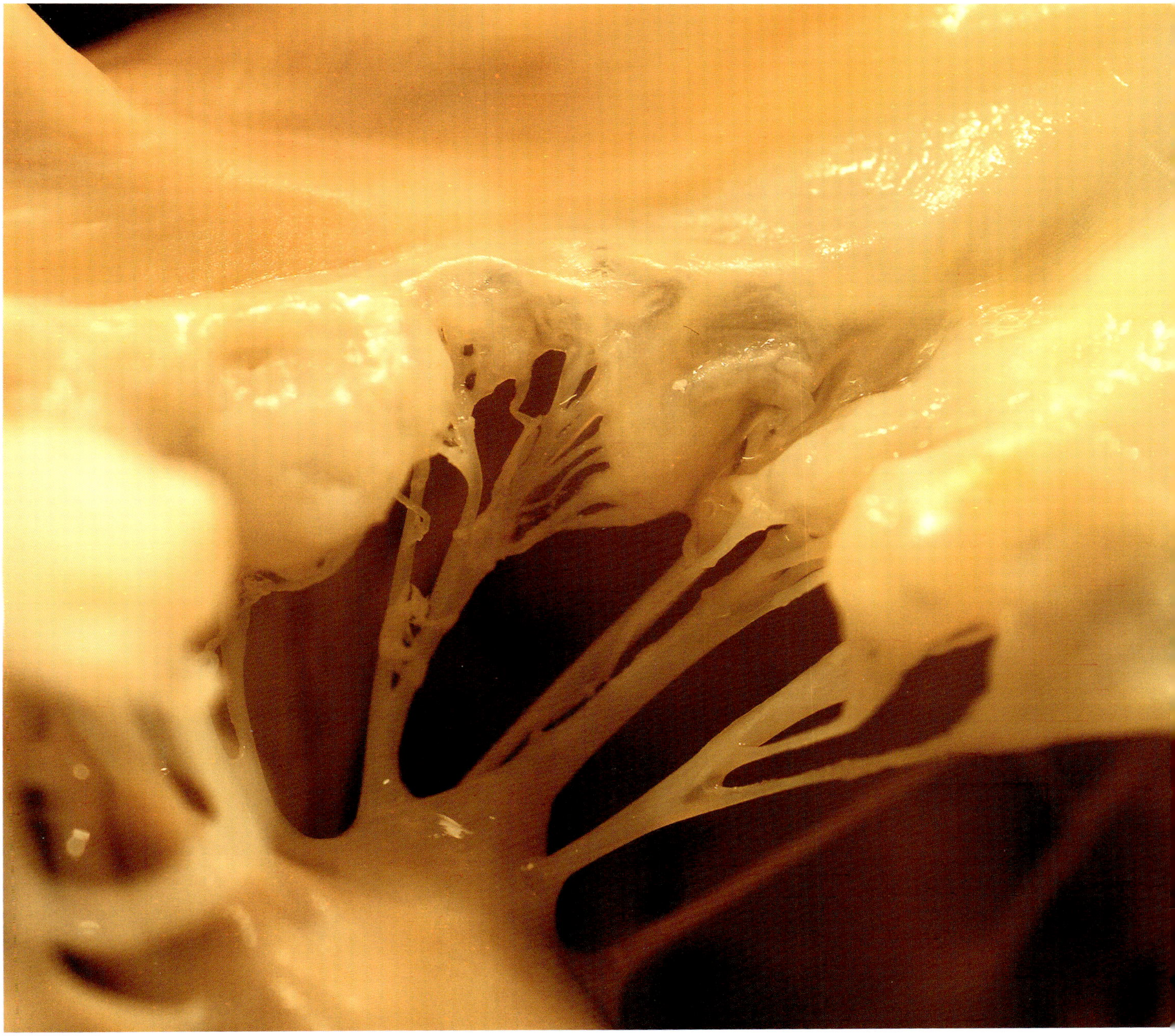

Figure 15. The enlargement of the left ventricular cavity, the flattening of the papillary muscles and greater distance between them, together with the dilation of the valve annulus may cause incompetent closure of the mitral valve.

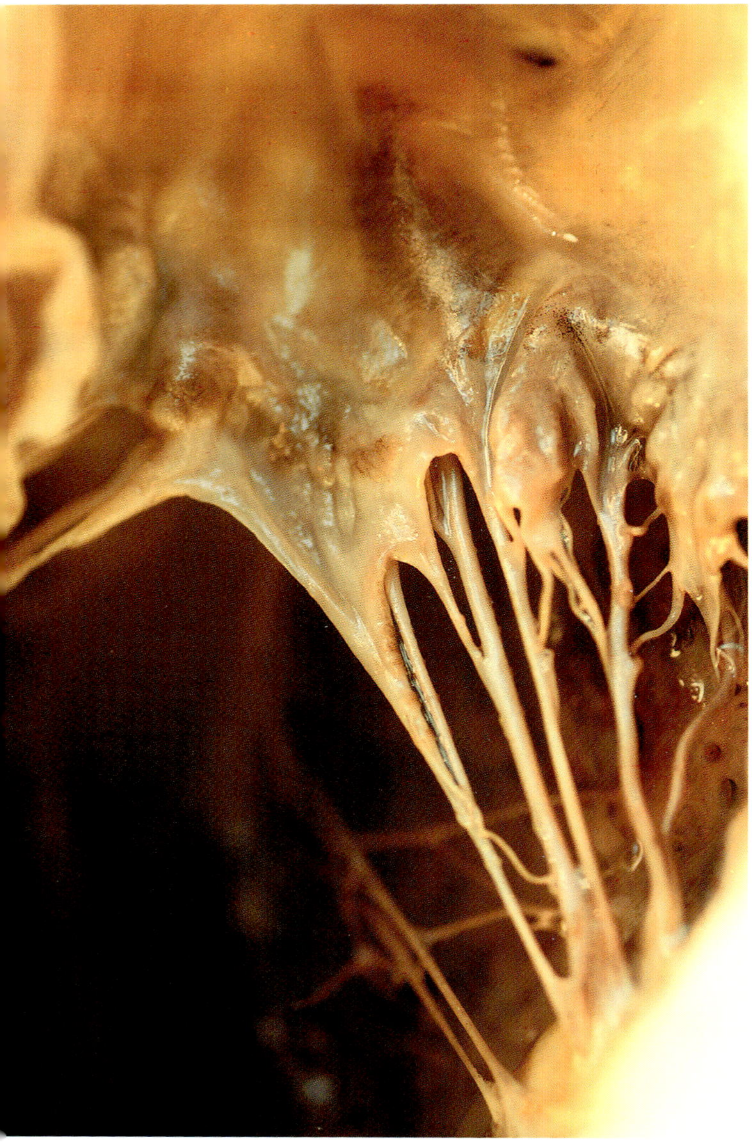

Figure 16. Image of the cranial leaflet of the mitral valve. It is also frequent to find elongation of the chordae tendineae, as well as distended moderator bands.

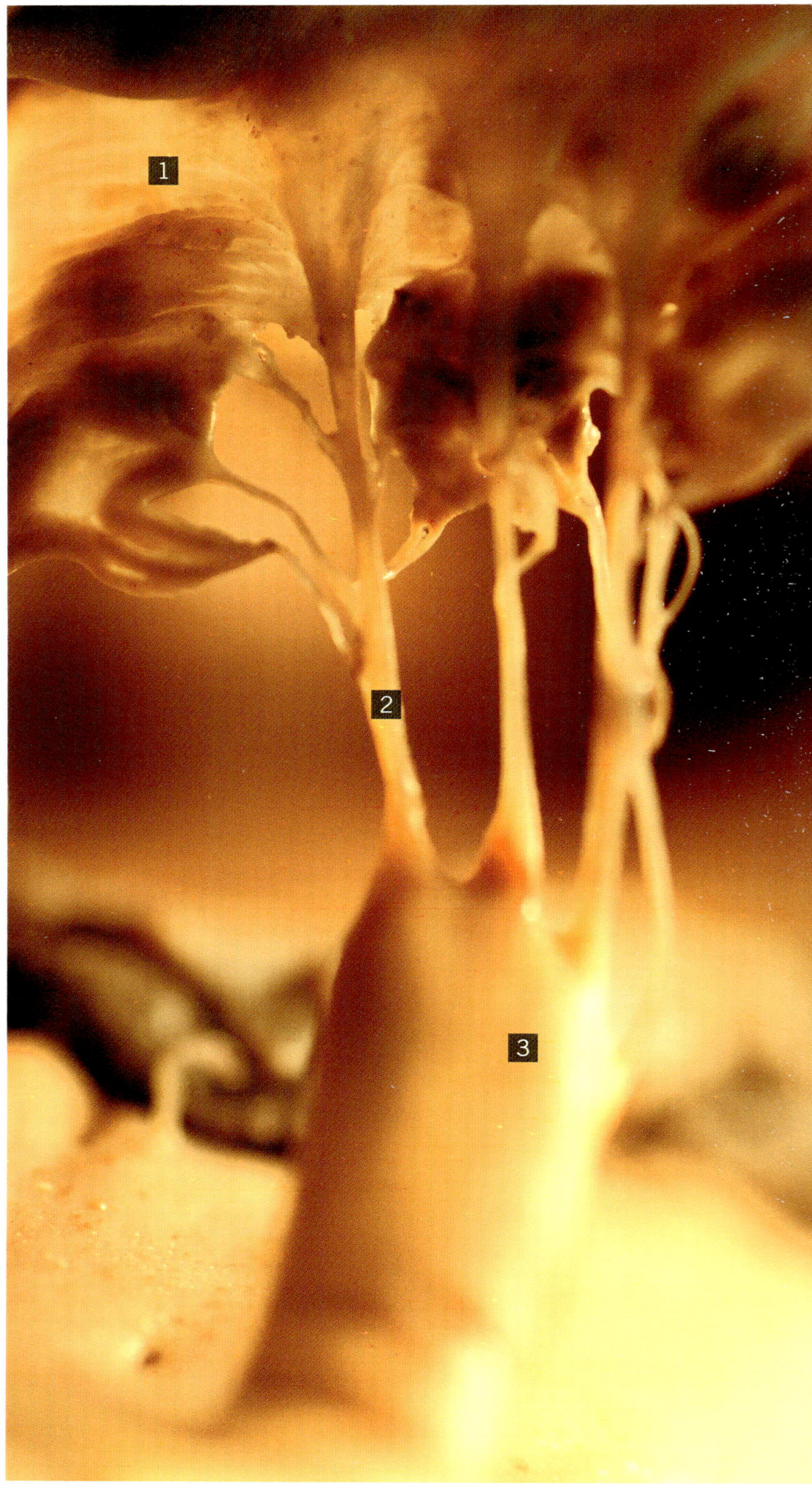

Figure 17. In the tricuspid valve, we can also find elongation of the chordae tendineae and a certain degree of elongation of the papillary muscles.

[1 Mural leaflet]

[2 Chordae tendineae]

[3 Papillary muscle]

Figure 18. The dilation of the ventricular cavity can also be observed in the outflow tract of the left ventricle.

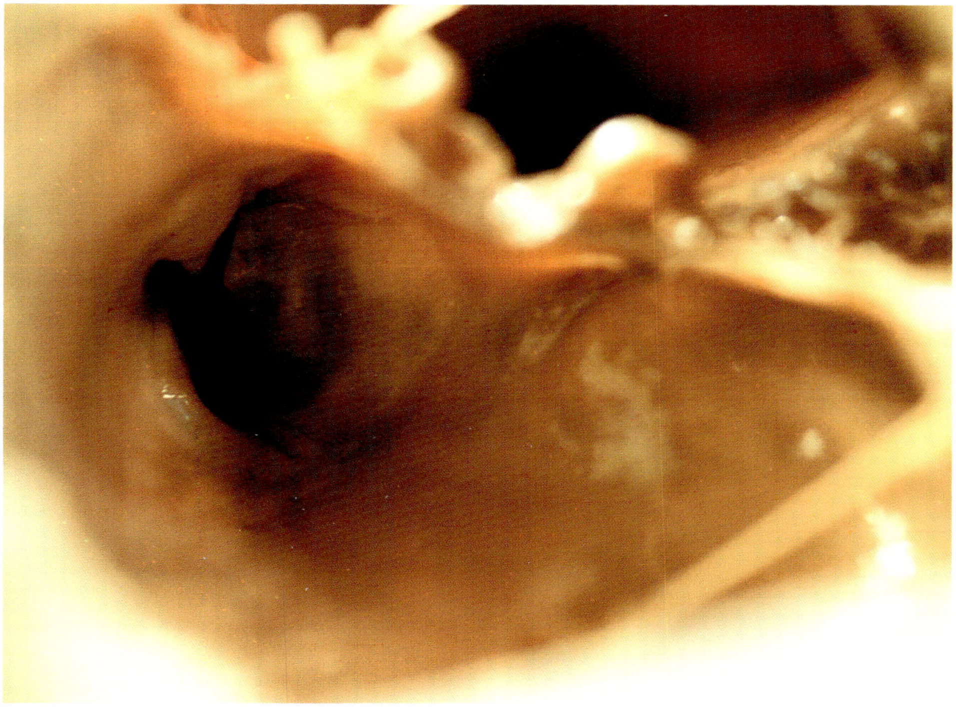

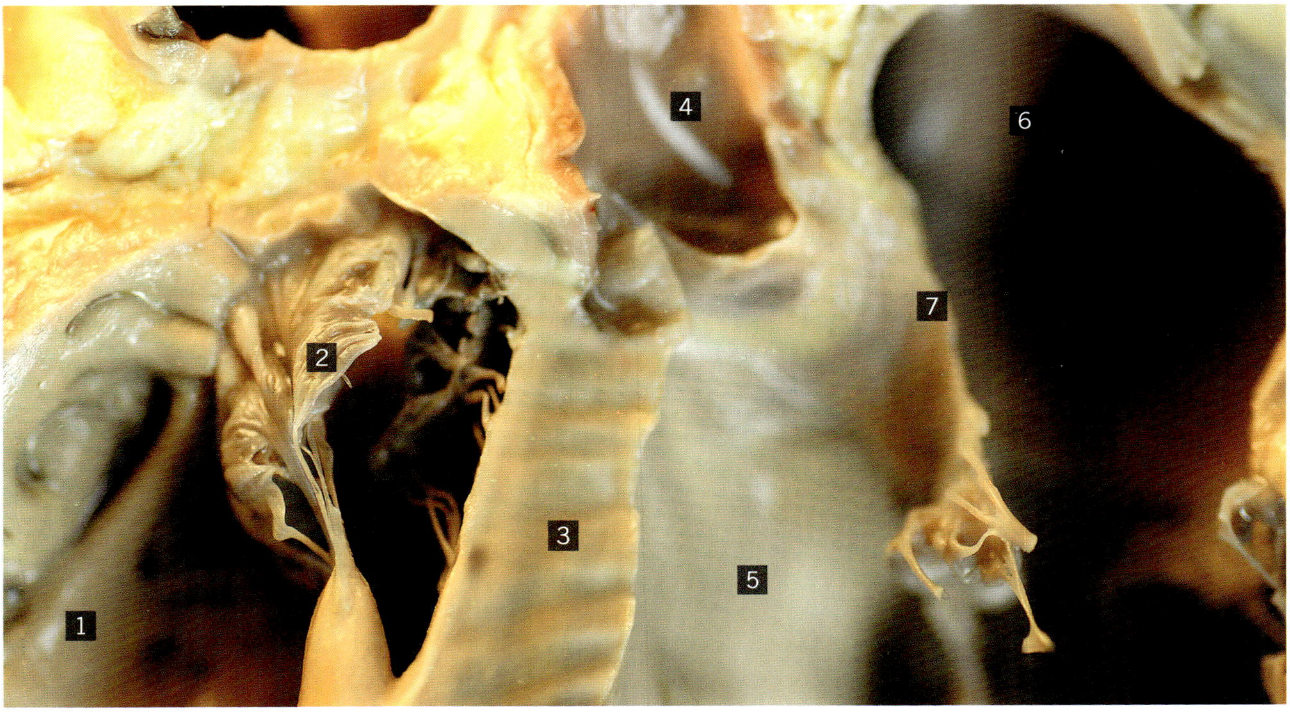

Figure 19. Dilated cardiomyopathy.

[1 Right ventricle]

[2 Tricuspid valve]

[3 Interventricular septum]

[4 Aorta]

[5 Outflow tract of the left ventricle]

[6 Left atrium]

[7 Cranial leaflet of the mitral valve]

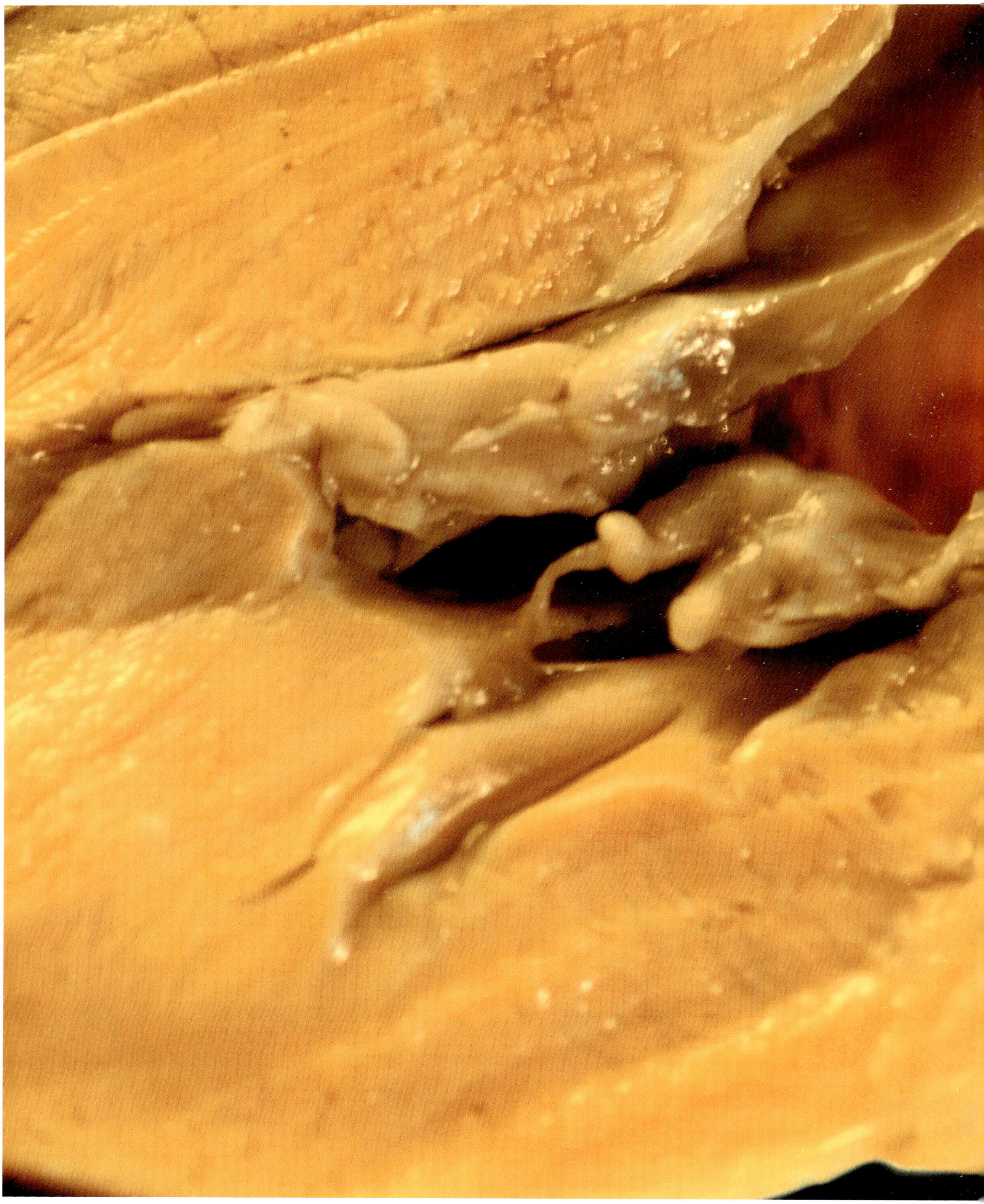

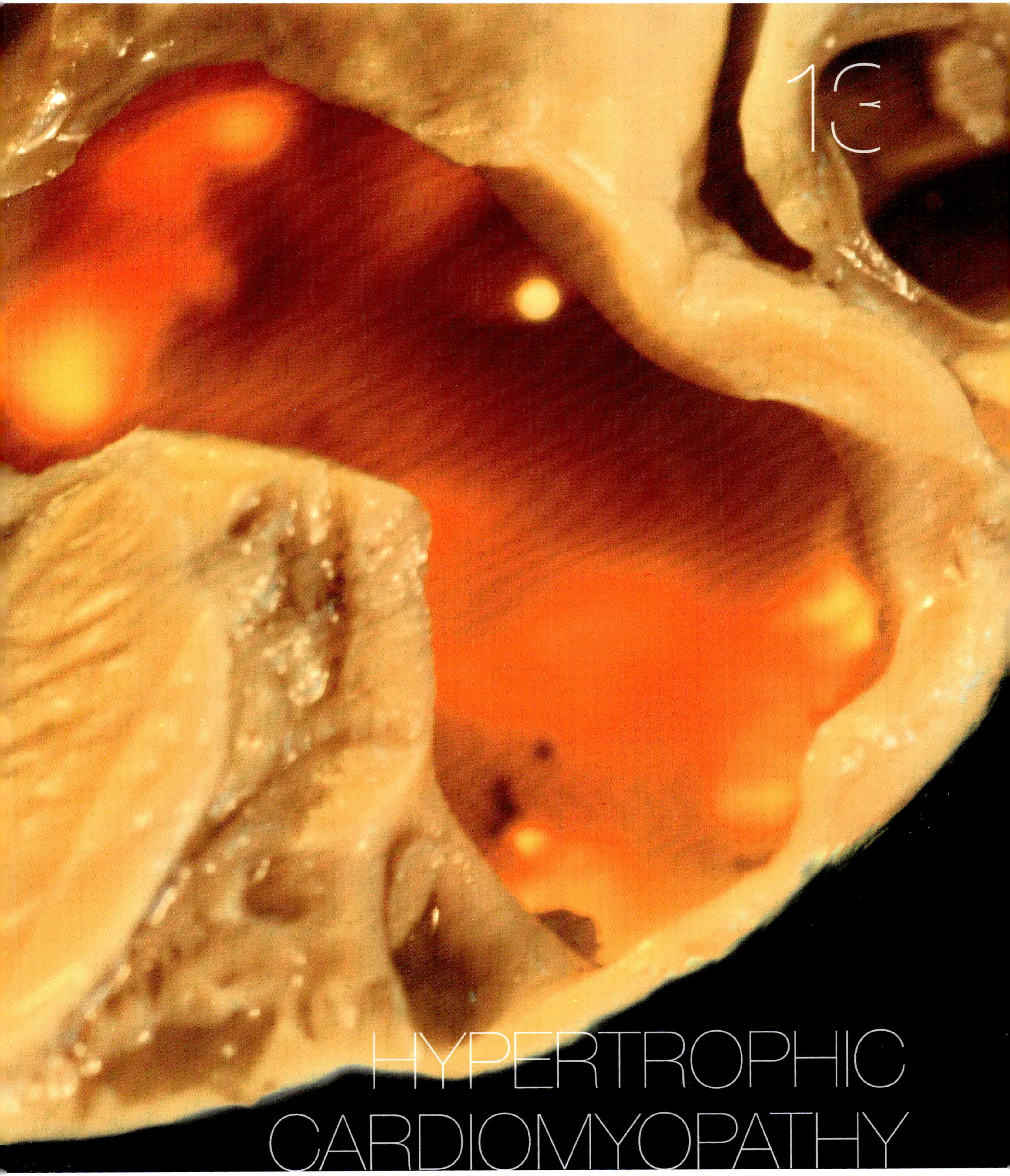

13

HYPERTROPHIC CARDIOMYOPATHY

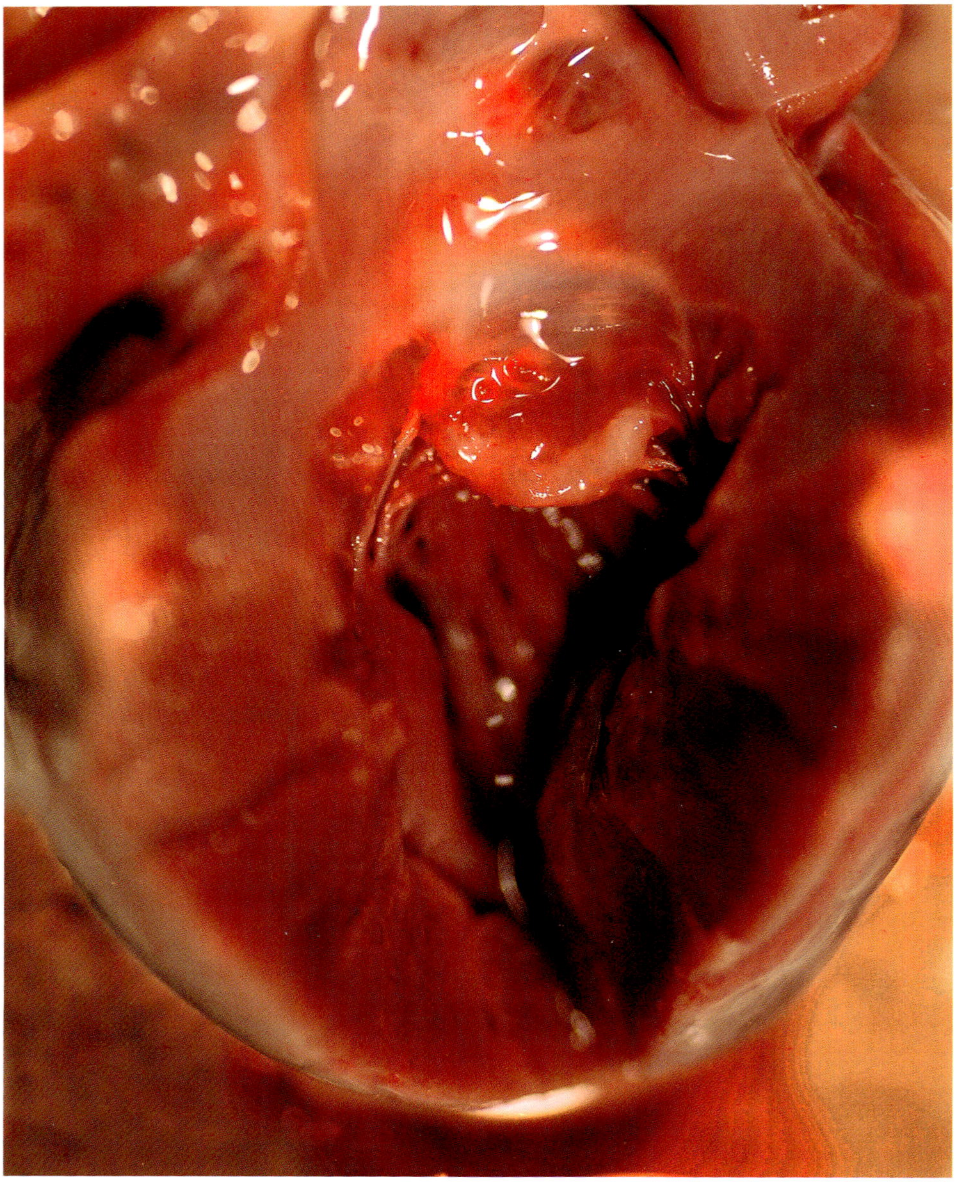

Figure 1. Hypertrophic cardiomyopathy in a Boston Terrier. Although it is uncommon, this disease can also be found in dogs.

Hypertrophic cardiomyopathy is a disease of the myocardium that is characterised by ventricular concentric hypertrophy with no primary cause, such as hypertension, hypothyroidism or aortic stenosis.

It is the most frequent myocardial disease in cats, although it can also be observed in dogs on rare occasions.

It essentially affects middle-aged to senior cats and is more often observed in males. A genetic form of the disease has been described in the Maine Coon breed and there seems to be a family predisposition in Persian, Ragdoll and Cornish Rex cats, although it has also been found in crossbred cats.

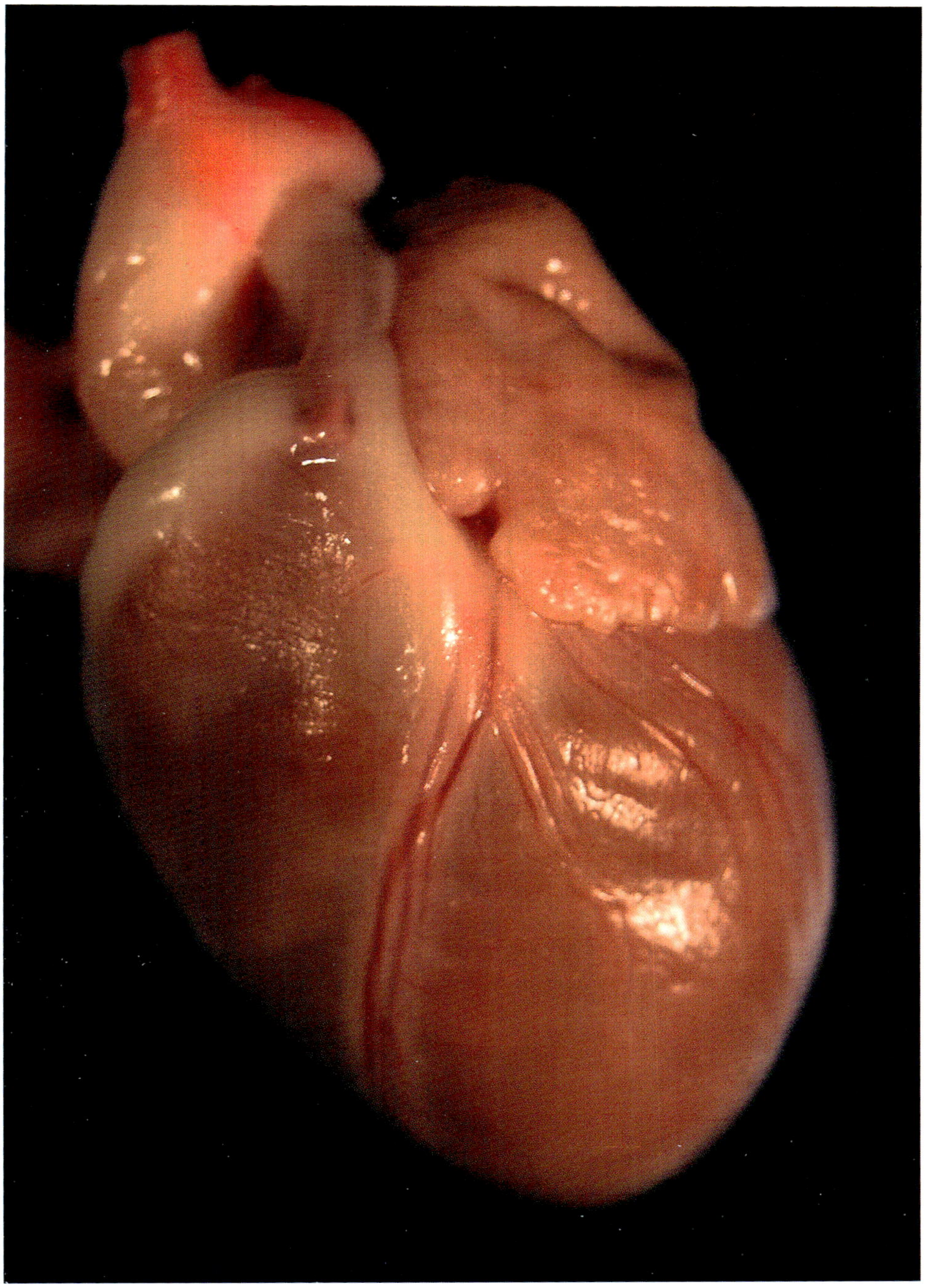

Figure 2. Hypertrophic cardiomyopathy in a cat. It is possible to observe a great enlargement of the left atrium.

The essential characteristic of the disease is the concentric hypertrophy of the left ventricle that affects the interventricular septum, free wall and papillary muscles, although not always to the same extent, and that may give rise to an asymmetric form (with greater involvement of the septum or free wall) or to a symmetric form.

The hypertrophy of the papillary muscles is generally very marked.

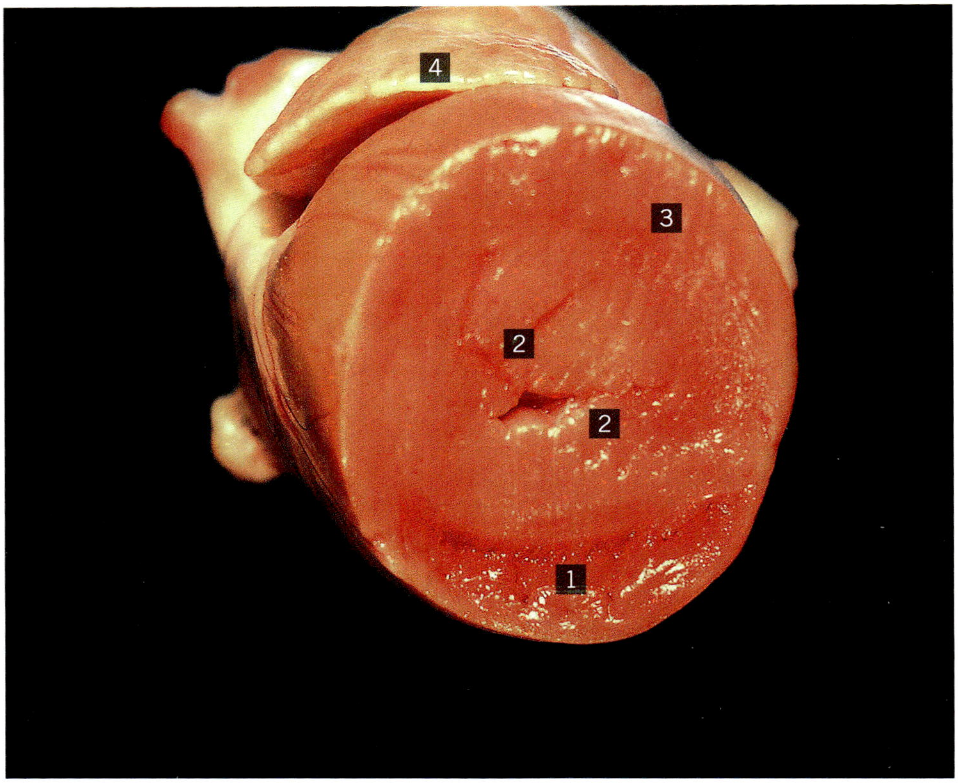

[1 Interventricular septum]

[2 Papillary muscles]

[3 Free wall of the left ventricle]

[4 Left atrial appendage]

Figure 3. The concentric hypertrophy of the left ventricle is the main characteristic of this disease. In this case, in the cross-section, we can see that the interventricular septum, papillary muscles and free ventricular wall are affected.

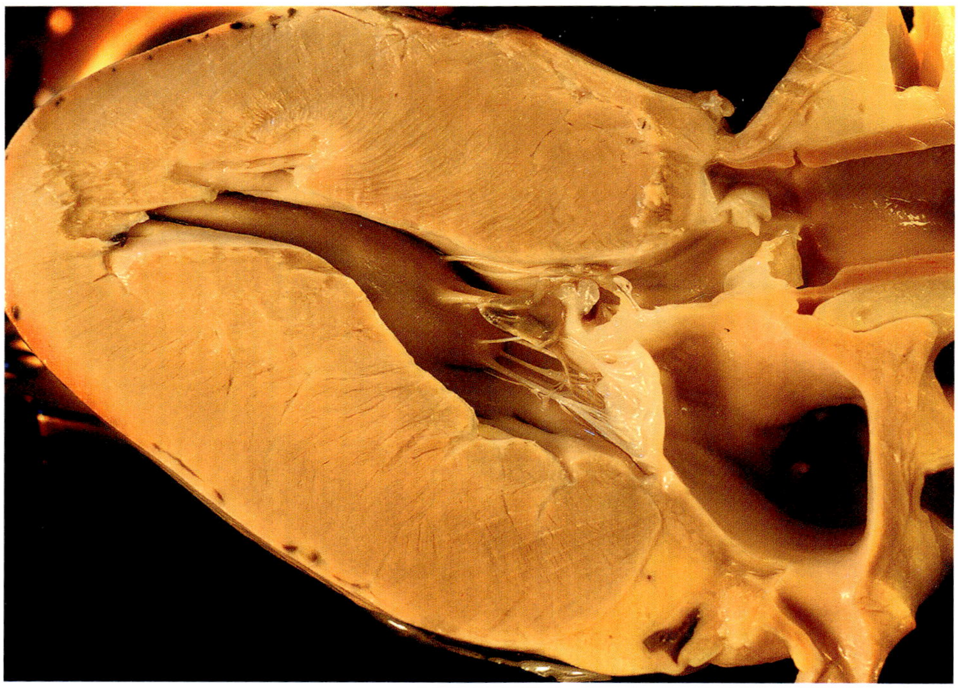

Figure 4. Symmetric hypertrophic cardiomyopathy, both the interventricular septum and free wall are affected to the same extent.

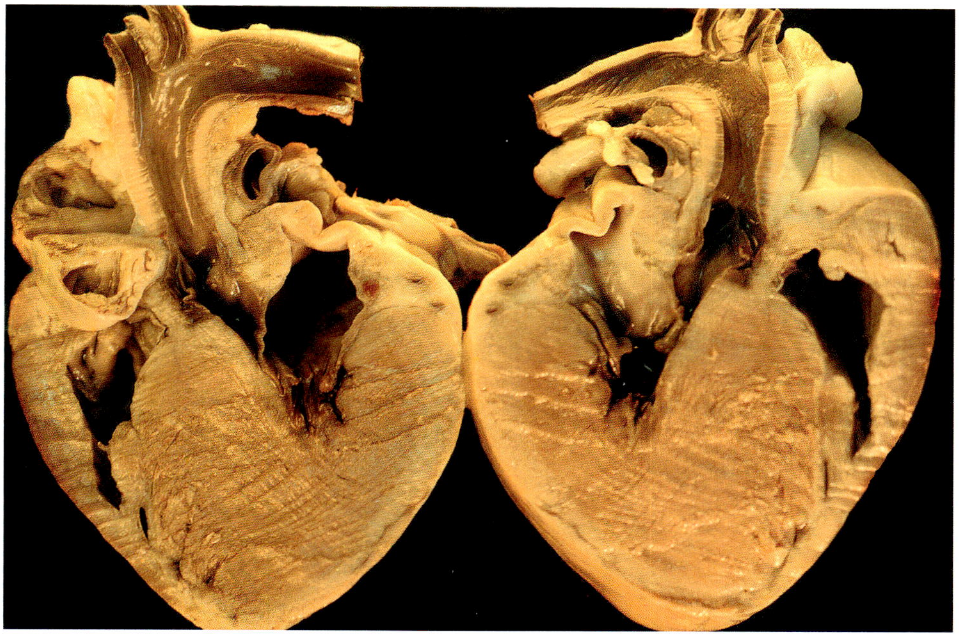

Figure 5. Asymmetric hypertrophic cardiomyopathy; the interventricular septum is much more affected than the free wall.

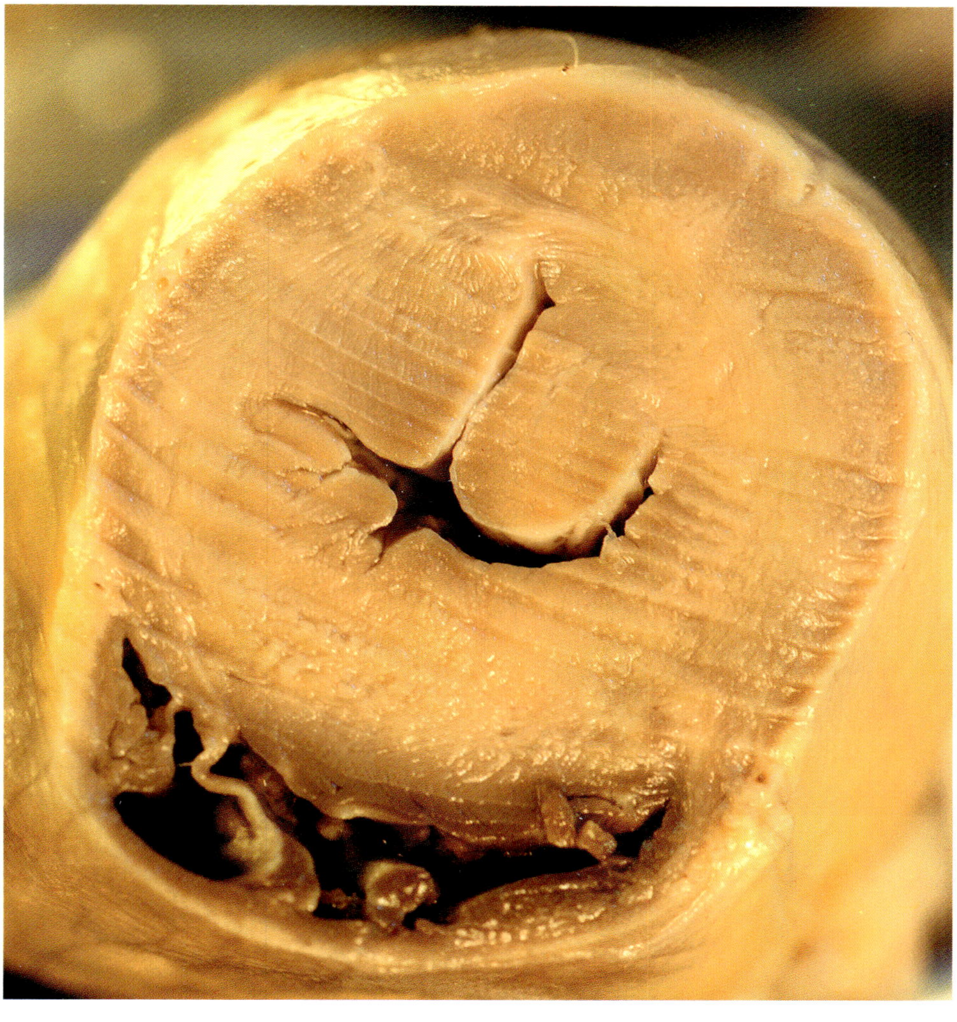

Figure 6. Another common characteristic of both symmetric and asymmetric hypertrophies is the considerable reduction of the ventricular cavity as it is invaded by the hypertrophied myocardium.

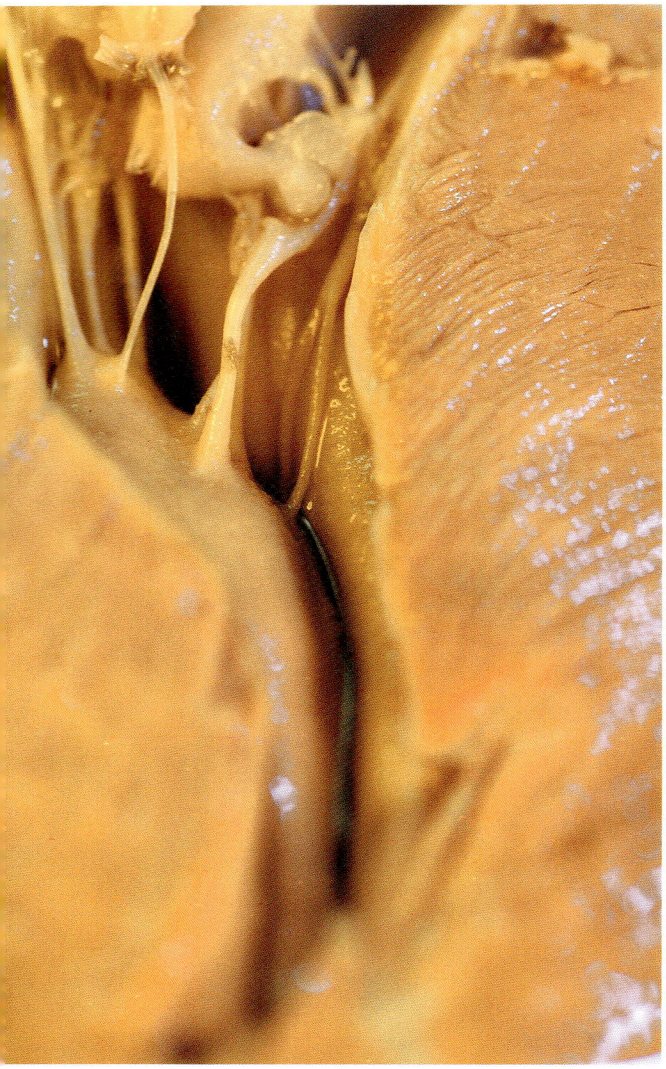

Figure 7. The hypertrophy of the papillary muscles is usually marked. This results in the chordae tendineae being closer to the leaflets, thus contributing to the functional alteration of the mitral valve apparatus.

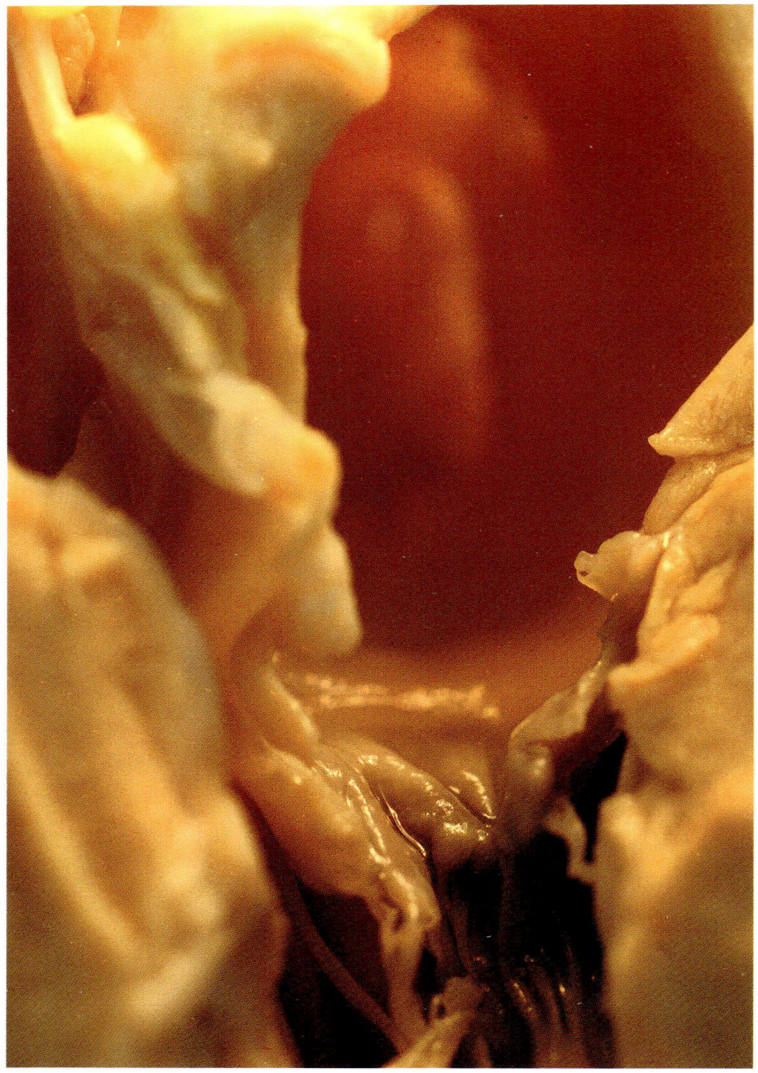

Figure 8. Diastolic dysfunction is going to cause an increase in the pressure of the left atrium, which will in most cases lead to significant atrial dilation.

In all the cases, the ventricular cavity is considerably reduced as it is invaded by the hypertrophied myocardium; although there is usually some ventricular contraction after death in cats with hypertrophic cardiomyopathy, and the thickness of the wall in necropsy samples is therefore closer to the one observed at the end of systole when the animal is alive.

The hypertrophy of the myocardium, associated fibrous lesions and ischaemia related to the decrease in the coronary density/myocardial mass ratio lead to a deterioration of ventricular relaxation and to an increase in the rigidity of the walls of the ventricle. This results in diastolic dysfunction, which will cause an increase in the pressure of the left atrium with atrial dilation and hypertrophy.

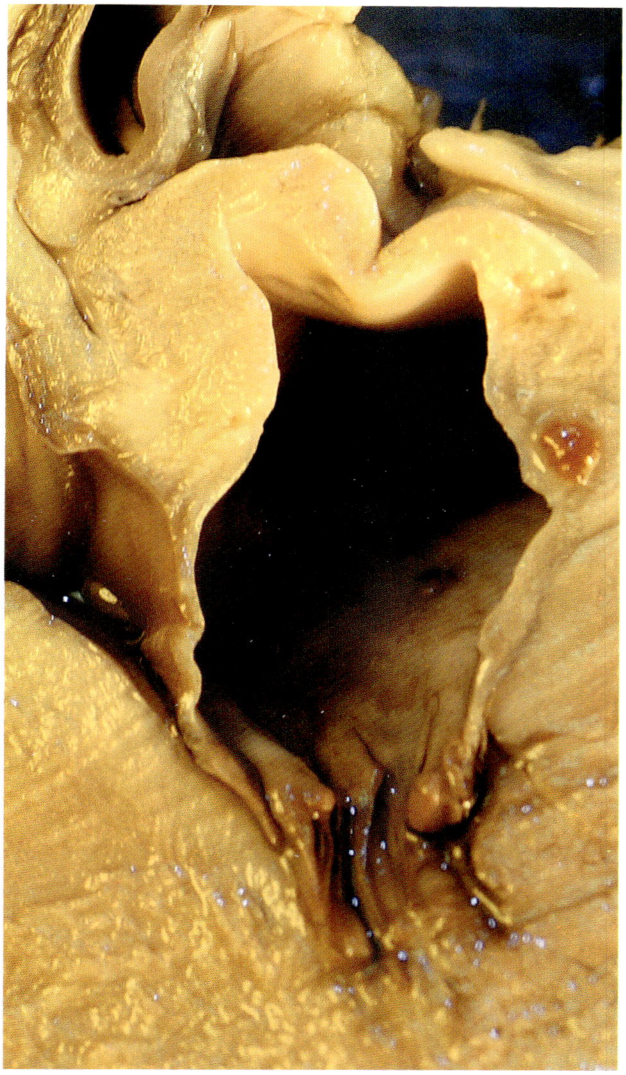

Figure 9. Some degree of hypertrophy can sometimes be found in addition to dilation of the atrial cavity.

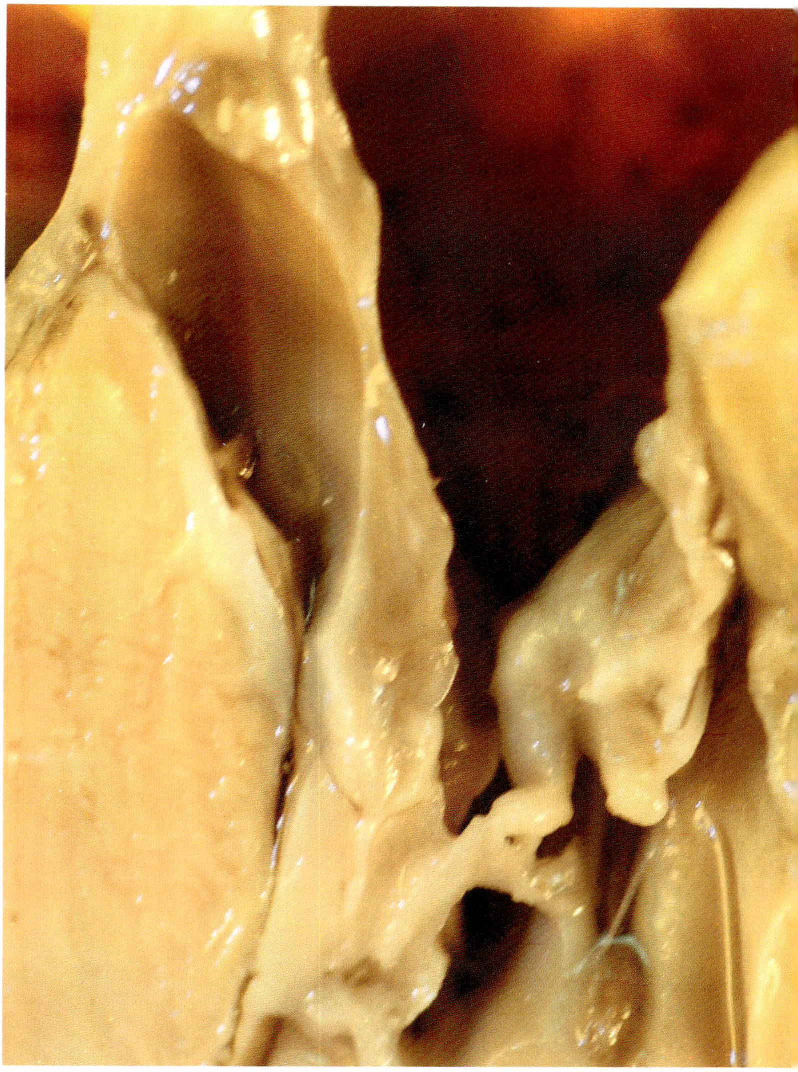

Figure 10. It is common to find thickened mitral valve leaflets.

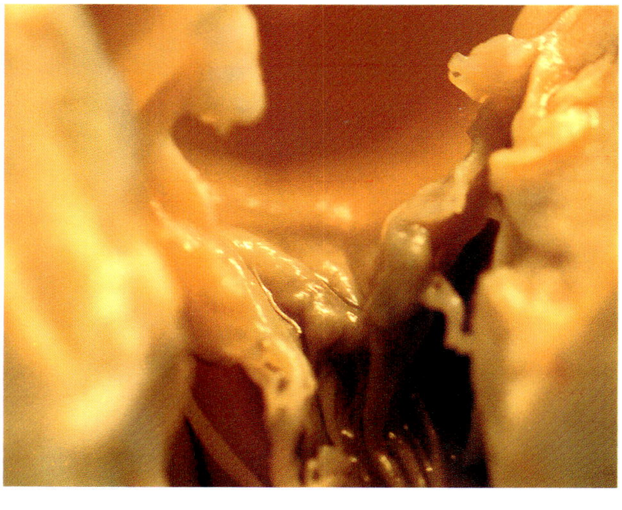

Figure 11. Thickened mitral valve leaflets.

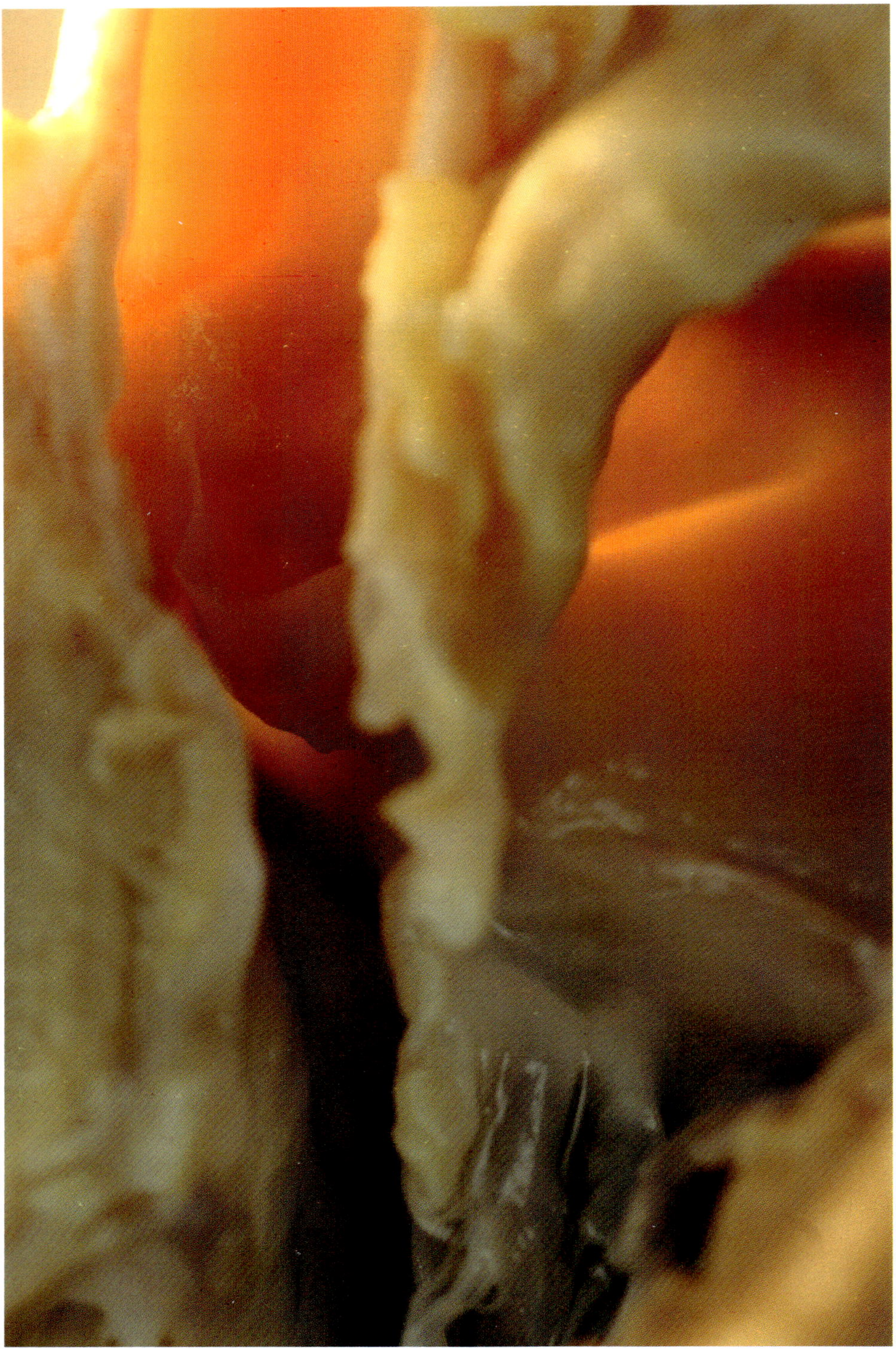

Figure 12. The geometrical alterations that take place in the left ventricle as a consequence of the hypertrophy of the septum, free ventricular wall and papillary muscles, together with atrial dilation, will lead to a dynamic obstruction of the outflow tract of the left ventricle and mitral regurgitation.

We often observe, during systole, a dynamic obstruction of the outflow tract of the left ventricle and mitral regurgitation, which contribute to the worsening of the heart failure.

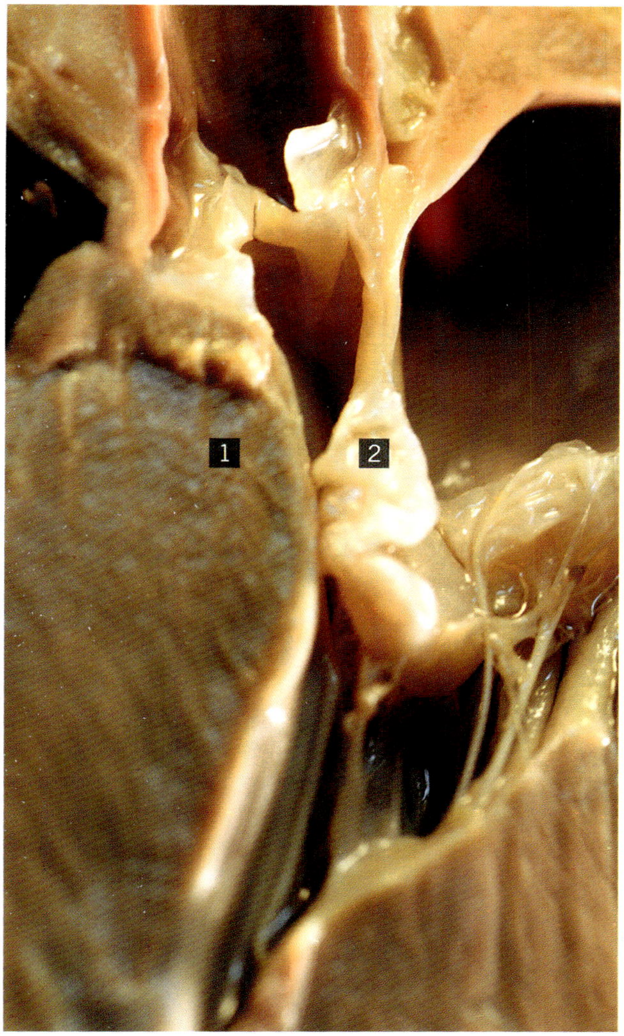

Figure 13. The dynamic obstruction of the outflow tract of the left ventricle will be originated by the thickening of the basilar region of the ventricular septum and the systolic anterior movement of the cranial leaflet of the mitral valve.

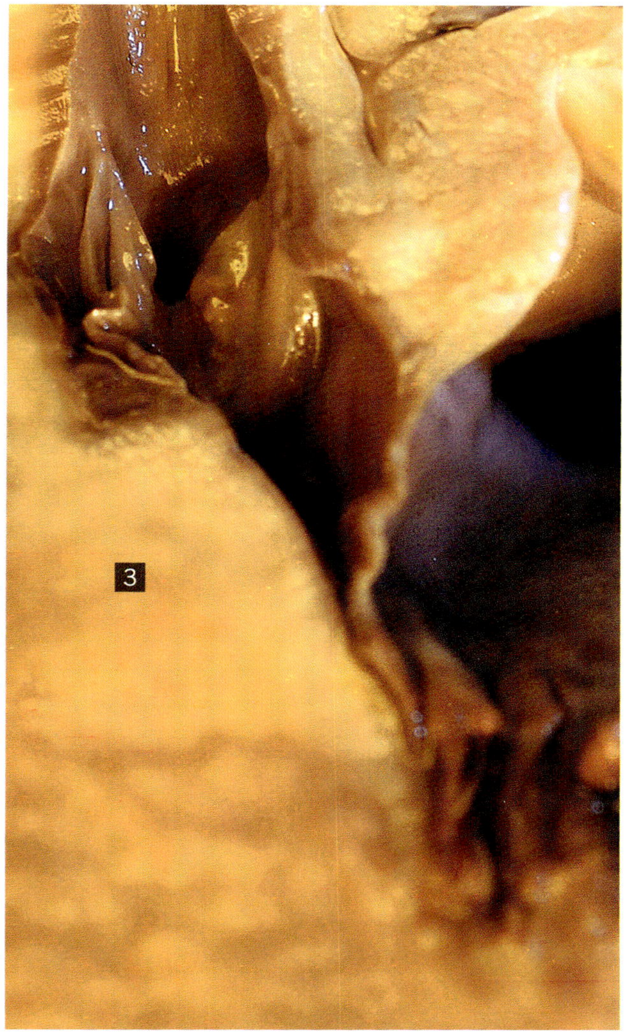

Figure 14. Marked thickening of the interventricular septum that invades almost the whole outflow tract.

[1 Interventricular septum]

[2 Cranial leaflet of the mitral valve]

[3 Basilar part of the interventricular septum]

These alterations are the direct consequence of geometrical changes in the left ventricle. On the one hand, there is an alteration of the structure that the mitral valve apparatus should occupy, due to the hypertrophy of the walls and papillary muscles and to the dilation of the left atrium; on the other hand, the chordae tendineae lie closer to the leaflets due to the hypertrophy of the papillary muscles and their main holding function is therefore altered to some extent. This will facilitate the systolic anterior movement of the mitral valve which, together with the marked thickening of the basilar part of the interventricular septum, will lead to the dynamic obstruction of the aortic outflow tract, which can be intermittent or continuous.

A thickening of the leaflets of the mitral valve may also sometimes be found.

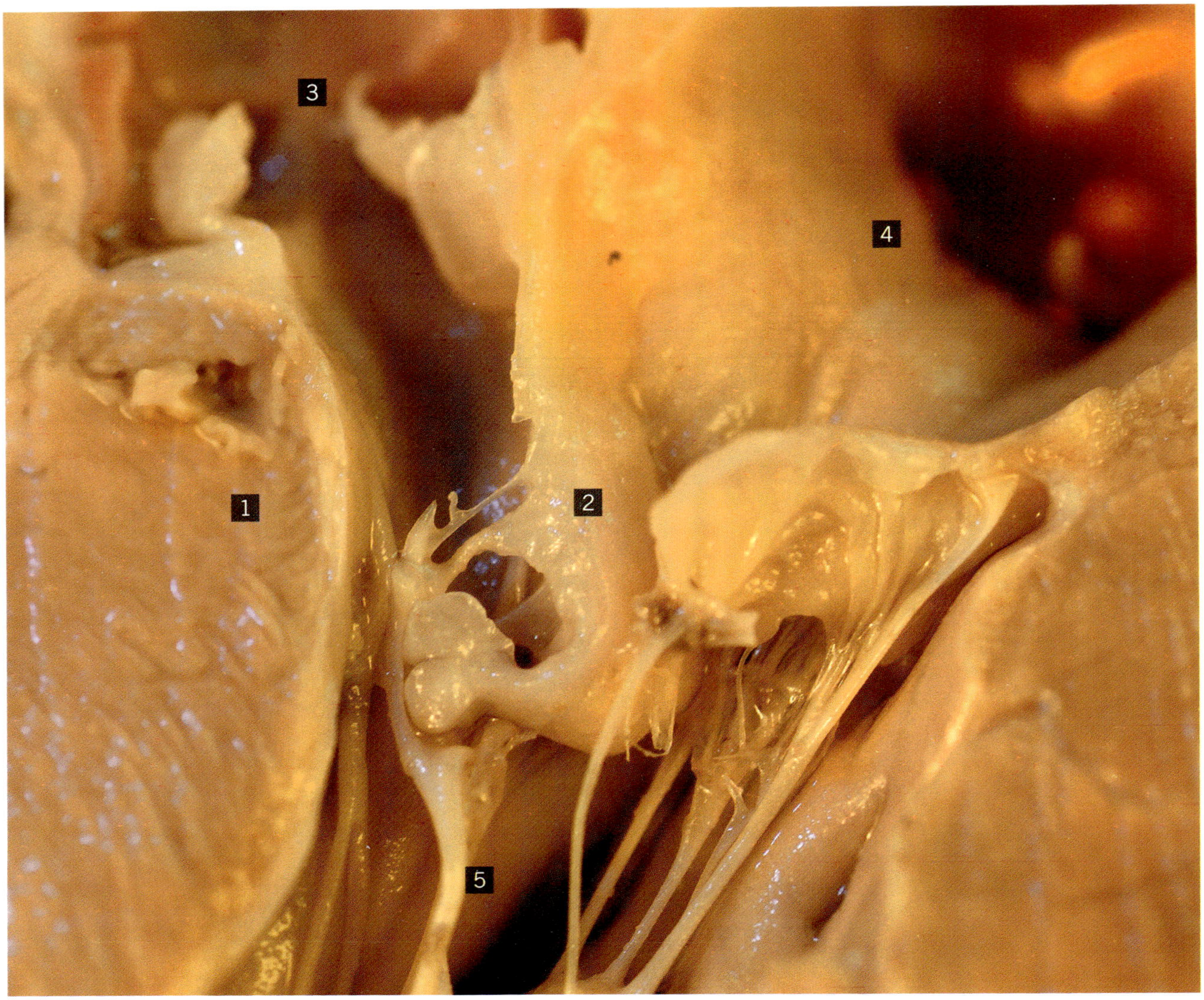

Figure 15. The systolic anterior movement of the mitral valve occurs due to the displacement of the papillary muscles caused by their hypertrophy, which leads to an incorrect tension of the chordae tendineae. The hypertrophy of the septum causes a narrowing of the ventricular outflow tract, which leads to an increased blood flow velocity at this point. This produces a Venturi effect that pulls the valve towards the outflow tract, which causes a dynamic obstruction.

[1 Septum]

[2 Cranial leaflet of the mitral valve]

[3 Aortic leaflet]

[4 Left atrium]

[5 Chordae tendineae]

The marked dilation of the left atrium causes alterations of the normal flow in it, as well as alterations of the atrial endothelium, with a possible release of cytokines that facilitate the appearance of thrombi. These thrombi may also occur, on occasions, in other areas of the heart that are predisposed to blood stasis, such as the apical region of the left ventricle.

These thrombi tend to cause systemic embolisation and frequently remain (90 % of cases) in the distal aortic trifurcation, causing ischaemic neuropathy of the hind limbs.

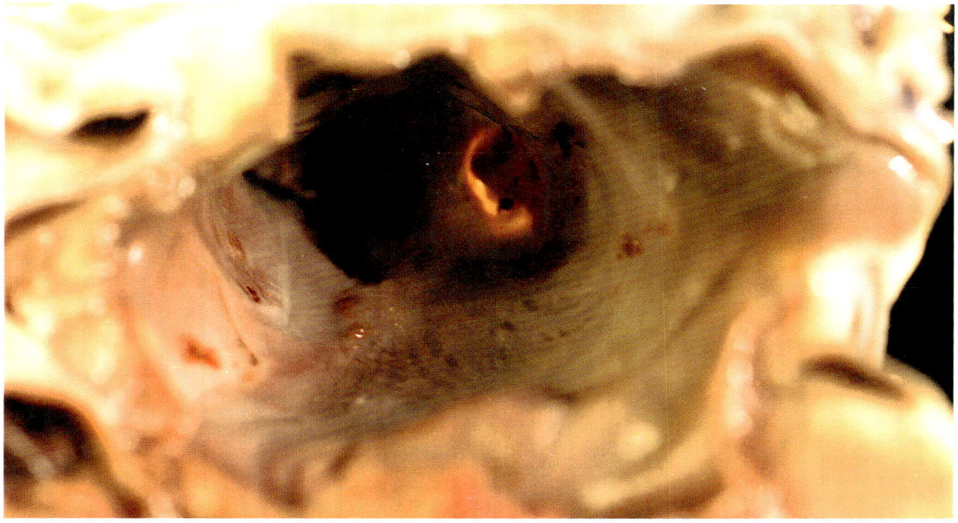

Figure 16. The marked dilation of the atrium leads to alterations of the flow in this chamber of the heart, as well as to the release of cytokines in the endothelium, which are going to favour the appearance of thrombi in this area.

[1 Site where more than 90 % of thrombi remain in cases of hypertrophic cardiomyopathy]

[2 Right iliac artery]

[3 Left iliac artery]

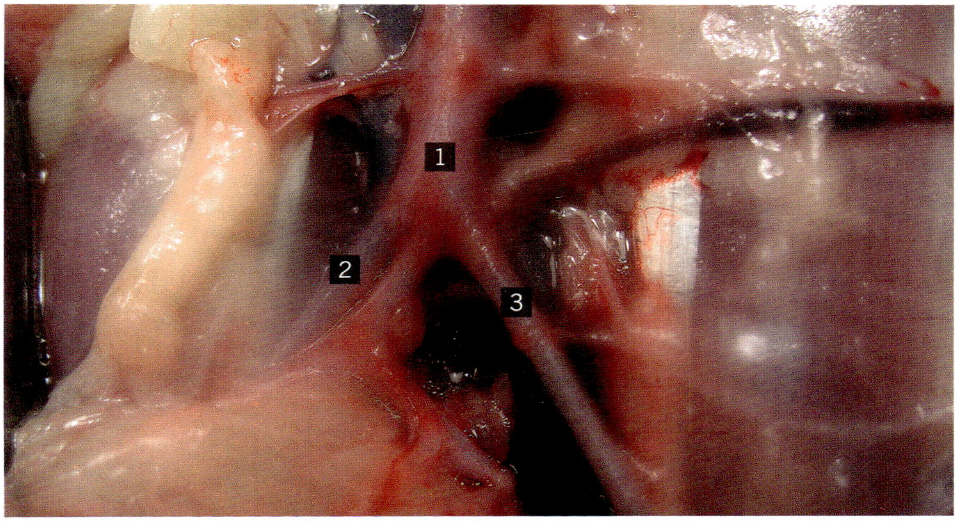

Figure 17. The thrombi that form tend to emigrate, the aortic trifurcation being the site where they most frequently remain.

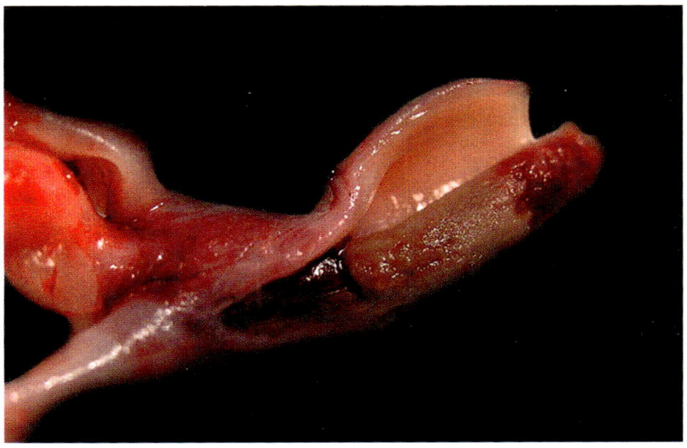

Figure 18. Thrombus in the aortic trifurcation in a cat with hypertrophic cardiomyopathy.

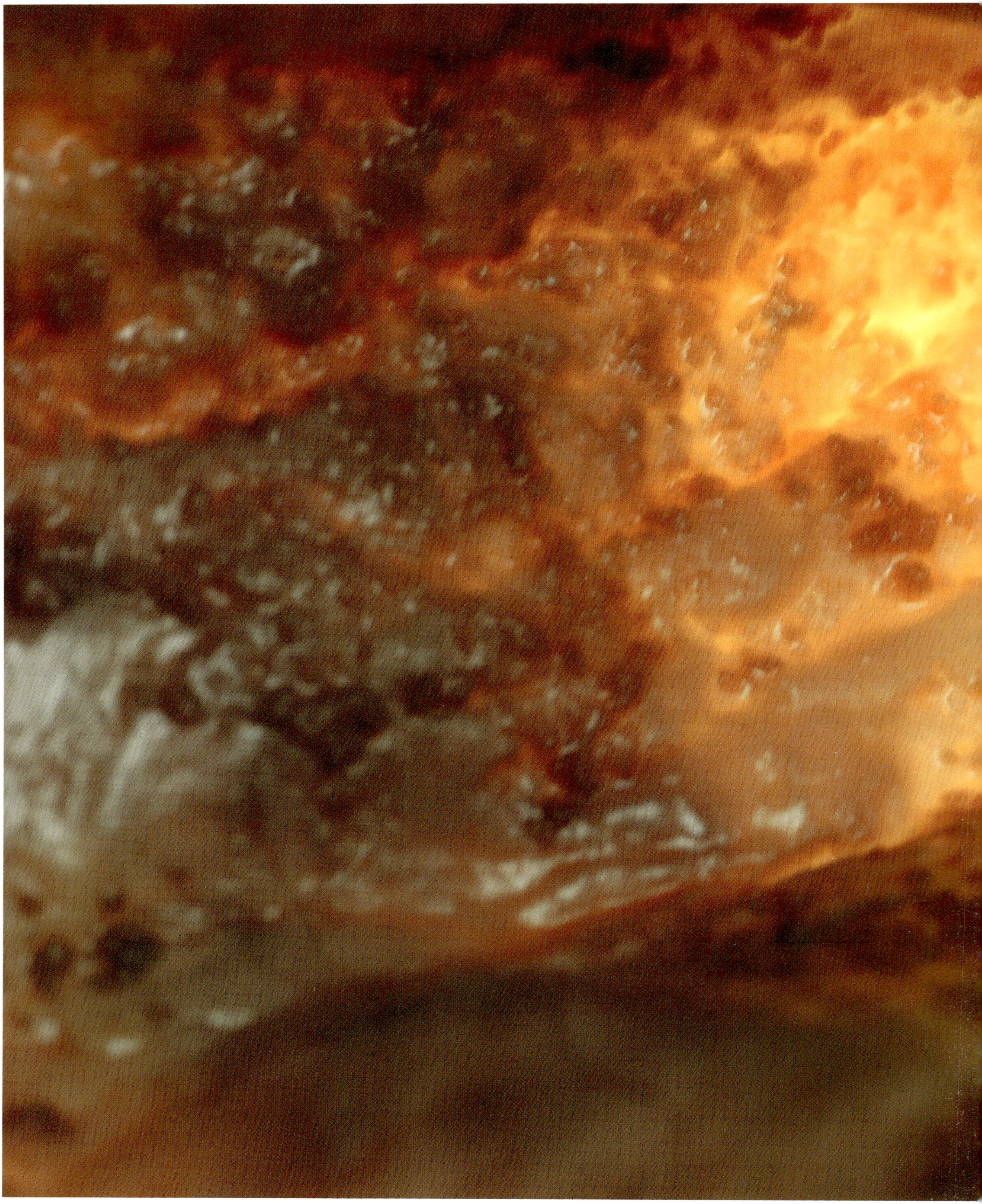

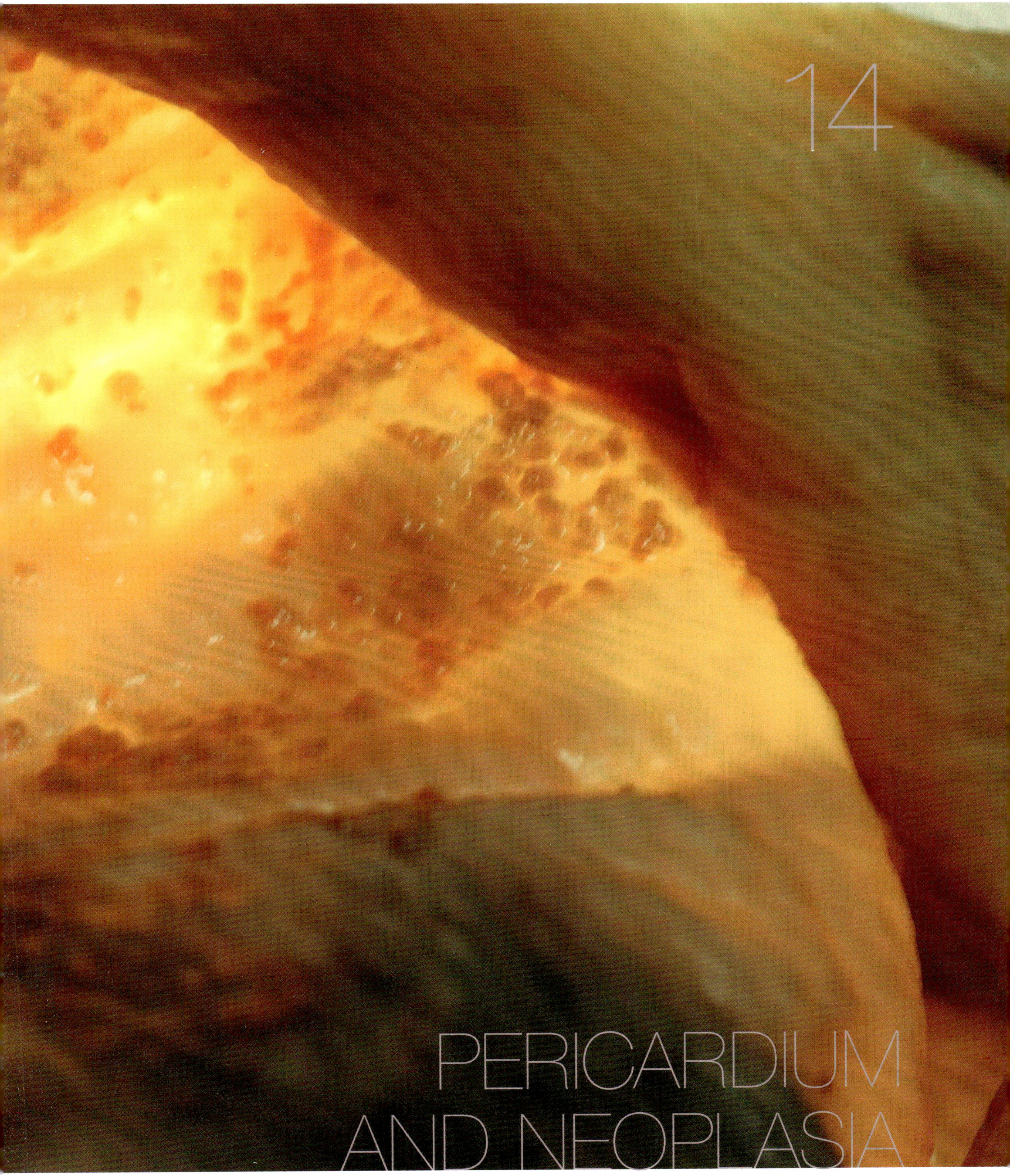

14

PERICARDIUM AND NEOPLASIA

The pericardium is the serofibrous sac that surrounds the heart. It is formed by an outer fibrous layer and an inner serous layer, which is in turn divided into two parts. One of them is directly related to the fibrous pericardium and the other, named epicardium, to the myocardium. The pericardial cavity, which contains a small amount of lubricating fluid, lies between these.

The diseases related to the pericardium that may be observed are: its congenital absence, intrapericardial cysts, peritoneal-pericardial hernia, constrictive pericarditis and pericardial effusions. Of all these, the two latter are, by far, the most frequently observed diseases.

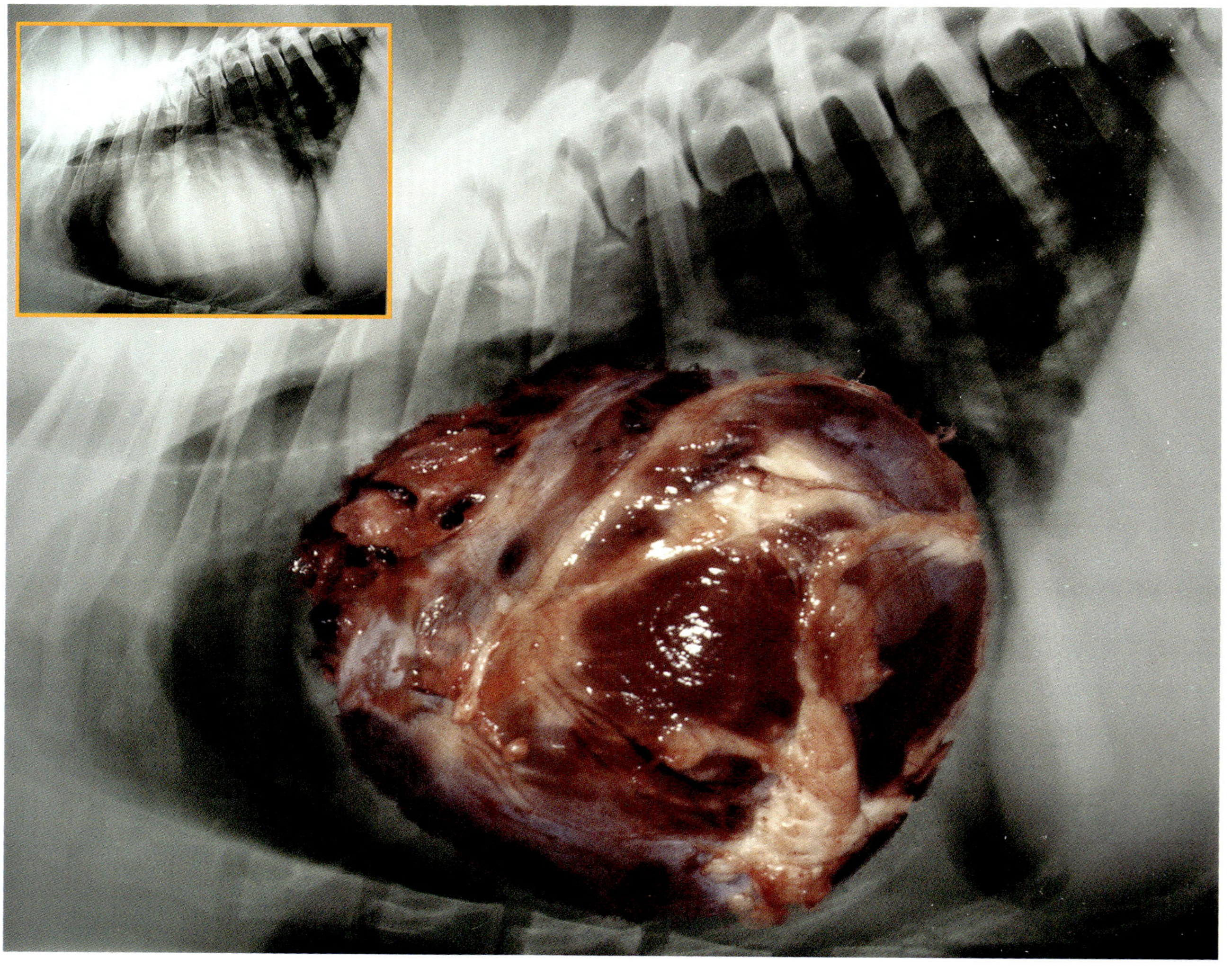

Figure 1. A marked increase of the cardiac silhouette, which acquires the aspect of a balloon, may be observed in radiographs of a heart with pericardial effusion. In this laterolateral projection, the anatomical image of a heart with marked pericardial effusion has been superimposed. As can be seen, this causes an elevation of the trachea, which occupies a large space in the thoracic cavity.

PERICARDIAL EFFUSION

A pericardial effusion corresponds to the presence of an excessive volume of fluid in the pericardial cavity.

The fast accumulation of fluid leads to an increase in intrapericardial pressure, which makes ventricular filling difficult, especially in the right ventricle, and causes a significant decrease of the cardiac output, leading to a stage known as cardiac tamponade.

Slow accumulations, on the other hand, cause a dilation of the fibrous pericardium and therefore an increase of the pericardial space. The increase in intrapericardial pressure is thus much lower, which delays the appearance of the cardiac tamponade.

Effusions may be transudative (cardiac failure, hypoproteinaemia), exudative (septic, inflammatory, neoplastic) and haemorrhagic (idiopathic, neoplastic).

Most pericardial failures are haemorrhagic, with a lower haematocrit than that of blood. They are characterised by an absence of coagulation.

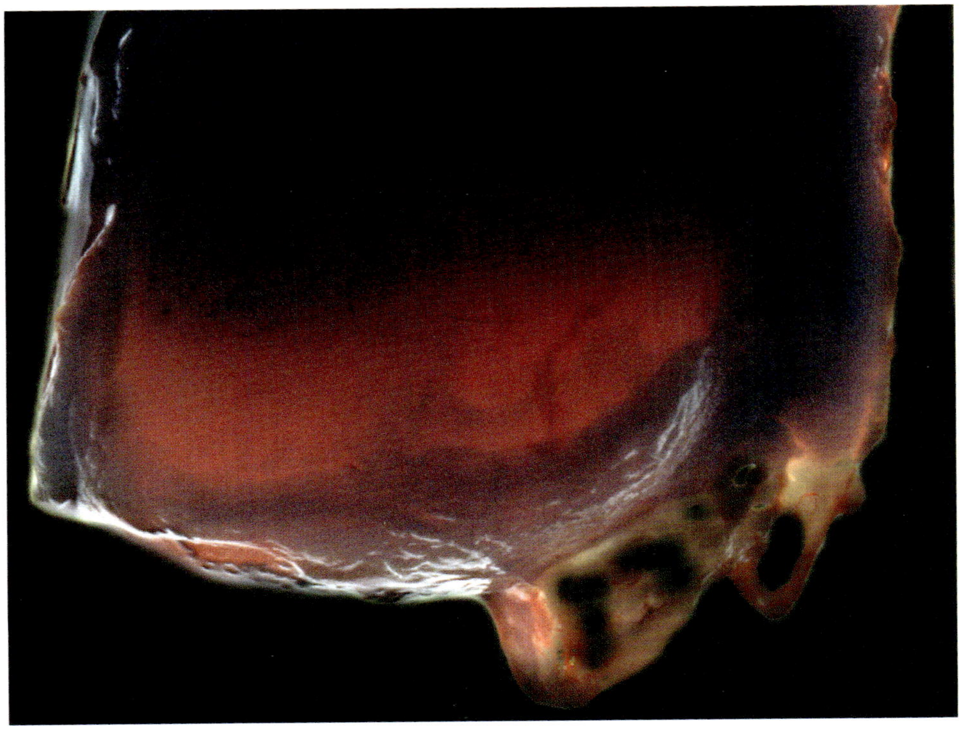

Figure 2. In pericardial effusions, large amounts of fluid may eventually accumulate in the pericardial sac. These accumulations, which may occur in a chronic or acute form, result in an increase in intrapericardial pressure, which causes a reduction of ventricular diastolic filling and therefore of the cardiac output. When intrapericardial pressure is the same as the right atrial and ventricular diastolic pressures, cardiac tamponade occurs.

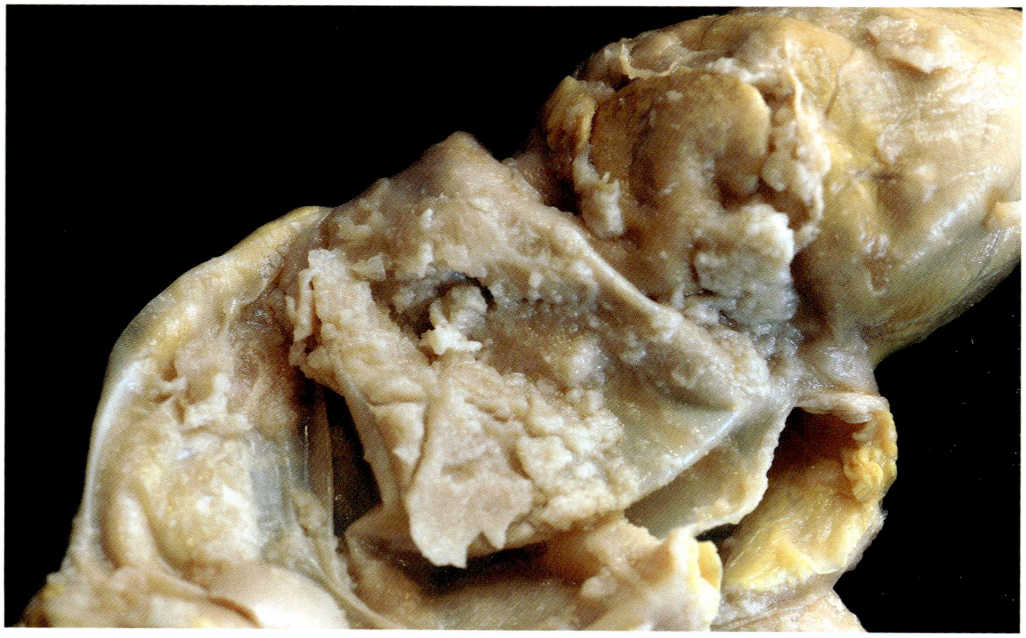

Figure 3. Septic pericarditis.

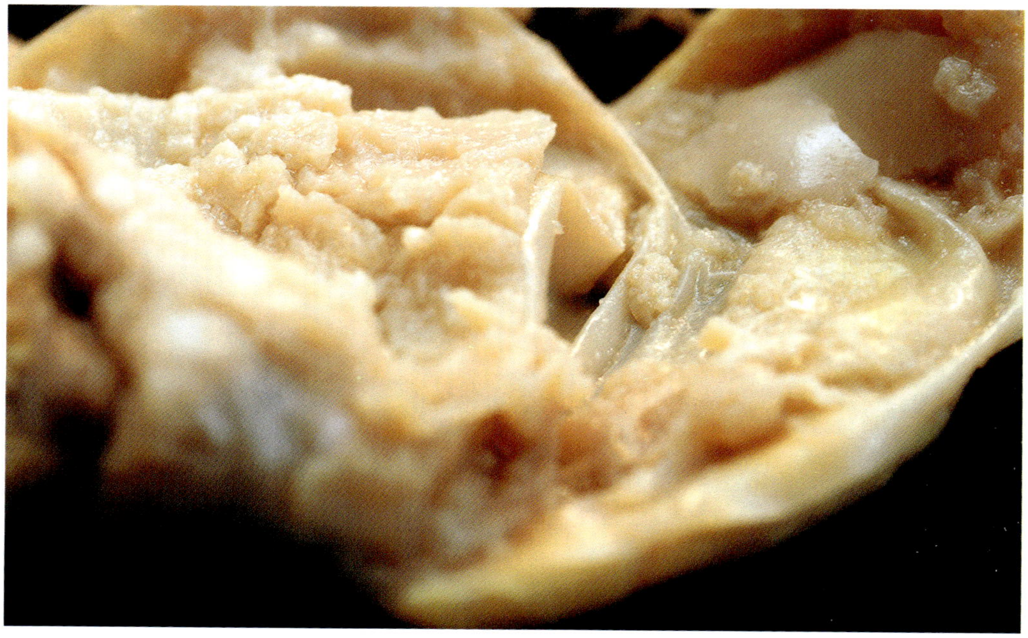

Figure 4. Detail of the effusion in a septic pericarditis.

Tumours are the main cause of pericardial effusion, as we will see later on. The second most frequent cause in dogs is idiopathic haemorrhagic pericardial effusion. Its aetiology, which is obviously unknown, may be related to viral and immune-mediated processes. Fluid accumulates slowly, which originates late signs of tamponade, and there is great dilation of the pericardial cavity. It may resolve spontaneously or be drained by pericardiocentesis or pericardiectomy. Recurrences of this type of effusion or a chronic evolution may lead to constrictive pericarditis.

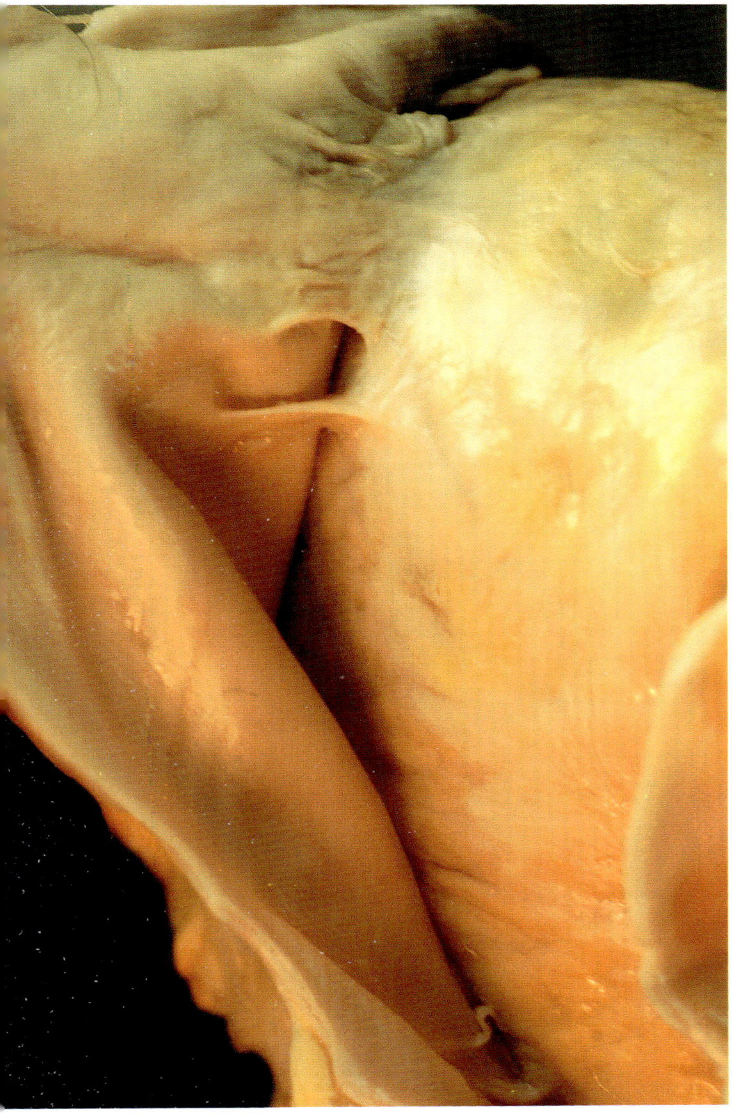

Figure 5. Constrictive pericarditis. The thickening of the pericardium and fibrous adherences between the epicardium and the pericardium may be observed.

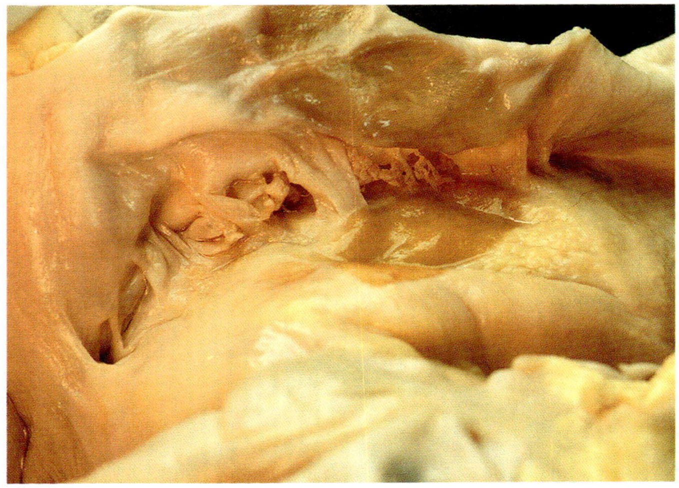

Figure 6. Constrictive pericarditis. Important adherences between the parietal pericardium and the epicardium.

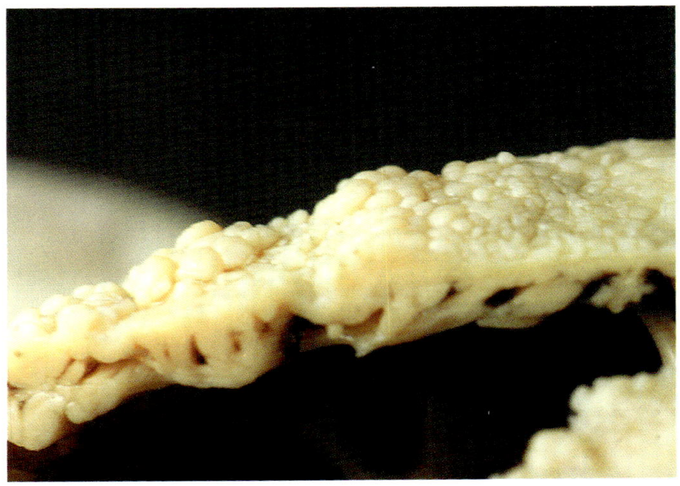

Figure 7. Constrictive pericarditis. In those cases in which the process is circumscribed and there is little fibrin, focal hyaline thickenings, known as milk spots, can be observed.

Constrictive perdicarditis causes a thickening of the pericardium. Adherences develop between the parietal and visceral layers and the distensibility of the pericardium decreases, which results in a reduction of the cardiac output. In addition, it is common to observe the presence of focal hyaline thickenings in the epicardium. Constrictive pericarditis may also occur due to infectious or neoplastic causes.

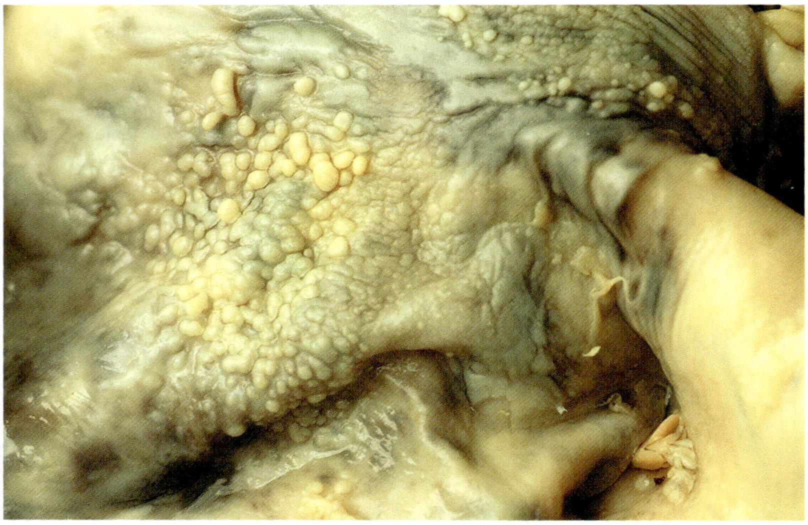

Figure 8. Constrictive pericarditis. Although hyaline thickenings are more frequently observed in the epicardium, they may also be found in the parietal pericardium.

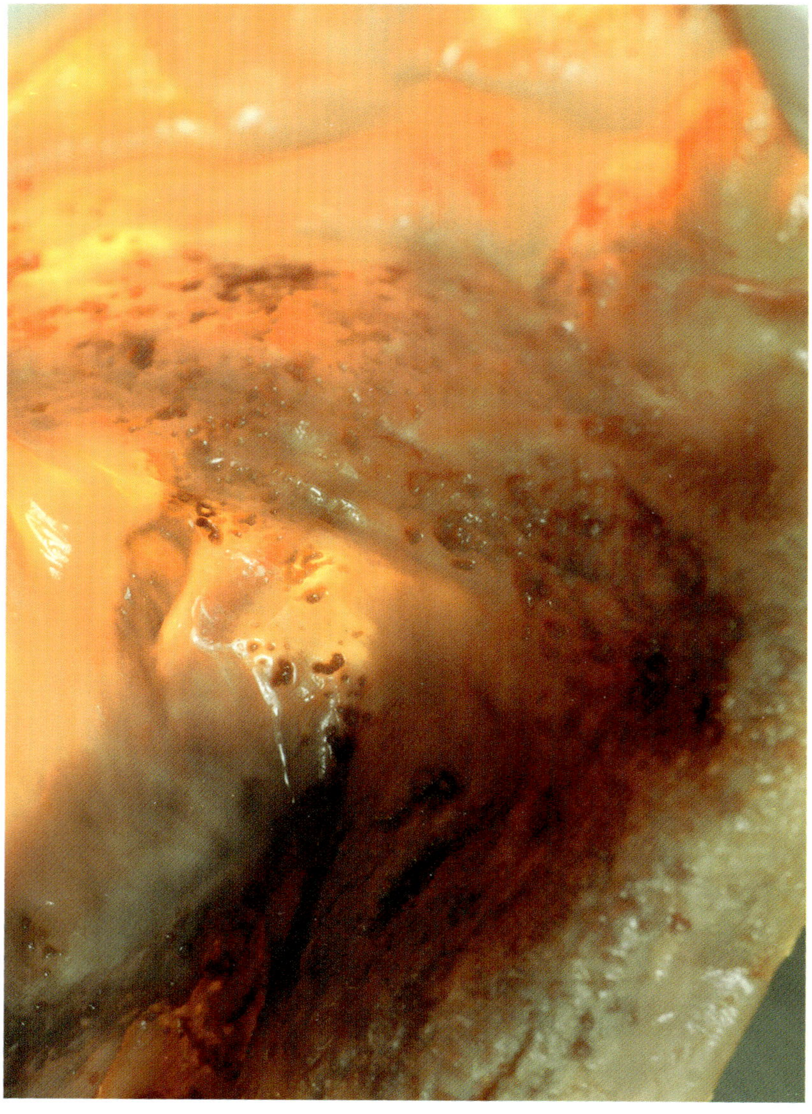

Figure 9. Constrictive pericarditis. Areas of hyaline thickening.

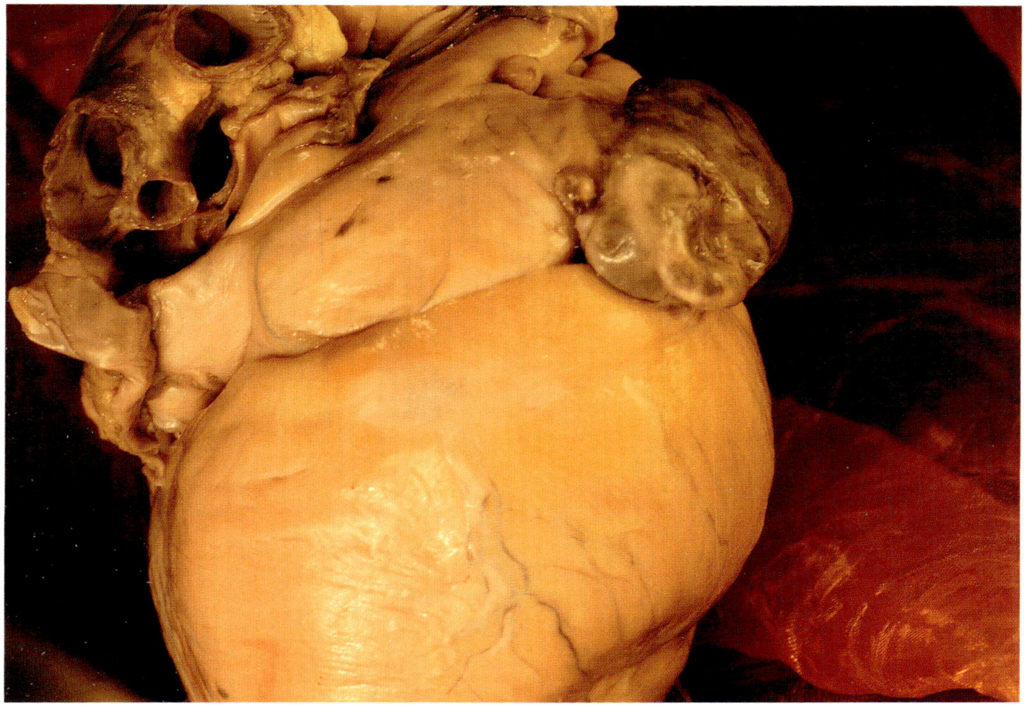

Figure 10. Haemangiosarcoma. The most frequent location of this type of tumour is the right atrial appendage. Note how the tumour extends on the right coronary sulcus.

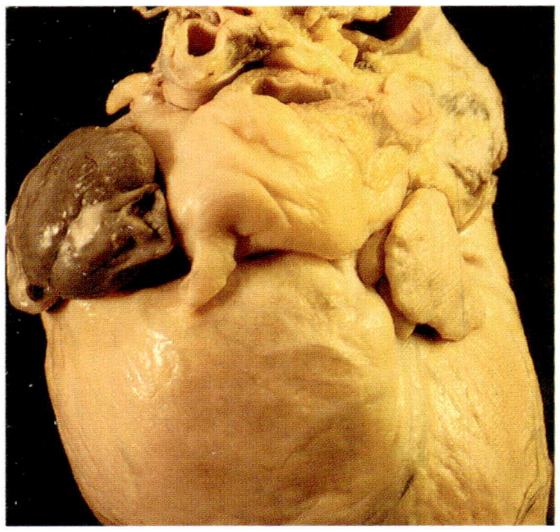

Figure 11. Same lesion as in the previous image in cranial view, where the right atrial appendage occupied by the haemangiosarcoma and the normal left atrial appendage can be observed.

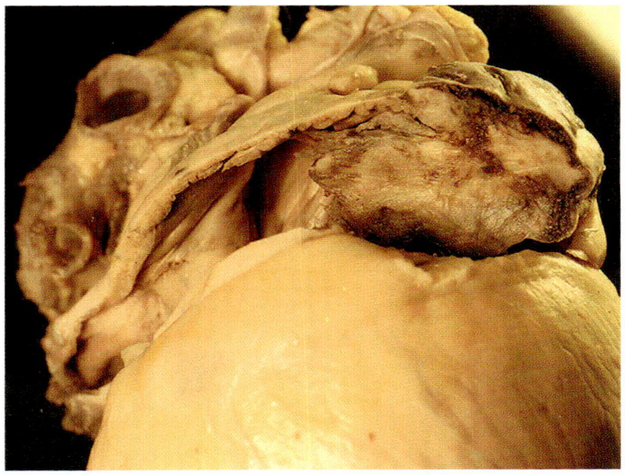

Figure 12. Section of the right atrial appendage in which the occupation of the cavity by the neoplastic tissue can be observed.

CARDIAC NEOPLASIA

Most cardiac neoplasia (more frequent in dogs than in cats) are located on the surface of the heart and between the great vessels and often cause pericardial effusions.

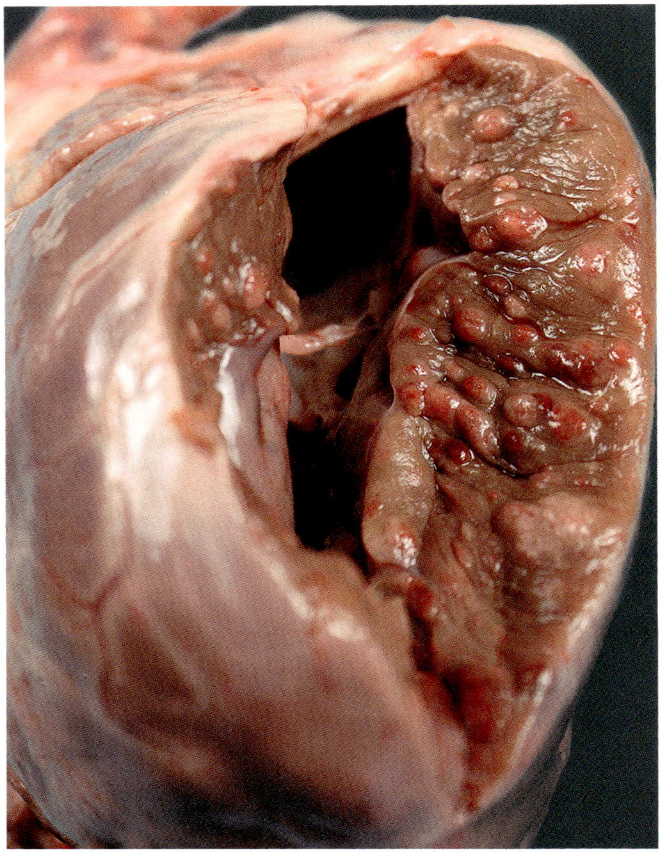

Figure 13. Haemangiosarcoma. Although it is rare, this type of tumour may sometimes be found with other presentations. In this case, the tumoral tissue practically invades all the myocardium, both atrial and ventricular.

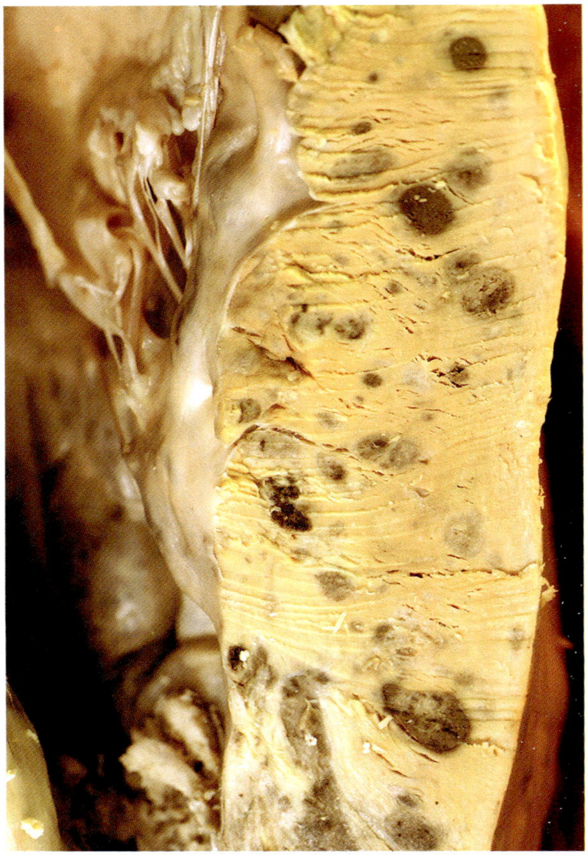

Figure 14. Haemangiosarcoma. Section of the free wall of the right ventricle of the previous anatomical structure after being fixed in formol, where the areas affected by neoplasia can clearly be seen.

In dogs, the most frequent cardiac neoplasms are haemangiosarcomas and heart base tumours; mesotheliomas are very rare. Neoplasms are rare in cats; lymphosarcomas are the most common tumours.

HAEMANGIOSARCOMA

They occur more frequently in the right atrial appendage or in adjacent tissues and often originate a haemorrhagic pericardial effusion, as they usually bleed. This effusion may be chronic or acute. On rare occasions, they may also affect both the atrial and ventricular myocardium. The presence of metastases at the time of their diagnosis is frequent.

Their incidence is greater in German Shepherds and Golden Retrievers.

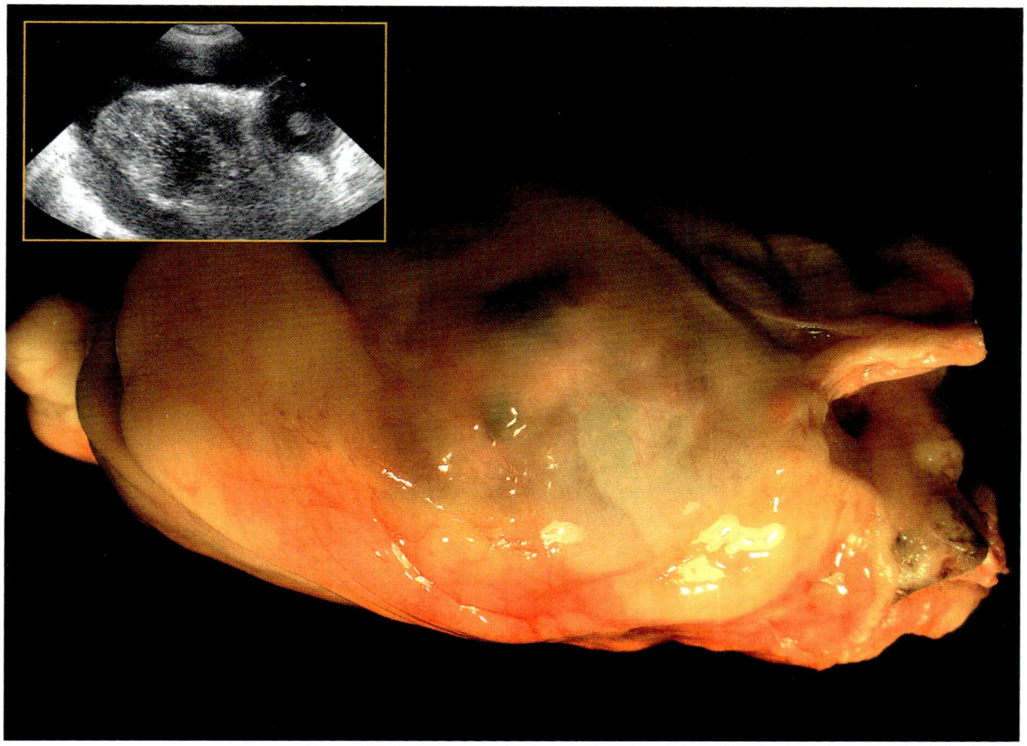

Figure 15. Haemangiosarcoma. In addition to the pericardial effusion, it is possible to see the presence of a cystic area with a small nodule in it in the ultrasound image. The location corresponds to the right coronary sulcus.

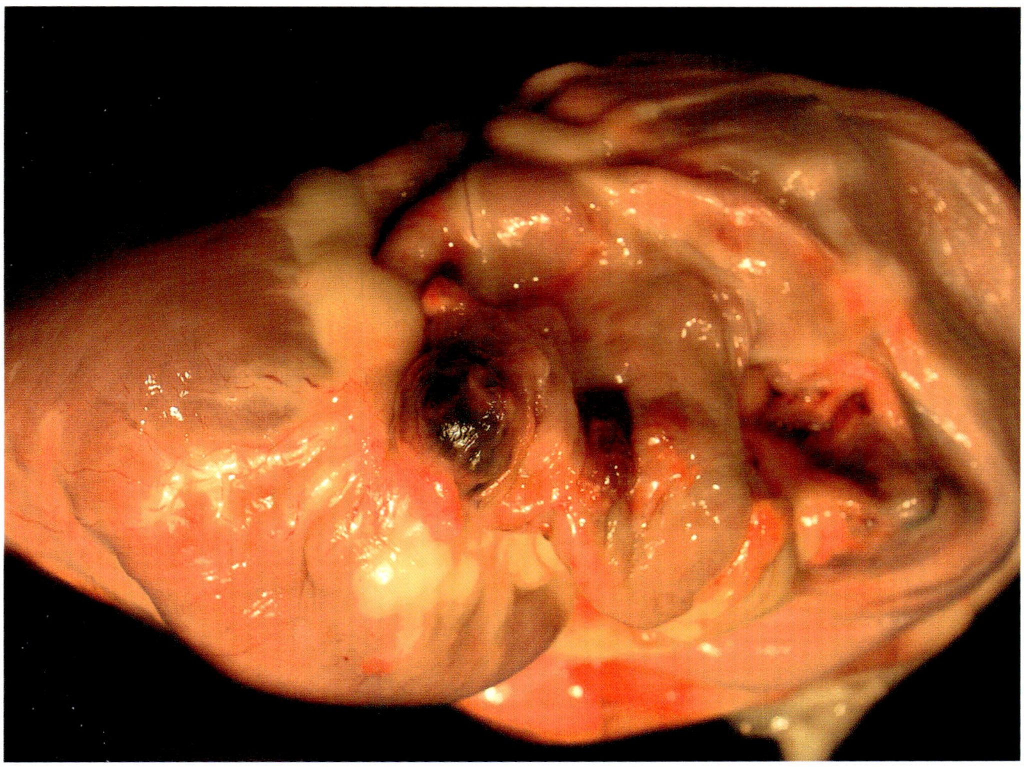

Figure 16. Once the effusion was drained, it was possible to see the capsule of the cyst with the nodule in it.

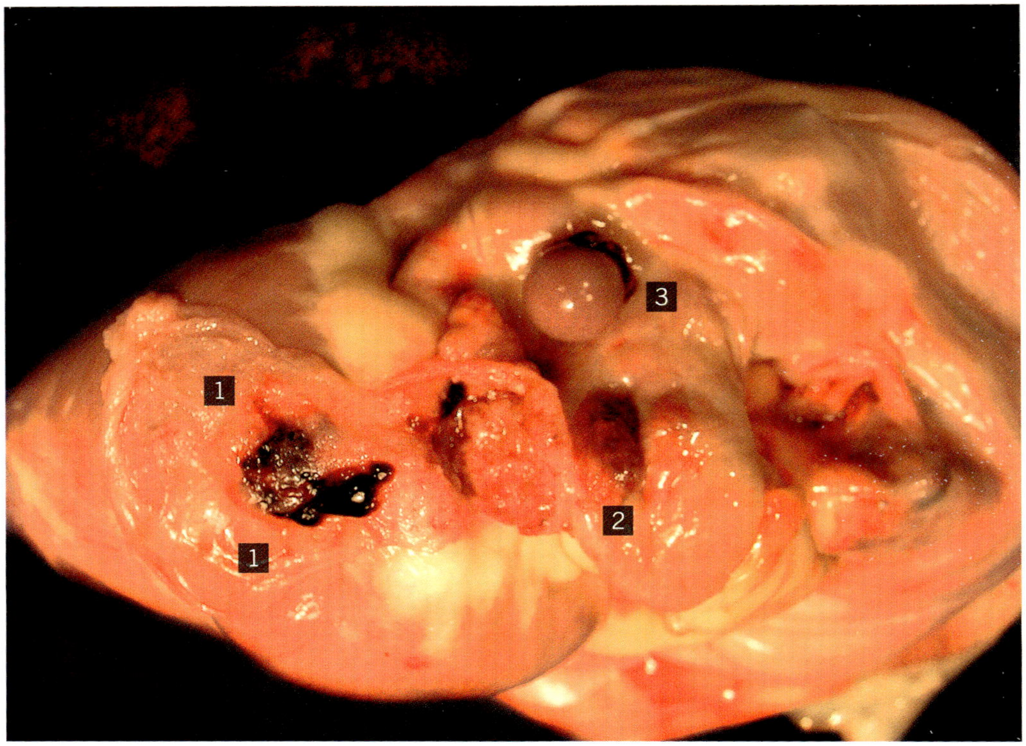

[1 Capsule]

[2 Right atrial appendage with area affected by haemangiosarcoma]

[3 Nodule]

Figure 17. The nodule was extracted by opening the capsule. Its anatomopathological examination revealed it was a haemangiosarcoma. The tumour cells had been growing from a central tissue nucleus, with a formation similar to that of a pearl. The base of the right atrial appendage, where the cyst originated, was also affected by the tumour.

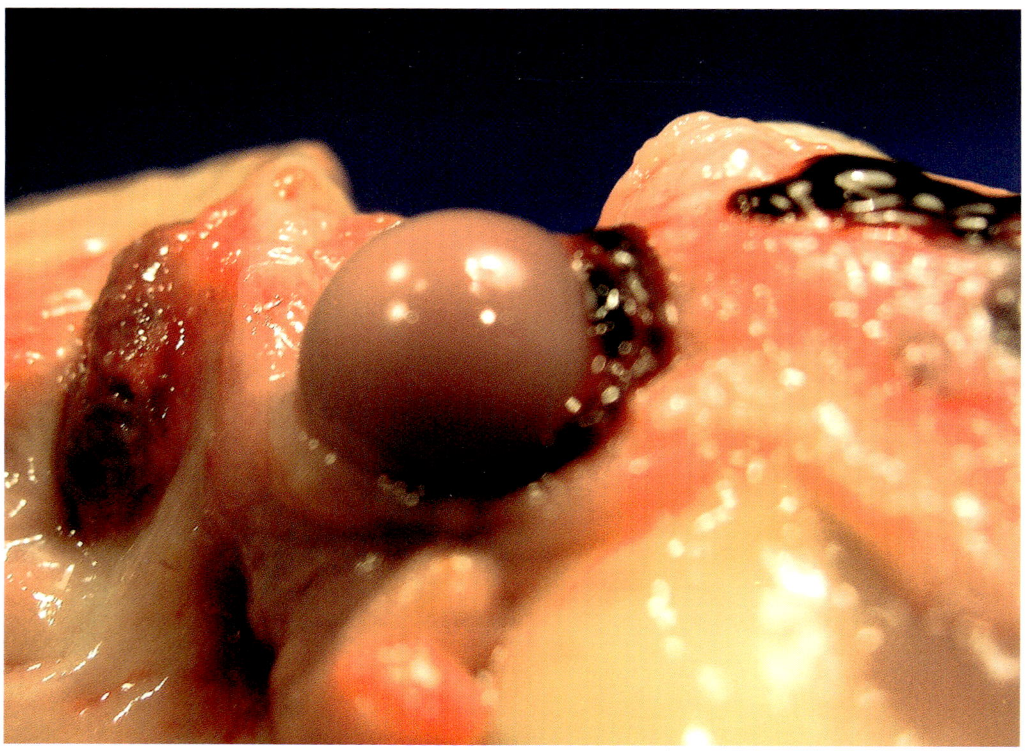

Figure 18. Detail of the nodule.

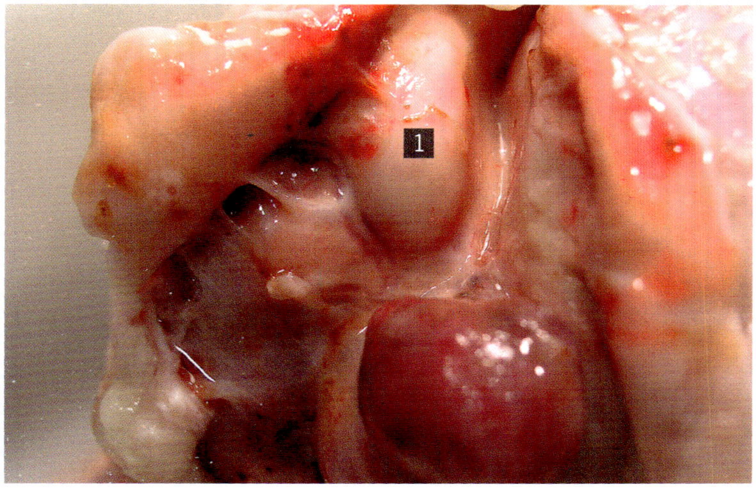

Figure 19. Heart base tumour. The aorta (1) is completely surrounded by tumoral tissue.

[1 Aorta]

[2 Pulmonary trunk]

[3 Aortic valve]

[4 Tumour surrouding the ascending aorta and pulmonary trunk]

[5 Left atrium]

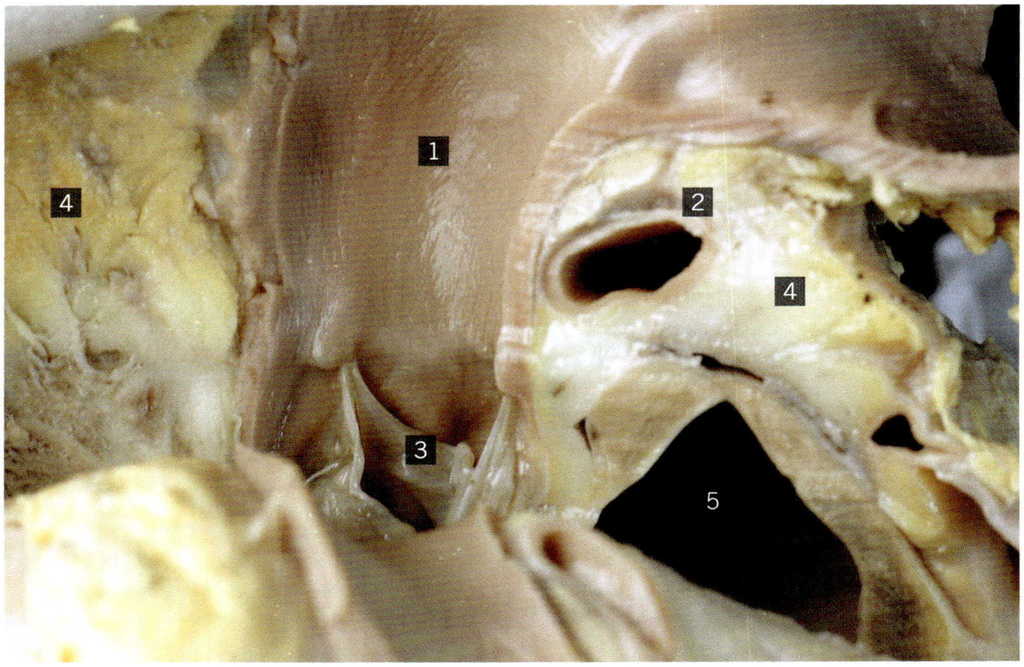

Figure 20. Heart base tumour, sagittal section at aortic level.

HEART BASE TUMOURS

Most heart base tumours usually derive from chemoreceptor cells (chemodectomas) located between the ascending aorta and the pulmonary trunk (aortic body tumour). Their growth is usually slow and the most common clinical sign is the presence of pericardial effusions, but there may also be a compression of adjacent vascular structures. They usually reach a large size, often before the appearance of symptoms. The presence of metastases is possible, although it generally occurs at a late stage.

Their incidence is greater in brachycephalic breeds.

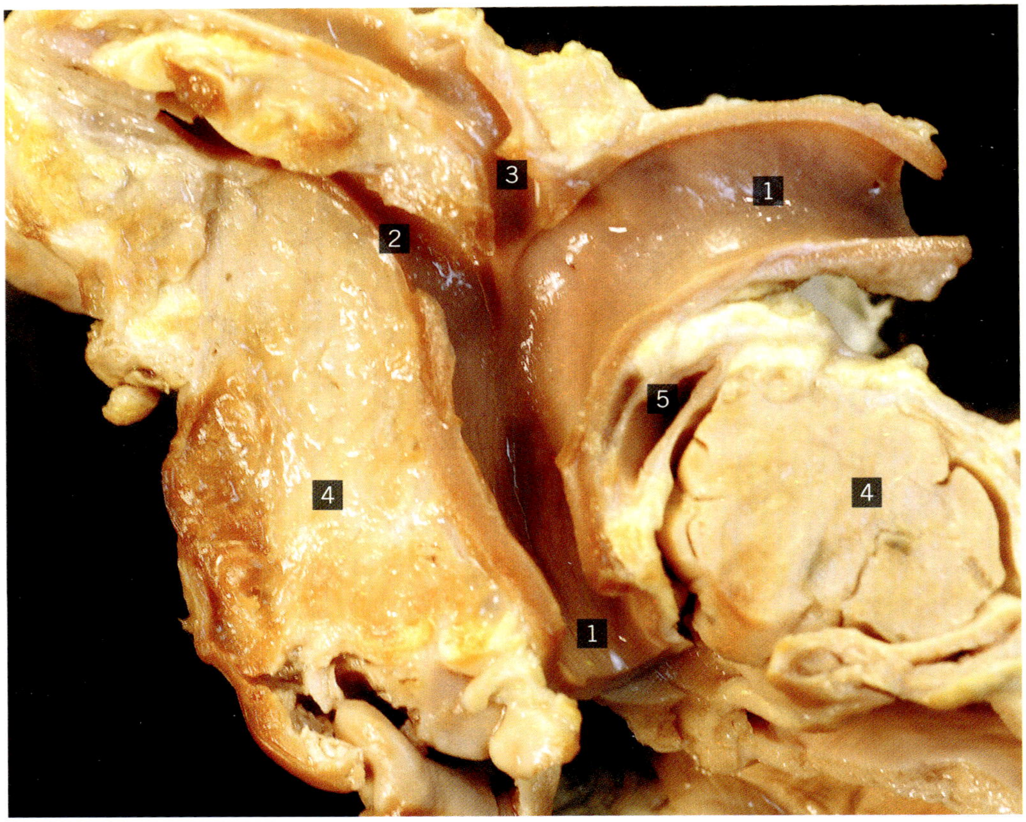

[1 Aorta]

[2 Brachiocephalic trunk]

[3 Left subclavian artery]

[4 Tumour]

[5 Pulmonary trunk]

Figure 21. Heart base tumour, sagittal section.

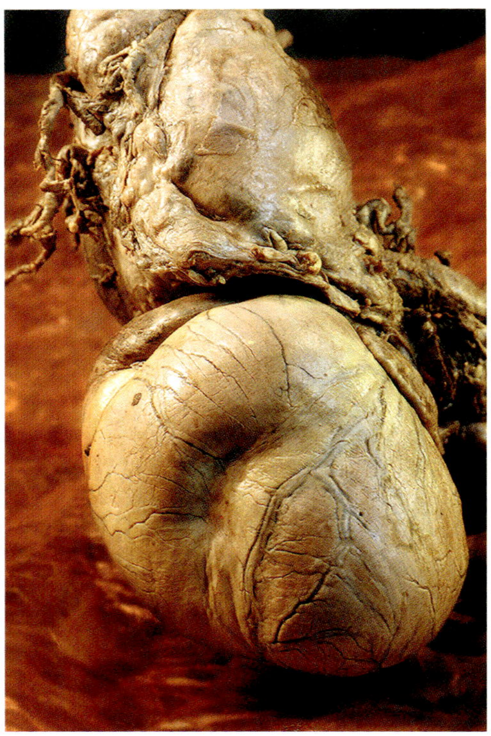

Figure 22. Heart base tumour, cranial view. It is possible to see how the size and location of the tumour hides the opening of the great cardiac vessels.

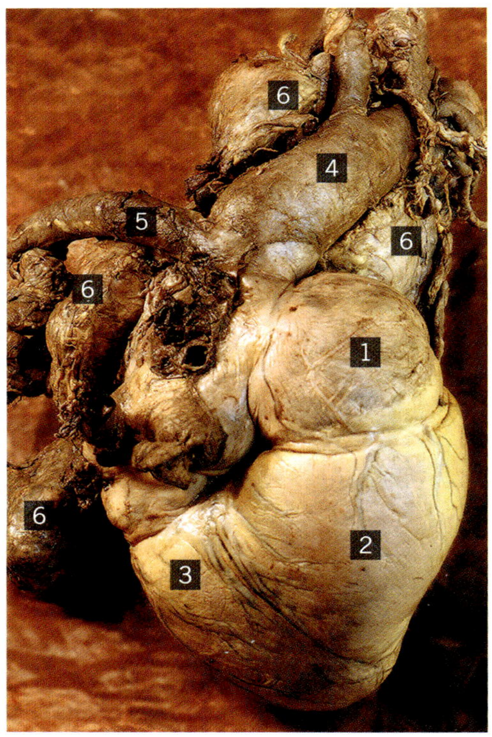

Figure 23. Heart base tumour. Right caudal view.

[1 Right atrium]

[2 Right ventricle]

[3 Left ventricle]

[4 Cranial vena cava]

[5 Azygos vein]

[6 Tumour]

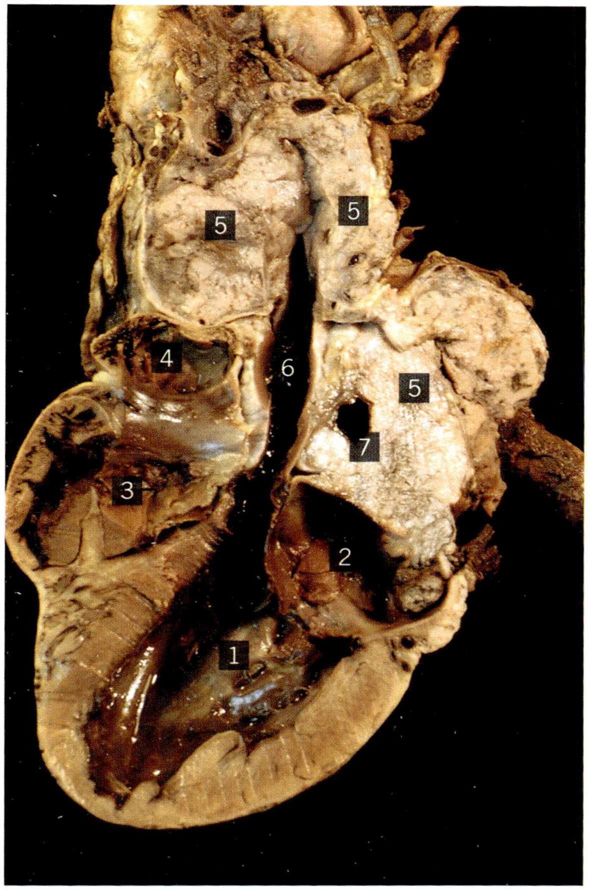

Figure 24. Heart base tumour, sagittal section.

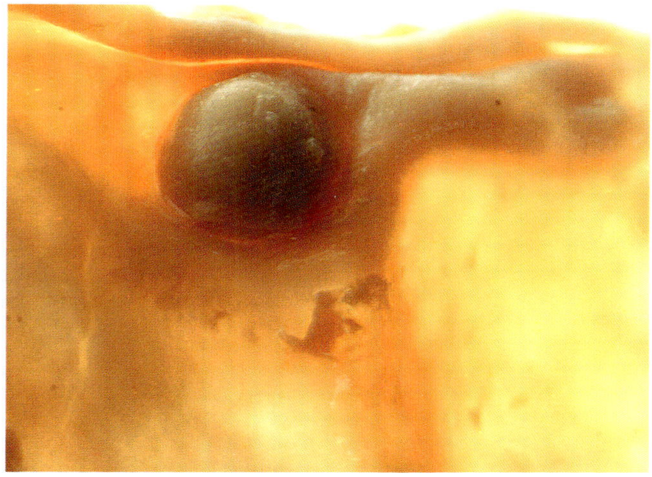

Figure 25. Heart base tumours may metastasise, although they usually do so at a late stage. The metastasis of one of these tumours in the pericardium may be seen in this image.

[1 Left ventricle]

[2 Left atrium]

[3 Right ventricle]

[4 Right atrium]

[5 Tumour]

[6 Aorta]

[7 Pulmonary trunk]

MESOTHELIOMA

This type of neoplasm derives from serous membranes such as the pleura or pericardium. It causes haemorrhagic effusion in the pericardium with no easily detectable masses.

It is difficult to diagnose since a cytological examination of the effusion will show a great number of reactive mesothelial cells, which are almost impossible to differentiate from tumour cells. A biopsy is required to establish a definitive diagnosis. These tumours carry a very poor prognosis.

LYMPHOSARCOMA

It is the most frequent cardiac tumour in cats and may affect both the myocardium and pericardium. Its diagnosis is established by means of cytology.

REFERENCES

1. Anderson RH, Razavi R, Taylor AM. Cardiac anatomy revisited. *J. Anat.*, 2004; 205:159–177.
2. Anderson WD, Anderson BG. *Atlas of Canine Anatomy.* Philadelphia. Ed. Lea&Febiger, 1994.
3. Bishop SP. Developmental Anatomy of the Heart and Great Vessels. In: Fox PR (ed.). *Canine and Feline Cardiology.* Churchill Livingstone, New York, 1988.
4. Bonagura JD. Chronic Valvular Disease in Dogs. In procedings of 14th ECVIM-CA. ESVC (Pre-congress day). Barcelona, 2004.
5. Bonagura JD. Congenital Heart Disease in Dogs and Cats. In procedings of 14th ECVIM-CA. ESVC (Pre-congress day). Barcelona, 2004.
6. Buchanan P. Persistent ductus arteriosus in the dog. Aetiology pathology. *Kleintierpraxis*, 1980; 25(1):40-41.
7. Dawes GS. The fetal circulation in the lamb. *J. Physiol*, 1954; 126:563.
8. Du Plesis LA, Marchand P. The anatomy of the mitral valve and its associated structures. *Thorax*, 1964 19:221-227.
9. Enriquez F. Anatomía y Fisiopatología de la válvula tricúspide. *Cir. Cadiov.*, 2005, 12(4):337-340.
10. Evans HE, Christensen GC. *Miller's Anatomy of the dog.* Ed. Saunders, 1979.
11. Fox PR. Feline cardiomyopathies. In: *Texbook of Canine and Feline Cardiology, principles and clinical practice.* Fox PR, Sisson D, Moise NS (eds.). WB Saunders Company, Philadelphia, 1999; 621-678.
12. Gross L, Kugel MA. Topographic Anatomy and Histology of the valves in the Human Heart. *Am. J. Pathol*, 1931, 7:445-473.
13. Gumbiner CH, Takao A. Ventricular Septal Defect. In: Garson AJ, Bricker Jt, McNamara DG (eds.). *The Science and Practice of Pediatric Cardiology.* Lea&Febiger, 1990.
14. Häggström J, Pedersen HD, Kvart C. New insights into degenerative mitral valve disease in dogs. *Vet Clin Small Anim*, 2004; 34:1209–1226.
15. Heyman MA, Iwamoto HS, Rudolph AM. Factors affecting changes in the neonatal systemic circulatión. *Ann. Re. Physiol*, 1981; 43:371-383.
16. Heyman MA, Iwamoto HS, Rudolph AM. Factors affecting changes in the neonatal systemic circulation. *Ann. Re. Physiol*, 1981; 43:371-383.
17. Ho SY. Anatomy of the mitral valve. *Heart*, 2002; 88:5-10.
18. Kittleson MD, Kienle, RD. *Small Animal Cardiovascular Medicine*. Ed. Mosby, 1998.
19. Lam JHC, Ranganathan N, Wigle ED, Silver MD. Morphology of the Human Mitral Valve: I. Chordae Tendineae: A New Classification. *Circulation*, 1970; 41:449-458.
20. Mucha CJ. Degeneración valvular mixomatosa. REDVET, 2007, Vol. VIII, Nº 7.
21. Netter FH. Embriology. In: Yonkman FF, Netter FH (eds.). *The Ciba Collection of Medical Illustration: The Heart*, 1974, vol. 5.
22. Oyama MA, Sisson DD, Thomas WP, Bonagura JD. Congenital heart diseases. In: Ettinger SJ, Feldman EC (eds.). *Texbook of Veterinary Internal Medicine*. 5th. WB Saunders, Philadelphia, 2005; pp. 972-1021.
23. Patterson DF. Epidemiologic and Genetic Studies of Congenital Heart Disease in the Dog. *Circ Res*, 1968; 23:171-202.
24. Tarrío R. Anatomía funcional de la raíz de la aorta. *Cir. Cardiov.*, 2005; 12(4):279-81.
25. Tildholm A, Jönsson L. Histologic Characterization of Canine Dilated Cardiomyopathy. *Vet Pathol,* 2005; 42:1–8.
26. Tilley LP. *Manual of Canine and feline cardiology.* Ed. Saunders, 2008.
27. Vick GW, Titus JL. Defects of the Atrial Septum including the atrioventricular canal. In: Garson AJ, Bricker Jt, McNamara DG. *The Science and Practice of Pediatric Cardiology.* Lea&Febiger, 1990.